M. Amiel A. Maseri H. Petitier N. Vasile

Coronary Artery Diseases

Diagnostic and Therapeutic Imaging Approaches

With Contributions by
W. Benicelli Ph. Brun P. A. Crean D. Crochet
G. J. Davis Ph. Gaspard Ph. Mikaëloff
A. L. Muir G. Pelle A. P. Selwyn P. Vignon

With 175 Figures and 15 Tables

Springer-Verlag
Berlin Heidelberg New York Tokyo 1984

Michel Amiel, M.D.
Director, Coronary and Congenital Cardiac Diseases Radiology Unit, Professor of Radiology, Cardiovascular Hospital and University of Lyon, F-69394 Lyon 03

Attilio Maseri, M.D.
Director, Cardiovascular Unit, Professor, Department of Cardiovascular Medicine, Royal Postgraduate Medical School, London – Hammersmith Hospital, Ducane Road, GB-London W12 OHS

Hubert Petitier, M.D.
Director, Hemodynamic Center and Thoracic Radiology Unit, Professor of Radiology, North Hospital and University of Nantes, F-44035 Nantes

Norbert Vasile, M.D.
Director, Radiology Unit, Professor of Radiology, Henri Mondor Hospital and University of Paris-Creteil, F-94010 Creteil

ISBN-13:978-3-642-69606-0 e-ISBN-13:978-3-642-69604-6
DOI: 10.1007/978-3-642-69604-6

Library of Congress Cataloging in Publication Data. Coronary artery diseases: Includes bibliographies and index. 1. Coronary heart disease – Diagnosis. 2. Radioisotope scanning. 3. Coronary arteries – Radiography. 4. Coronary heart disease – Treatment. 5. Radiology, Interventional. I. Amiel, Michel. [DNLM: 1. Coronary Disease – therapy. 2. Coronary Vessels – radiography. 3. Coronary Vessels – radionuclide imaging.
WG 300 C8196] RC685.C6C6324 1984 616.1'230757 84-5577

Softcover reprint of the hardcover 1st edition 1984

2127/3140-543210

Contents

List of Contributors

Contributors of Part I Nuclear Medicine Investigations

Benicelli, W., C. N. R., Clinical Physiology Laboratory, University of Pisa, Italy

Crean, P. A., M. D., Cardiovascular Research Unit, Royal Postgraduate Medical School, London – Hammersmith Hospital, Ducane Road, GB-London W12 OHS, Great Britain

Davies, G. J., M. D., Cardiovascular Research Unit, Royal Postgraduate Medical School, London – Hammersmith Hospital, Ducane Road, GB-London W12 OHS, Great Britain

Muir, A. L., M. D., Department of Medicine, Royal Infirmary of Edinburgh, Lauriston Place, GB-Edinburgh EH3 9YW, Great Britain

Selwyn, A. P., M. D., Cardiovascular Research Unit, Royal Postgraduate Medical School, London – Hammersmith Hospital, Ducane Road, GB-London W12 OHS, Great Britain

Contributors of Part II X-Ray and Ultrasound Investigations

Brun, Ph., M. D., Research Master, Health and Medical Research National Institutes, Ultrasonography Unit, University of Paris-Creteil, F-94010 Creteil, France

Crochet, D., M. D., Associate Director, Hemodynamic Center and Thoracic Radiology Unit, North Hospital, F-44035 Nantes, France

Gaspard, Ph., M. D., Assistant, Coronary and Congenital Cardiac Diseases Radiology Unit, Cardiovascular Hospital and University of Lyon, F-69394 Lyon 03, France

Mikaëloff, Ph., M. D., Director, Cardiovascular Surgery Unit, Professor of Surgery, Cardiovascular Hospital and University of Lyon, F-69394 Lyon 03, France

Pelle, G., M. D., University Assistant, Ultrasonography Unit, University of Paris-Creteil, F-94010 Creteil, France

Vignon, P., M. D., University Assistant, Ultrasonography Unit, University of Paris-Creteil, F-94010 Creteil, France

Introduction

The pathology of the coronary arteries is dominated by atheroma or atherosclerosis, which is responsible for the affection now usually referred to as "coronary artery disease". Other affections – congenital, inflammatory, infectious, metabolic or tumorous – involving the coronary arteries alone or in association with the heart have a special interest because of their singularity and infrequency of occurrence.

The clinical history of coronary artery disease as it is understood today probably began on 21 July 1768, when William Heberden's famous communication about angina pectoris was presented before the College of Physicians in London. Coronary atheroma was anatomically identified around 1793 during autopsies performed by Edward Jenner and John Hunter. However, the pathological mechanisms responsible for angina and myocardial ischaemia remained obscure for a long time. In the twentieth century, stricter clinical observation, the recording of meticulously analysed pathological observations and the establishment of solid clinicopathological correlations have contributed to the rapid progress in our knowledge of coronary artery disease. The greatest advance has been the advent of coronary arteriography, the only method capable of providing reliable in vivo anatomical diagnosis of the disease. The pioneers of this technique merit special mention: Radner, Di Guglielmo, Arnulf, Paulin and, especially, Mason Sones, the developer of selective coronary arteriography, whose work permitted this technique to be introduced into routine clinical practice in 1962.

The atheroma which impairs the coronary arteries is indistinguishable in its histology and pathogenesis from that attacking other arteries. Said to be characteristic of the twentieth century and of an industrialized society with a high standard of living, this disease seems indeed to be related to European and North American ways of life and eating habits. It is infrequent in Asia, South America and Africa. Hyperlipaemia, systemic hypertension, the use of tobacco, excessive consumption of sugar and fats, obesity, sedentary life, professional and emotional stress and heredity are the identified risk factors. These factors are more or less determined from childhood on, so that prevention of the disease may today justifiably be regarded as a veritable paediatric problem.

Localization of atheroma in the coronary artery is second in frequency to that in the abdominal aorta. On the basis of autopsies performed on young subjects killed in accidents, it is known that atheroma is present in the coronary arteries of individuals as young as 25 years of age. The incidence of the disease increases with age. In France it is 3.5 per 1000 at 45 years and 10.5 at 60 years. The incidence is 2.2 times as high in Finland and 1.6 times as high in the United States, where around 100000 patients per year currently undergo myocardial revascularization surgery. At the present time, two major methods dominate diagnostic imaging techniques for coronary artery disease: radio-nuclide examinations and coronary and left ventricular radiography using contrast media.

Part I
Nuclear Medicine Investigations

I Radio-Nuclide Explorations: Diagnostic Use of Radioisotopes in Coronary Disease

The clinical applications of nuclear medicine in cardiology have rapidly expanded since the development of imaging cameras and short-lived isotopes suitable for practical use. Indeed, cardiovascular nuclear medicine is often available not only in specialized centres but also in peripheral hospitals. The reasons for this rapid expansion are multiple and reflect the remarkable spread of sophisticated technology in medicine and cardiology. The possibility of investigating pathophysiological problems from a new angle, the appeal of using techniques that have proved useful in research, the attraction of non-invasive methods and the pressure from industry have all played a role in the establishment of the present state of affairs.

Capital investment, running costs and radiation exposure necessitate a careful assessment of the merits of nuclear medical techniques with respect to the actual clinical demand and to the available alternatives. The transfer of new technology from research to routine has been rather hasty and, in several instances, it took place before a clear demonstration of its practical advantages had been obtained. This is certainly true of its use in the field of coronary artery disease for the detection of transient myocardial ischaemia, of acute infarction and of myocardial scar.

1 Detection of Transient Myocardial Ischaemia

When thallium scintigraphy of the myocardium became available, it was immediately used during exercise stress testing with the hope that it might detect non-invasively the presence or absence of coronary atherosclerosis. A large number of comparisons with coronary angiography were reported, with conclusions about the specificity and sensitivity of scintigraphy.

The same occurred with gated blood pool imaging of the left ventricle, when it was found that acute transient myocardial ischaemia is always associated with a severe impairment of ventricular function. Yet it was not sufficiently appreciated that these techniques should be used to detect ischaemia, not anatomical features. Sensitivity and specificity should be calculated on the basis of the actual presence or absence of ischaemia rather than on the presence or absence of atherosclerotic obstructions. The figures reported for sensitivity and specificity in detecting stenoses are highly influenced by the prevalence in the group of patients studied of severe coronary lesions not adequately compensated by collaterals (with respect to the sensitivity), and the prevalence of ischaemia caused by transient reduction of supply such as acute vasoconstriction (with respect to the specificity).

This attitude derives from the assumption that coronary atherosclerosis is the only possible determinant of therapy and prognosis. Yet it is obvious that a negative exercise test is not falsely negative if it indicates correctly that no ischaemia developed, even if atherosclerotic narrowings are present. Indeed, it shows that obstructions are not severe enough or are adequately compensated by collaterals for the level of myocardial demand generated during the test. Conversely, a positive test is not falsely positive if ischaemia is caused by coronary vasoconstriction or by other dynamic factors in the absence of critical organic coronary obstructions. A variable development of collaterals and a variable susceptibility to dynamic stenoses can largely account for the discrepancy between severity of coronary atherosclerosis and the development of ischaemic syndromes.

It is thus important to appreciate that exercise stress testing is not only important for the detection of the development of ischaemia but also for the assessment of the extent to which the coronary flow reserve is limited (i.e. by the balance between severity of coronary atherosclerosis on the one hand and adequacy of collateral development and function on the other). In the absence of a practical standard for the detection of ischaemia it seems reasonable to assume that a positive diagnosis of ischaemia can provisionally be made in the presence of the combination of at least two diagnostic elements:

1. Typical chest pain associated with transient ECG changes or with transient changes of ventricular function or of myocardial perfusion or metabolism
2. Typical changes on the ECG, even without pain, associated with transient changes of ventricular function or of myocardial perfusion or metabolism.

This applies not only for exercise stress testing but also for any other condition in which transient myocardial ischaemia may occur.

Patients who report pain occurring during exertion should be submitted to exercise stress testing. In the presence of a normal resting tracing, the test is diagnostic if it reproduces the symptoms with transient ischaemic ECG changes. If maximal heart rate is reached without signs or symptoms of ischaemia, there is little advantage in using techniques more sophisticated than the ECG; moreover, the test indicates that the patient has a good coronary flow reserve (if coronary atherosclerotic obstructions are present, they are not severe enough or they must be adequately compensated by collaterals). If such a patient gives a convincing history of angina, this is more likely to be caused by dynamic than by fixed stenoses. Studies of ventricular function, myocardial perfusion or metabolism should be reserved for those who during the test develop pain but no diagnostic ECG changes or ischaemic-like ECG changes without pain, or for when abnormalities are already present on the resting tracing and prevent the reliable assessment of changes.

Conversely, patients who complain of anginal pain occurring spontaneously and for levels of exertion usually well tolerated should be investigated with ambulatory ECG monitoring when the episodes are frequent, or with provocative tests, performed in specialized centres, when the episodes are infrequent. The detection of transient changes of the ECG on the Holter tape *during* an episode of pain is diagnostic. Accordingly, the transient development of typical ECG changes and pain or of changes in ventricular function or myocardial flow and metabolism during provocative tests is diagnostic.

The actual sensitivity of these nuclear medical techniques in detecting transient ischaemia is unknown. It appears that for thallium scintigraphy three-dimensional reconstruction does improve the sensitivity. The specificity for detecting transient ischaemia is strongly influenced by the threshold accepted for the recognition of the abnormality and it is also unknown. Because of the lack of a standard it can be best assessed by appropriate reproducibility studies.

2 Detection of Acute Myocardial Infarction and of Scar Tissue

Two options are generally available for the study of acute infarction:

1. Hot spot indicators, taken up into the necrotic tissue only (typically ^{99m}Tc-pyrophosphates) and showing the infarcted area
2. Cold spot indicators, not taken up by the necrotic tissues but only by the intact myocardium (typically thallium-201), and showing the infarcted area as a defect.

The first type of indicator is specific; the second type is non-specific because it does not allow a distinction of necrotic myocardium from scar tissue and from old ischaemia.

These two approaches (with their inherent limitations) do find diagnostic application only when the ECG and the serum enzymes are non-diagnostic. They can indeed provide an indication of the location of the infarction and a rough quantitation of its extension. Ventricular angiography does not provide good information on its extension and separation from viable but non-contracting myocardium. Gated contrast computerized axial tomography provides the best assessment of ventricular wall thickness because of its spatial resolution and three-dimensional presentation. Two-dimensional echocardiography would be able to provide useful information if its resolution were improved.

Tracers that are taken up by the myocardium theoretically lend themselves to the identification of scar tissue (which does not take up tracer). However, gated three-dimensional reconstruction, which is now becoming available, has a resolution of only about 15 mm at best, and two-dimensional imaging provides only gross information. Radioisotopic imaging can therefore provide only semi-quantitative data, Thallium (or any other tracer taken up by the myocardium with a good organ to background ratio) is suitable. Its combined use with ventricular volume studies by radioangiographic techniques can be useful in patients with enlarged hearts (but no diagnostic history or ECG) for the differential diagnosis between dilated cardiomyopathy and localized postinfarction scar tissue. It can also be used in patients with old infarction to try and define the fraction of total left ventricular myocardium replaced by scar (as stated above), but the spatial resolution of the technique limits the accuracy of this assessment.

3 Perspectives

Radio-nuclides have considerably helped in our understanding of coronary disease and of the potential of other techniques for the study of patients. I believe that future developments will largely depend on positron tomography. The resolution of single-photon tomography is unlikely to be improved to 1 cm, whereas that of positron tomography should reach 0.5 cm. Cyclotron production of ultra-short-lived nuclides will give us insight into pathophysiological mechanisms and into clinical syndromes. Correlation with the results obtained from other more widely available techniques and with clinical observation should also allow diagnostic advances, independent of the availability of expensive equipment, which should be confined to the field of research until its diagnostic yield is proved worthy of the cost.

II Radio-Nuclide Explorations: Short-Lived Radio-Nuclides: Present and Future Applications to the Study of Perfusion and Metabolism in the Heart

1 Introduction

The clinical methods available can provide useful estimates of ventricular function and detection of myocardial ischaemia in situations where the information may aid the management of the condition. Nevertheless, these widely available methods have a limited ability to quantify and measure the determinants of cardiac physiology that are essential prerequisites to normal ventricular function, and which are disturbed at the onset of myocardial ischaemia (i. e. coronary blood flow and myocardial metabolism).

This section aims to present the progress that has been made with nuclides that emit twin photons (positron emission) and tomographic detection (i. e. ring detection of a slice through tissues or organs), and then to discuss whether this approach could be used to improve diagnosis, help to understand available methods, objectively assess new treatments and, perhaps, look at pathophysiological disturbances in regional myocardial perfusion and metabolism in different disease states [1].

2 Detection of Radio Tracers in the Heart

The attractive prospect of using isotopes and non-invasively measuring cardiovascular physiology started with the single probe. These provided the time course or transit time of tracers through the circulation and measured cardiac output and later ventricular function. This did not give any regional or spatial localization of organ function. The gamma camera later provided a two-dimensional representation of the heart with some impression of the third dimension (i. e. depth) by recording different views. Single photon tracers and individual tissue densities are important reasons that a gamma camera cannot be developed to measure the true concentration of tracer in tissues. This fact limits resolution and will always prevent the determination of measurements by physiological units.

If the isotope emits twin photons (each of 511 keV) at 180° and these are detected in coincidence by a pair of crystals, the pathway can be localized. If this process is repeated and multiple pathways recorded by a ring of detectors arranged in pairs, the plane or tomogram gives the distribution of activity in the slice of tissue within the field of view. An external ring source of activity can be used to identify the individual tissue densities and attenuation of radiation. This will overcome many of the problems of the gamma camera in trying to record a more quantitative estimate of tracer concentration in tissues. These ring detectors (positron tomograph) can record the distribution of a radio-nuclide in the tissues with linear sensitivity and calibration to µCi/ml in a well counter [1–3]. These substantial advantages are counterbalanced by limited spatial resolution (1.5–2.0 cm), the problem of cardiac motion and the systematic underestimation with decreasing object size, beginning at 3 cm^3 (partial volume effect). The sensitivity (time taken to record adequate counts), use of cardiac gating, spatial resolution and an independent assessment of wall thickness are all areas that require improvement and research. Further benefit may be gained by timing the arrival of each photon and estimating not only the flight path but also the point source of the annihilation (time of flight) [3, 4].

3 Tracers and Their Clinical Applications

3.1 Detection of Myocardial Ischaemia

A variety of nuclides can be given by peripheral intravenous injection and these will distribute to the myocardium according to the cardiac output and coronary blood flow. The regional myocardial concentration achieved depends on coronary blood flow and extraction or metabolic trapping of the tracer, and also on wall thickness. If the concentration in the heart can be measured and standardized to the delivered dose, the signal is sensitive to changes in regional myocardial perfusion and/or extraction. Nitrogen-13-labelled ammonia has been shown to provide a signal in the myocardium proportional to regional myocardial perfusion, and has demonstrated in patients with angina and coronary disease the inhomogeneous regional myocardial perfusion that results when dipyridamole is given to these patients [5]. Similarly, the myocardial uptake of carbon-11-labelled palmitate will demonstrate regional abnormalities in the early phases of acute myocardial infarction (Fig. 1) [6]. The relative contribution of perfusion and impaired β-oxidation has not been determined. Fluorine-18-labelled deoxyglucose is taken up by the myocardium but is not metabolized like natural glucose. Transient regional myocardial ischaemia is thought to cause a temporary preference for glucose in the metabolism of the affected myocardium. Schelbert et al. have demonstrated regional increases in glucose uptake in segments of myocardium in patients with coronary artery disease [7].

The intravenous use of rubidium-82 is free from the constraints of working online to a cyclotron (Fig. 2). During a continuous intravenous infusion the short half-life allows the calculation of the delivered arterial activity. Standardized uptake can be measured after infusion in each region of the myocardial tomograms in patients with coronary artery disease. This information has shown evidence of transient ischaemia following exercise or cold pressor tests and as a spontaneous event with no apparent cause. All of these transient ischaemic episodes have been recorded with chest pain and in the absence of chest pain and also with and without electrocardiographic evidence. The evidence of ischaemia following exercise tests using the tomograms is prolonged and lasts at least two to three times longer than the electrocardiographic signs of ischaemia.

These measurements of uptake in tomograms provide a mixed signal of flow and extraction. The inverse relation between these two parameters will dampen the response of the signal to flow but should demonstrate directional changes in perfusion. Perhaps more importantly, the signal responds to the disturbances produced

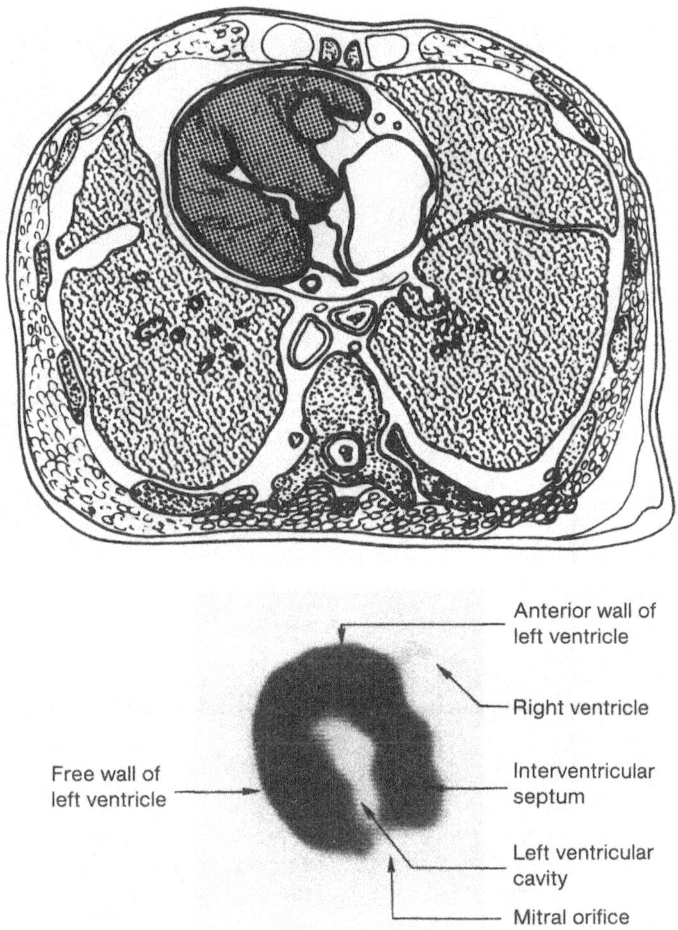

Fig. 1. The diagram shows the tissues exposed by a transaxial slice through the chest. The heart is shown in cross-section, and this anatomical slice shows how external detection by tomography will display the heart. An emission tomogram from a normal subject shows the cardiac structures that can be recorded non-invasively. There is concentrated activity in the myocardium following a peripheral intravenous injection of ^{11}C-acetate (used in the Krebs cycle to produce adenosine triphosphate)

by transient ischaemia. This may help in the more precise diagnosis of chest pain, investigation of the time course and character of transient ischaemia, silent ischaemia, ST segment changes without symptoms and the effects of treatment [8, 9].

3.2 Regional Myocardial Perfusion

The further investigation of transient ischaemia and any other metabolic events in the heart requires a more specific measure of regional myocardial perfusion at the same time. Oxygen-15-labelled CO_2 can be inhaled continuously or as a bolus, and

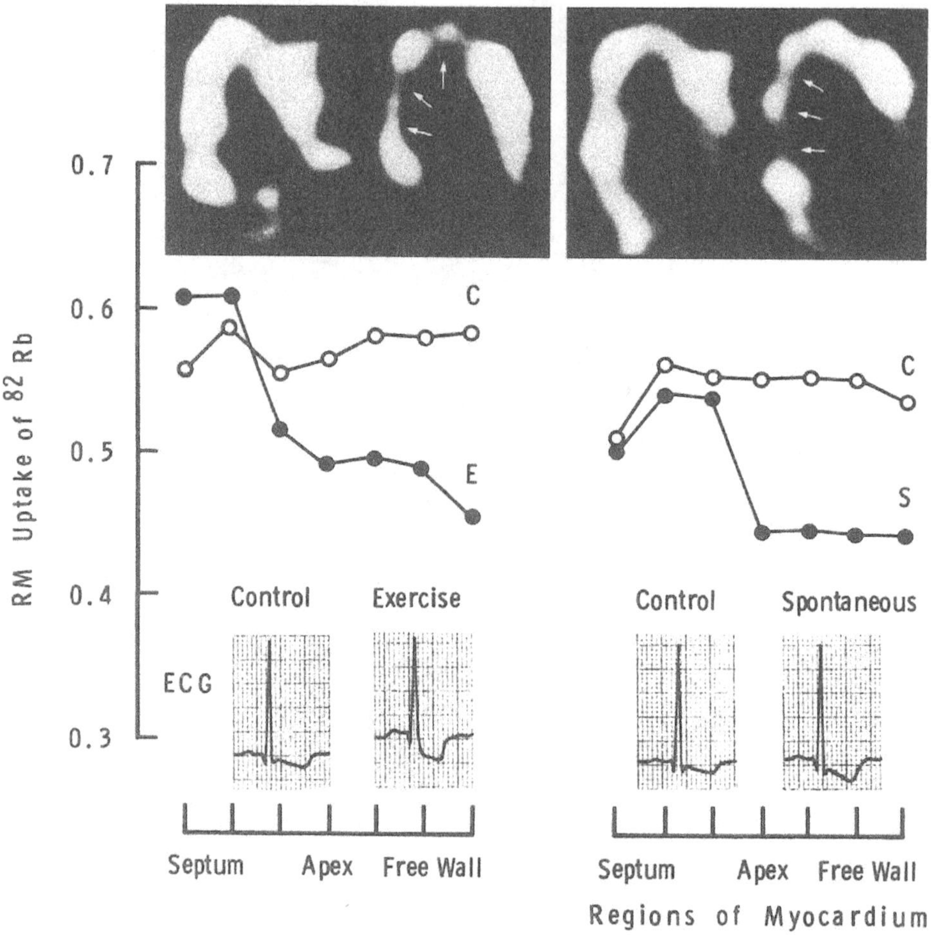

Fig. 2. These serial tomograms are from a patient with angina on stress and at rest. The regional myocardial *(RM)* uptake of ^{82}Rb (a cation-like potassium) changes and shows the transient ischaemia that underlies the chest pain following exercise and the silent transient ischaemia that occurs for no obvious reason. The familiar ECG changes and attempts to quantify the tomographic data are shown *below*

the tissue concentration achieved is related to perfusion. However, the quantitation of regional myocardial perfusion in this way requires subtraction of the blood pool, partial volume correction and a measure of the arterial input. The bolus inhalation of oxygen-15-labelled CO_2 or intravenous injection of oxygen-15-labelled water can also be used, and will have the advantage or more rapid acquisition of data than the steady state approach. Any attempt to use this method for quantification will still face the problems listed above [10].

The left atrial injection of radio-labelled microspheres represents a reference measure of regional myocardial blood flow but cannot be easily adapted for use in patients. Biodegradable albumin microspheres can be labelled with positron-emitting isotopes and can be injected into the left atrium or left ventricle. The regional myocardial activity is recorded non-invasively using positron tomography, and the arterial reference can be withdrawn for well counting. Gallium-68-labelled microspheres have been used in this way in experiments, but the radio-chemical bond between nuclide and spheres is not ideal. A new radio-chemical procedure binding carbon-11 ($t_{1/2}=20$ min) to microspheres is stable, providing a tracer that will allow the application of a rigorous principle to measure regional myocardial blood flow in patients. This complex and elaborate method will not be widely used. However, in clinical research it will provide a sound measure of changes in coronary blood flow in different pathological states. It may also represent a useful in vivo reference standard to enable new or less invasive or elaborate methods to be checked [11].

3.3 Regional Myocardial Metabolism

Arterial and coronary sinus blood sampling with an estimate of flow represents the traditional approach to the study of myocardial metabolism in patients. Because this cannot provide direct or regional information from the myocardium, the prospect of using tracers and then the external detection of regional myocardial metabolism is attractive. Short-lived positron-emitting isotopes (e.g. carbon-11 and fluorine-18) can be included in natural substrates usually involved in oxidative metabolism (e.g. palmitate, acetate, glucose), protein metabolism (amino acids) and drugs (carbon-11 and fluorine-18-labelled chlorpromazine, L-dopa and amphetamines). Following a peripheral intravenous injection, the regional myocardial concentration and clearance of these tracers can be measured in patients using positron tomography. The appearance and clearance of the tracer in the myocardium can be related to the dose and blood activity, and a variety of models are being tested which are designed to use carbon-11-labelled palmitate and carbon-11-labelled acetate to try and assess aerobic oxidative and anaerobic metabolism. Analogues of glucose (deoxyglucose) and fatty acids (methyl fatty acids) are taken up by the myocardium but are not catabolized. These tracers and their physiological models are being tested using positron tomography and investigated for their ability to measure glucose utilization and free fatty acid utilization by the myocardium [7, 12].

On a clinical level, carbon-11-labelled acetate has been given to patients with angina and ischaemic heart disease. Acute transient regional myocardial ischaemia is shown by a failure of uptake when the tracer is given following exercise. Conversely, if carbon-11-labelled acetate concentrates in the myocardium and exercise is then used to produce transient ischaemia, the clearance of this natural substrate from the ischaemic segment is delayed, suggesting impaired aerobic metabolism [12]. The regional myocardial uptake of fluorine-18-labelled deoxyglucose varies in patients according to the nutritional state. However, Schelbert et al. have demonstrated regional increases in the myocardial uptake of glucose in patients with ischaemic heart disease, suggesting that the compromised myocardium uses more glucose and possibly less fatty acid than the surrounding normal tissue [7]. Measurements of amino acid uptake in the myocardium are being tested in the same way and models are being developed for the assessment of protein turnover in the heart. Similarly, radio-labelled drugs and possibly monoclonal antibodies are being developed so that, if these molecules are used as tracers, the pharmacokinetics of the drug in the target organs can be studied. Physiological experiments must still be used to test these models.

The multiple metabolic pathways of many of these tracers and the spatial resolution of the system will considerably limit the chemical interpretation of the signal obtained by external scanning. Simple tracer models and an accompanying measure of flow are required in validating experiments before these tracers can be used in patients to study myocardial metabolism.

4 Conclusion

Positron tomography can give a three-dimensional measure of tracers in the myocardium in patients. This represents improved quantitation but is still being developed to improve resolution, sensitivity and an understanding of the effects of object size. So far the tracers can give information about regional myocardial cation uptake, perfusion and different aspects of myocardial metabolism. Once again, the physiological models must be validated in experiments to ensure that the clinical interpretation of the signal is correct. The clinical application of these methods has so far provided some improvement in the quantitation of myocardial infarction, detection and study of transient ischaemia in patients with angina and the regional myocardial uptake of fluorine-18-labelled deoxyglucose, which is increased in ischaemic segments of muscle. Rubidium-82 has demonstrated transient ischaemia in many different physiological states which are also frequently asymptomatic and prolonged in nature. The whole approach requires a parallel effort in the areas of technical development, physiological validation and clinical application in patients. It will not be used for routine diagnosis, to confirm infarction, ischaemia or metabolic derangement. It is more likely to be useful in the future in helping to unravel the pathophysiological sequence of changes in regional myocardial perfusion and/or metabolic function that underlie transient ischaemia in coronary disease and heart muscle failure of unknown cause. It could also be used to improve the understanding of more widely available but less direct methods used in clinical practice, such as the electrocardiogram. Finally, if it is possible to measure these functions in the myocardium, then the effects of new treatments can be objectively assessed before the stage of large-scale clinical trials.

III Radio-Nuclide Explorations: Thallium-201 for Myocardial Perfusion Imaging

1 Introduction

Thallium-201 is an isotope which is produced by the reaction ^{203}Tl (p, 3n) ^{201}Pb 201_{Tl}. It is prepared as thallous chloride and has a half-life of 73 h, emitting mercury X-rays with a 69–83 keV photopeak in 98% abundance (and gamma rays of 135 keV and 167 keV in very low abundance). Thus it is suitable for imaging with the standard scintillation camera using a low-energy, high-sensitivity parallel-hole collimator. The relatively long half-life renders it widely available and facilitates its use in unpredictable circumstances such as spontaneous angina.

The initial distribution of ^{201}Tl to the heart following intravenous administration is proportional to the fraction of the cardiac output perfusing the myocardium. However, as for potassium tracers in general, this situation exists only for the time during which a balance is maintained between the amount of tracer not extracted during the first circulation and the amount which re-enters the myocardium on recirculation [13]. This condition is achieved only transiently during the initial 2 min and is followed by progressive myocardial uptake for at least 20 min. Ten minutes after injection, arterial ^{201}Tl concentration is reduced to approximately 0.8% and myocardial uptake is increased by 20% relative to the level between 20 and 120 s [13].

The final equilibrium of distribution of ^{201}Tl, as of the other potassium tracers, will tend to be proportional to the potassium pool of the various organs. Therefore, scintigrams recorded soon after the injection of ^{201}Tl will reflect predominantly the regional myocardial perfusion, whereas later images will reflect the distribution of myocardial muscle mass. If ischaemia is relieved within 1 or 2 min of ^{201}Tl injection, when arterial tracer concentration is still high, the regional differences in concentration will rapidly disappear due to the high blood-tissue tracer gradient in the ischaemic areas. Conversely, when ischaemia persists longer, the initial regional differences will be maintained for longer periods. Regional myocardial perfusion can be evaluated by comparing scintigrams taken 5–20 min after injection with images recorded:

- 3 h later or more, when redistribution of tracer is complete, or
- several days later following the injection of an equal dose of ^{201}Tl in the absence of symptoms or acute electrocardiographic changes.

The actual differences in flow between ischaemic and non-ischaemic regions will be underestimated in early scintigrams because:

- potassium tracer clearance is greater at low flow [14], and
- when flow is restored before imaging begins, the previously ischaemic tissue has a larger net extraction than normal tissues.

Furthermore, the two-dimensional nature of the images inevitably results in overlap between ischaemic and non-ischaemic regions, accentuated by the cyclical change in cardiac shape.

The interpretation of transient defects should take into account the following factors:

1. Myocardial uptake, although related to the absolute level of myocardial blood flow, is dependent on the fraction of cardiac output distributed to the myocardium and surrounding organs and tissues.
2. Ventricular dilatation alone may lead to an apparent expansion of areas of decreased activity due to old myocardial infarction.
3. As non-uniformity of tracer distribution occurs in normal subjects, regional differences of less than 20% cannot be declared significant.
4. Overt ECG changes occur when flow is reduced to 50%–75% of requirements.
5. Over an intermediate range of myocardial blood flow (100–250 ml/min per 100 g myocardium) a 100% increase in flow leads to only a 40% increase in ^{201}Tl uptake [13].

Thus it follows that massive defects (hardly distinguishable from surrounding background) are most likely caused by a substantial absolute reduction in perfusion [15]. This is particularly likely to be the case when no increase in heart rate or blood pressure precedes the attack, these being the most important parameters determining the level of myocardial oxygen demand.

2 Technique

The arterial pressure (cuff manometer) is monitored together with either single or multiple ECG leads. If changes have been detected on a previous ECG recorded during pain or during stress, then the appropriate leads are monitored. At the onset of ECG change or pain, occurring spontaneously or induced by provocative tests (such as exercise, cold pressor, ergometrine injection), 1–2 mCi ^{201}Tl is injected via an indwelling venous cannula. Ischaemia should be allowed to persist for at least 2 min; it is therefore important to detect the earliest ECG change, which may precede the symptoms by 90 s or more. If effort is used as the provocative agent, then it may be necessary to continue the exercise for up to 2 min following the onset of ECG changes, but it is usually possible to reduce the load. The cold pressor test is generally performed by immersing one hand or forearm in iced water for a period of a min. The ergometrine test is performed by giving incremental doses (0.025 mg, 0.05 mg, 0.1 mg, 0.2 mg) intravenously at intervals of 6 min. It is important to begin with the very small dose of 0.025 mg in case the patient is very sensitive to its effects. It is also important to exclude patients with a severely limited exercise tolerance or diffuse coronary disease with poor left ventricular function and those experiencing

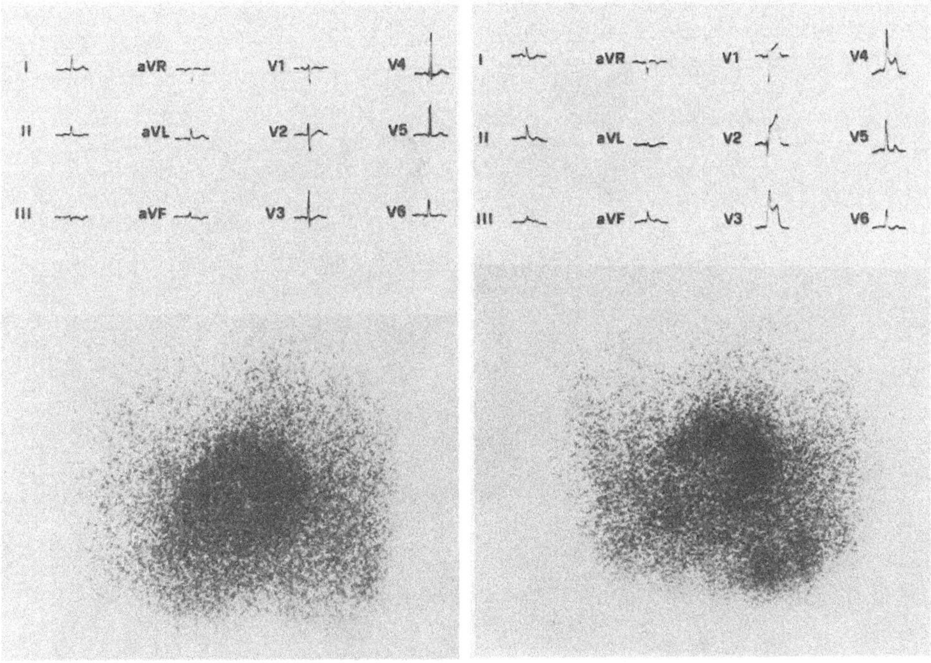

Fig. 1. Thallium-201 myocardial scintigrams (45° left anterior oblique projection) and corresponding 12-lead ECGs taken in the basal state *(left)* and during ergometrine-induced angina *(right)*. The ST segment elevation in the anterior and inferior leads is associated with a massive deficit of tracer uptake in the inferior and anterior left ventricular wall

frequent spontaneous episodes of angina at rest. Under no circumstances should ischaemia be allowed to persist beyond 5 min; it should be relieved by the administration of nitrates or verapamil. Nitrates can be given by inhalation of amyl nitrite, or by sublingual administration of glyceryl trinitrate or intravenous injection of isosorbide dinitrate (2.5 mg). Verapamil should be administered intravenously in a dose of 5 mg. Ergometrine testing should be performed only in specialized centres.

Imaging is commenced within 6–10 min of injection of isotope, starting with the 45° left anterior oblique projection and followed by the anteroposterior and left lateral projections. These three views should if possible be obtained within 20 min of ^{201}Tl injection, as beyond that time redistribution of tracer will have occurred to an important degree. When the redistribution process has reached equilibrium, 3–4 h after injection, control images are recorded in the same projections. If necessary, for instance when a defect persists without clinical evidence of old myocardial infarction, control images can be obtained 1 week later, using a second ^{201}Tl injection at rest, in the absence of acute ECG changes or symptoms. Imaging is performed with a gamma camera fitted with a high-sensitivity collimator to reduce imaging time. Using 1.5 mCi ^{201}Tl, approximately 120 s would be required for each view, obtaining 100000 counts within a 14 × 14 cm field of view centred on the heart. The images can be recorded in analogue form on polaroid or X-ray film and can also be converted to digital form for computer processing and storage.

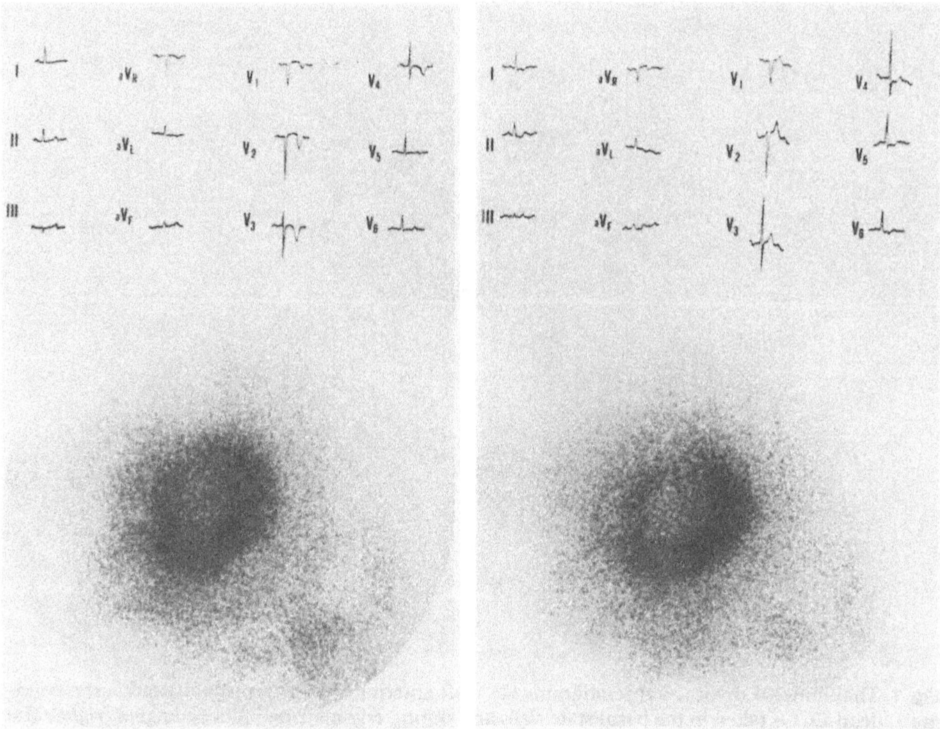

Fig. 2. Thallium-201 myocardial scintigrams (left anterior oblique projection) and corresponding ECGs taken in the basal state *(left)* and during a spontaneous attack of angina *(right)* associated with normalization of previously negative T waves in the anteroseptal leads. Coronary arteriography during an attack revealed severe, diffuse narrowing of the left anterior descending artery with delayed filling and run-off

The scintigrams, either in analogue or digital form, should be analysed by at least two independent, experienced observers, all projections being considered. Scoring can be carried out using a scale from 0 to 3 (0 = no defect detectable; 1 = doubtful; 2 = evident defect, but small; 3 = large defect). Some inhomogeneity of myocardial ^{201}Tl distribution is found in normals; the image of such inhomogeneity can be accentuated by computer processing, so that caution is necessary in the interpretation of computer-processed scintigrams. In fact, computerized analysis of ^{201}Tl scintigrams was found to agree closely with visual analysis both in normals and in patients with old myocardial infarction, suggesting that little is to be gained from computer processing of ^{201}Tl scintigrams.

3 Diagnostic Use

The sensitivity of the technique in detecting myocardial ischaemia depends on the causal mechanism of the ischaemia, i.e. to what extent it is caused by an absolute reduction in regional myocardial blood flow as opposed to an increase in myocardial oxygen demand.

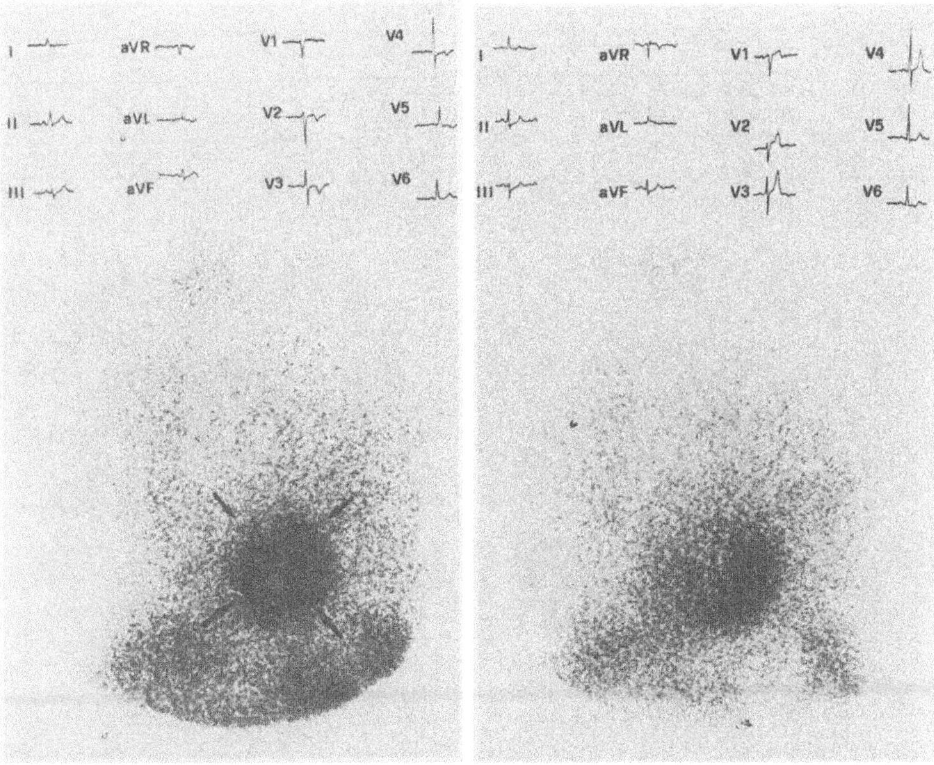

Fig. 3. Thallium-201 myocardial scintigrams (left anterior oblique projection) and corresponding ECGs. The basal scintigram *(left)* shows even distribution of activity in the left ventricle; the T waves are inverted in the anterior precordial leads. Normalization of the T waves with ST segment elevation is associated with a marked reduction in thallium activity in the anteroseptal wall due to a massive reduction in perfusion

3.1 Angina at Rest

Thallium-201 scintigraphy is invariably positive in the presence of ST segment elevation (Fig. 1) or normalization of previously negative T waves (Figs. 2 and 3) [16]. The defects are well defined and transmural, and are usually associated with transient complete occlusion of a major coronary vessel, either in the presence or in the absence of underlying atherosclerotic coronary stenosis. The site of the perfusion defect corresponds to that of the ST segment or T wave changes on the ECG. In over 90% of the patients with ST segment depression occurring spontaneously at rest abnormalities can eventually be seen on the scintigram (Figs. 4 and 5), although the defect is less well defined than in the case of ST elevation or normalization of T waves, indicating non-transmural and less severe ischaemia. Furthermore, the site of the perfusion defect does not necessarily coincide with that of the ECG changes (Fig. 6). Such patients often have more severe atherosclerotic coronary disease with collateral vessels [17], and coronary arterial spasm seen in these cases is often less extensive or subocclusive.

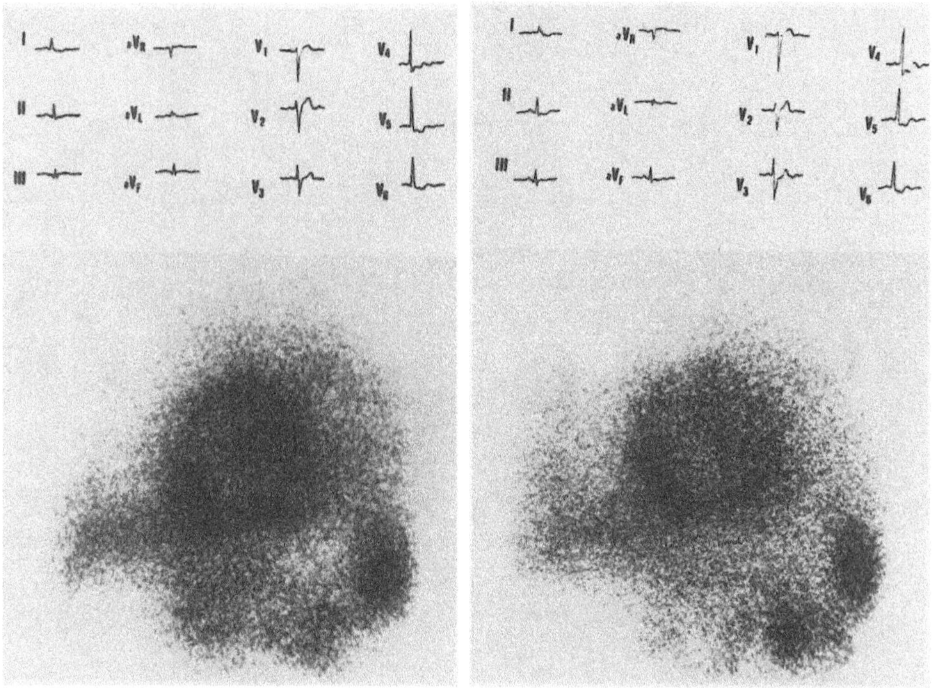
I aVR V1 V4
II aVL V2 V5
III aVF V3 V6
I aVR V1 V4
II aVL V2 V5
III aVF V3 V6

Fig. 4

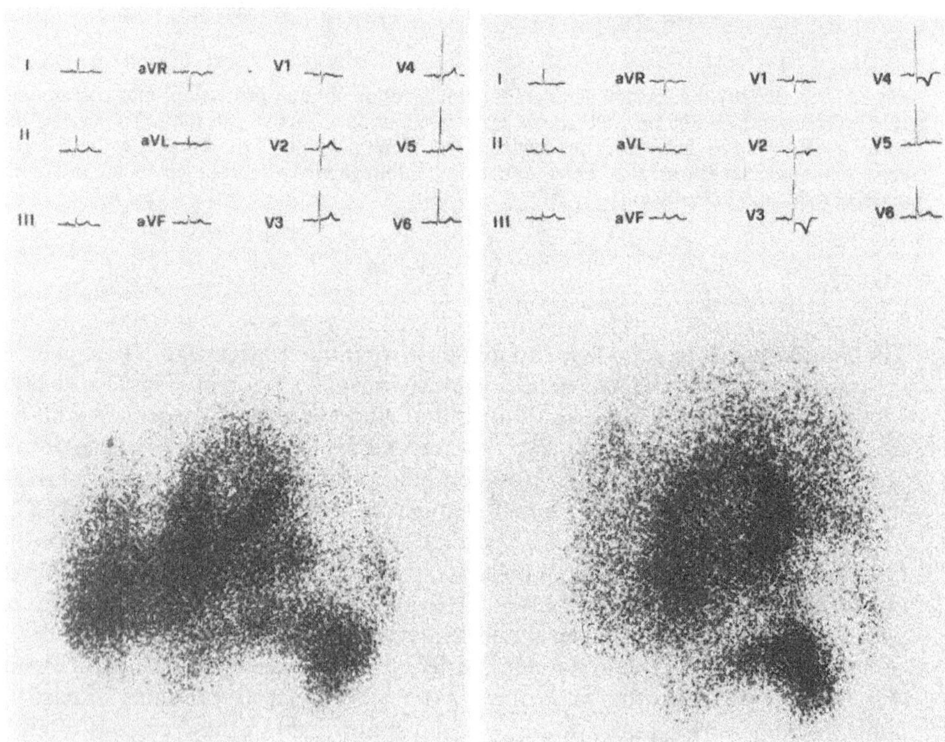
I aVR V1 V4
II aVL V2 V5
III aVF V3 V6
I aVR V1 V4
II aVL V2 V5
III aVF V3 V6

Fig. 5

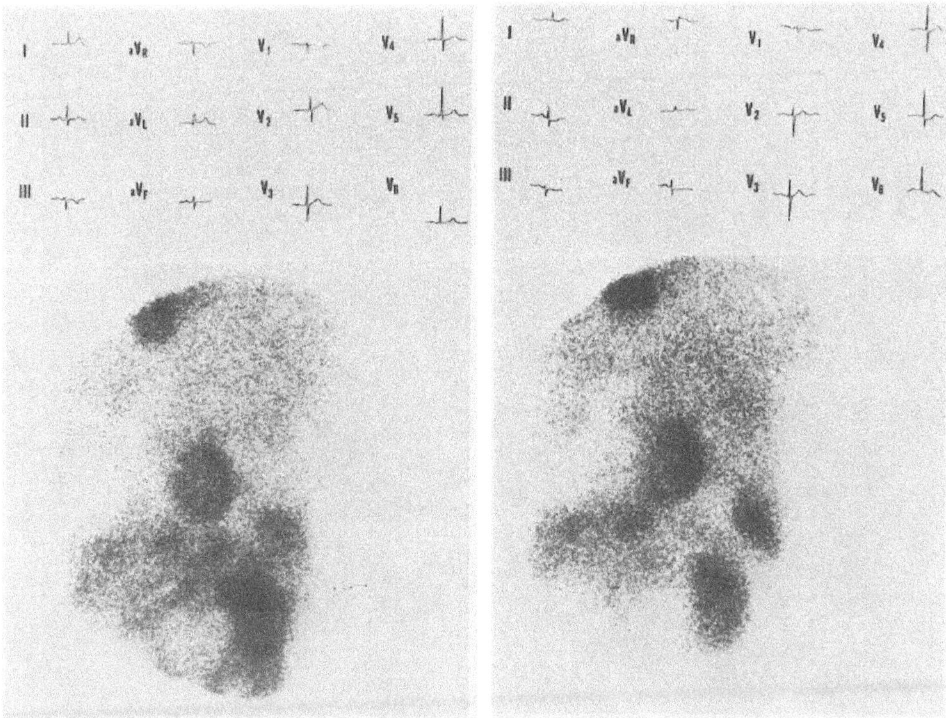

Fig. 6. Thallium-201 myocardial scintigrams (45° left anterior oblique projection taken during spontaneous angina at rest *(right)*, characterized by ST segment depression in the lateral precordial and inferior leads. Comparison with the basal scintigram *(left)* reveals a localized reduction in tracer uptake in the anteroseptal wall

◁ **Fig. 4.** Thallium-201 myocardial scintigrams with corresponding ECGs taken in the basal state *(left)* and during spontaneous angina characterized by ST segment depression *(right)*. Further ST segment depression in lead V^5 is associated with diffuse reduction in tracer uptake at the base and in the lateral wall of the left ventricle. The patient had severe triple-vessel disease, and coronary arteriography performed during a similar episode of ischaemia showed diffuse narrowing of a large obtuse marginal branch with poor, delayed filling and luminal reduction of the diagonal branches

◁ **Fig. 5.** Thallium-201 myocardial scintigrams (45° left anterior oblique projection) taken in the basal state *(left)* and during ergometrine-induced angina *(right)* associated with ST segment depression and T wave inversion in the precordial leads (V_2–V_4). A transmural defect in activity is seen in the inferior wall together with a reduction in activity in the anteroseptal wall. The inferior leads do not show signs of ischaemia in spite of the obvious defect in inferior wall activity on the scintigram

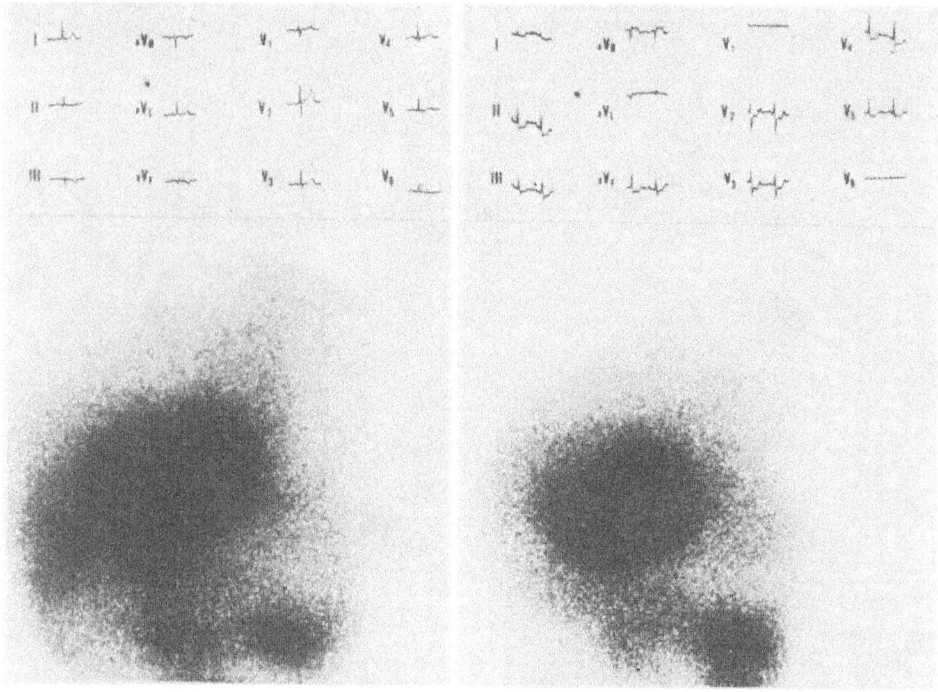

Fig. 7. Basal scintigram (left anterior oblique projection) taken in a patient with effort angina, showing even distribution of activity in the left ventricle *(left)*. During exercise *(right)* there is anterior ST segment depression associated with a marked perfusion defect in the posterolateral wall

The development of these scintigraphic defects, in the absence of changes indicating an increase in myocardial oxygen demand (such as tachycardia and elevation of arterial pressure), strongly suggests a primary reduction in blood supply as the cause of the anginal attack. Coronary arteriography may indicate that this reduced supply is due to arterial spasm.

3.2 Effort Angina

Abnormal scintigrams are almost invariably obtained in the presence of ST elevation or normalization of T waves (Fig. 7) [16]. Some of these patients also have attacks of angina at rest, so that it is probable that an absolute reduction in perfusion is partly responsible for the ischaemia. Indeed, coronary arterial spasm has been documented by arteriography in some cases with exercise-induced ST segment elevation. As in rest angina, the site of the defect corresponds to the location of the acute ECG changes and a major vessel is usually involved.

Effort angina with ST segment depression (Fig. 8) is not necessarily associated with a defect of perfusion, detectable by thallium scintigraphy [16]. In fact, scintigraphic findings are positive in only a little over half the patients (Fig. 9). This is probably due to several factors:

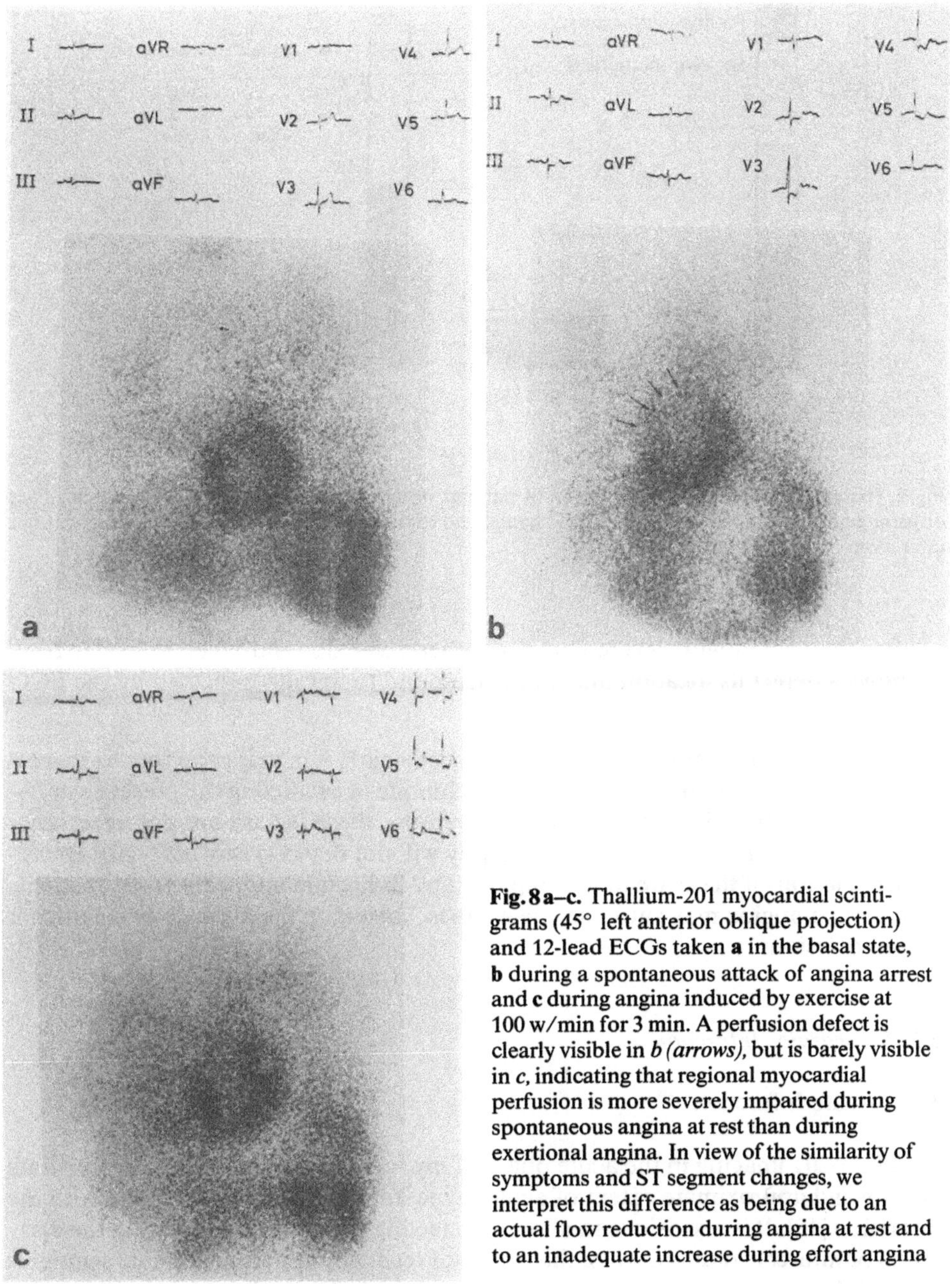

Fig. 8 a–c. Thallium-201 myocardial scintigrams (45° left anterior oblique projection) and 12-lead ECGs taken **a** in the basal state, **b** during a spontaneous attack of angina arrest and **c** during angina induced by exercise at 100 w/min for 3 min. A perfusion defect is clearly visible in *b (arrows)*, but is barely visible in *c*, indicating that regional myocardial perfusion is more severely impaired during spontaneous angina at rest than during exertional angina. In view of the similarity of symptoms and ST segment changes, we interpret this difference as being due to an actual flow reduction during angina at rest and to an inadequate increase during effort angina

1. The ischaemia is subendocardial.
2. The flow probably does not decrease in the ischaemic region, the ischaemia being relative to an increased requirement.
3. Superimposition of ischaemic and non-ischaemic regions is more likely than in the case of transmural ischaemia. As in the case of rest angina, ST depression is

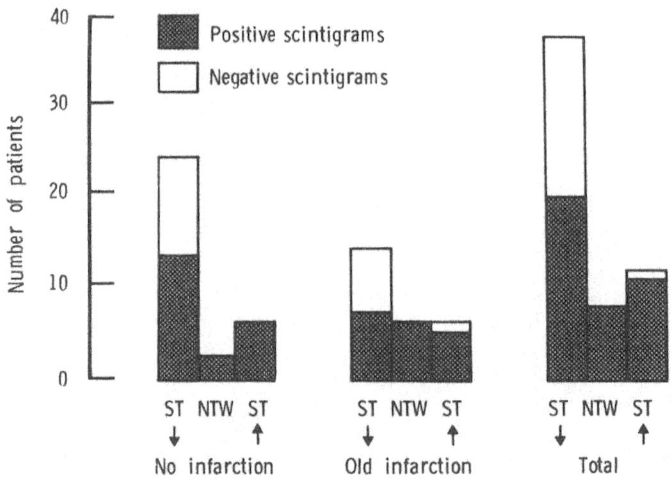

Fig. 9. Histogram showing the proportion of patients in whom scintigraphic findings are positive, distributed according to the type of ECG change and to the presence or absence of old myocardial infarction

often associated with severe coronary atherosclerosis, and when the scintigram shows a defect its location may not correspond to the site indicated by the ECG changes.

As defects of ^{201}Tl uptake are related to "ischaemia", it is inappropriate to discuss the "sensitivity" and "specificity" of this technique in predicting the presence or absence of coronary atherosclerotic lesions because these lesions are not necessarily related to ischaemia. Thus ^{201}Tl scintigraphy will not detect severe coronary atherosclerotic lesions if these are unaccompanied by ischaemia and, conversely, patients with variant angina may suffer severe acute ischaemia in the absence of significant coronary lesions.

3.3 Myocardial Infarction

3.3.1 Acute Infarction

Thallium-201 imaging in the acute phase of myocardial infarction will demonstrate the site and approximate extent of acute myocardial ischaemia associated with the infarction [18]. It is a sensitive method of detecting such ischaemia during the early hours of infarct evolution, when the results of technetium pyrophosphate scintigraphy will be negative and the serum creatine phosphokinase level has not begun to rise. Of course, in the majority of cases the ECG will show the classic changes of acute myocardial infarction, and thus the diagnosis will be established with ease and little financial burden. The technique is particularly useful, however, where the ECG is difficult to interpret, such as in the presence of left bundle-branch block and in some cases of partial-thickness infarction. Once discovered, however, the perfusion defect is not necessarily recent but may be related to myocardial scar tissue due to old infarction. The technique is therefore more useful in patients with no history of cardiac problems. Imaging later in the course of acute infarction reveals a tendency for the perfusion defects to become smaller [19].

3.3.2 Old Infarction

Even when an old myocardial infarct is definitely present, as assessed by clinical, enzymatic and ECG (pathological Q waves) criteria, the thallium scintigram may be negative [20]. Indeed, it is positive in only approximately 55% of these patients. Not surprisingly, large infarcts are more likely to be detected than small ones. In the recent series by Uthurralt et al. [20], scintigraphy produced positive results in all eight patients with extensive anterior infarction, but scintigraphic findings were positive in only three of ten patients with anteroseptal infarction and in five of 13 with inferior infarction. When the findings are positive, however, ^{201}Tl scintigraphy often localizes and delineates the infarction with greater precision than the ECG.

4 Conclusion

Myocardial perfusion imaging using ^{201}Tl is of value in the detection of acute myocardial ischaemia, particularly when this occurs spontaneously at rest or is induced by provocative tests. Its use in effort-induced ischaemia should be reserved for patients in whom ECG changes are equivocal or when the ECG is difficult to interpret due to left bundle-branch block, left ventricular hypertrophy, old myocardial infarction or the effects of drugs. It is an insensitive method for the detection of old myocardial infarction. However, in acute infarction, even at the onset of the clinical events, it invariably reveals the zone of acute ischaemia as a cold area. The defect corresponds to an unpredictable extent to necrosis, surrounding ischaemia and old scar tissue, if present. Comparison with previous scintigrams allows the identification of scar tissue. Comparison with subsequent scintigrams allows the distinction of necrosis from ischaemia, which should no longer be present after the acute phase of infarction.

IV Radio-Nuclide Explorations: Pyrophosphate Myocardial Imaging

1 Introduction

A variety of radio-pharmaceuticals have been used to identify myocardial infarction. Most have been based on substances, such as fluorescein or tetracycline, that were known to concentrate in infarcted muscle and which were labelled with gamma-emitting radio-nuclides [21]. The observations of Shen and Jennings [22] indicating that calcium is deposited in crystalline or subcrystalline form in irreversibly damaged myocardial cells led Bonte and colleagues [23] to speculate that technetium-99m pyrophosphate (^{99m}Tc PYP) might prove suitable for infarct imaging. They reasoned that the PYP would complex with the calcium in the damaged cells. Their observations showed that the technique was a sensitive means of demonstrating damaged myocardium.

2 Pathophysiological Mechanisms

After experimental coronary artery occlusion, cells show mitochondrial swelling with marked myofibril hypercontraction and distortion of cell architecture. The development of abnormal myocardial fluid retention and loss of cell volume regulation appear to precede the development of extensive myocardial necrosis, as judged by both ultrastructural and biochemical criteria. Muscle cells within the damaged region then begin to demonstrate changes indicative of irreversible cellular injury, including flocculent densities, marked mitochondrial calcification and severe myofibril disruption. Mitochondrial inclusions containing electron-dense spicular materials represent relatively advanced stages of mitochondrial calcification in myocardial infarction. Such calcification appears to be explained by the dual requirements of cellular injury and persistent tissue perfusion, which allow delivery of plasma calcium to the injured area. Histological and ultrastructural studies of experimental infarcts also show that discrete calcium deposits occur in the peripheral zones of the infarct. Buja et al. [24] found the highest ^{99m}Tc PYP concentration ratios in the periphery of experimentally induced infarcts (25 times that of normal myocardium), while the concentration in the centre was only 1.7 times the normal. It has been suggested that the concentration may be dependent on hydroxyapatite crystals formed within the mitochondria, but in cell fractionation studies Dewanjee and Kahn [25] found uptake in the soluble and nuclear fractions and only a small percentage of PYP in the mitochondria. Further, Kronenburg et al. [26] showed that adjacent to infarcted muscle there was marked ^{99m}Tc PYP uptake but very modest creatine kinase depletion. Certainly, the uptake of ^{99m}Tc PYP seems to be closely related to coronary flow. Zaret et al. [27] demonstrated that maximal PYP uptake decreased in ischaemic regions, where blood flow as measured by the microsphere technique was 30%–40% of normal. In low flow areas PYP uptake was predominantly epicardial, and border zones between normal and deeply ischaemic areas sequestered PYP. The question of the border zone is intriguing and the definition of cell death often difficult. Buja et al. [28], using tritiated diphosphonate, showed uptake in the border zone, but although there was absence of conventional histological evidence of irreversible damage, the cells were swollen, were loaded with lipid and had other features of cellular disarray. The ultimate fate of these border zone cells that take up the tracer is still uncertain.

3 Clinical Use

Although there is still uncertainty about the precise mechanisms of PYP uptake, the time course of events is much clearer. Infarcted myocardium accumulates ^{99m}Tc PYP within 6 h of coronary occlusion, and there is a progressive uptake for the next 24–72 h. The uptake remains abnormal for up to 6 days and then diminishes. The time course in man seems to be very similar to that observed in animal studies, but in some patients positive results may be obtained for many weeks after infarction [29]. Although uptake begins at about 6 h, the scan is unlikely to yield positive results before 12 h, and the optimal period is usually 24–48 h after infarction (Figs. 1–3). Scanning more than once over this time period can increase the yield, as there are inter-patient variations in the optimal scanning period. A negative scintigram 12–24 h following suspected acute myocardial infarction does not exclude myocardial infarction, and the procedure should be repeated 48–72 h following the acute event.

3.1 Scanning Technique

In practice, good-quality imaging can be obtained if 500 mBq ^{99m}Tc PYP are injected intravenously and scintigrams are taken after the blood pool has cleared and before there is intense bone uptake. We scan 2 h after injection of PYP, but if there is a diffuse pattern the patient is rescanned 2 h later to determine whether further clearance has taken place. Imaging should be conducted using a low-energy, all-purpose parallel-hole collimator coupled to the gamma camera. We accumulate 500 000 counts in each view (anterior, 45° left anterior oblique and left lateral). When a mobile gamma camera is used at the bedside, it is often more convenient to record the images on a radiographic film, but when it is used in the department digital data are stored in a computer for subsequent analysis. A gated ventriculogram can also be constructed in the first 5 min after injection of ^{99m}Tc PYP and before there is significant loss from the blood pool. The radiation exposure of target organs (skeleton, kidney and bladder) has been calculated at about 0.13 rad per organ.

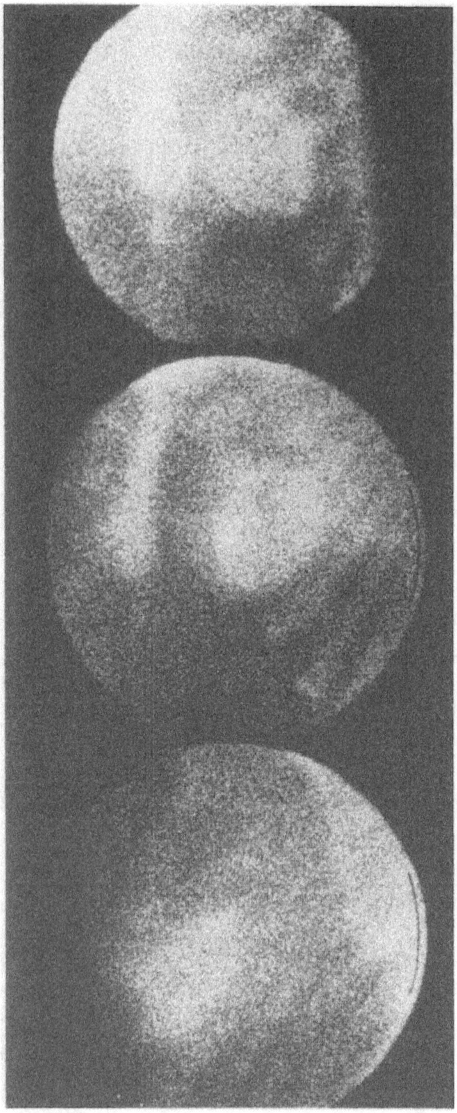

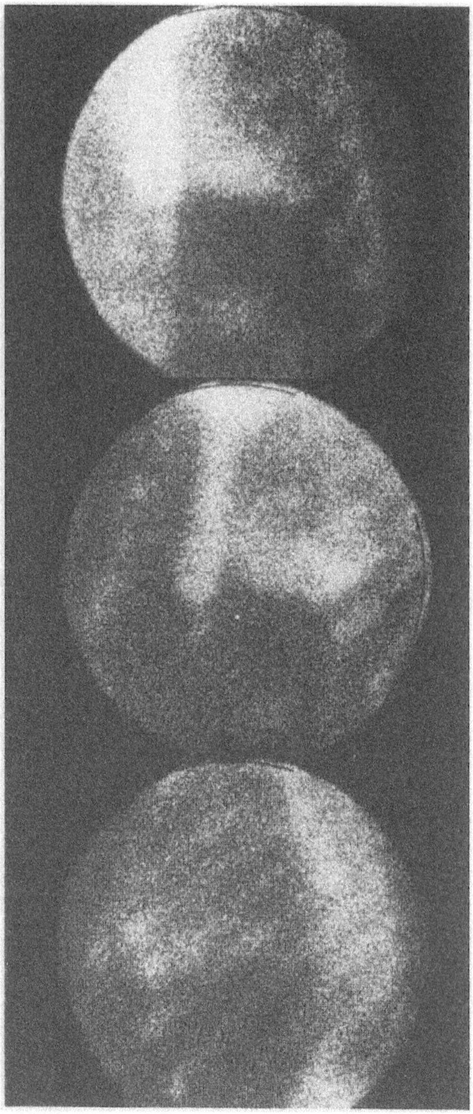

Fig. 1 *(left)*. Anterior myocardial infarction demonstrated by ^{99m}Tc PYP scintigraphy. The images were acquired 36 h after infarction and are, in descending order, anterior, left anterior oblique and lateral views

Fig. 2 *(right)*. Anterior, left anterior oblique and lateral views in a patient with inferior myocardial infarction

3.2 Technical Considerations

Unbound ^{99m}Tc may remain in the blood pool or diffuse out into the extravascular space to cause either false positive results or high background activity: the amount of free ^{99m}Tc should not exceed 5%. Reduced hydrolysed ^{99m}Tc forms a colloid which accumulates in the liver. Both the amount of free ^{99m}Tc and the reduced hydrolysed ^{99m}Tc can be checked by thin-layer chromatography, but an easy clinical guide to the quality of the scintigram is the outline of the rib cage. If the skeleton is not well delineated, it suggests either that there was a delayed clearance secondary to intrinsic renal disease or dehydration or that the in vivo binding of ^{99m}Tc PYP was inadequate.

3.3 Interpretation

When the images are read, scintigraphic abnormalities are usually classified firstly as localized or diffuse, and the intensity of the pattern is compared to that of the ribs [23, 30].

Greater intensity than bone	4+
Equal to bone	3+
Moderate but less than bone	2+
Slight	1+
None	0

When the activity in the myocardium is equal to or greater than that in bone, the result is unequivocally positive (i.e. 3+ and 4+). Likewise, focal uptake graded at 2+ represents infarcted tissue, but diffuse uptake at this level of intensity is more difficult to interpret and has been graded by Berman et al. [31] as "equivocal". This is the system that we follow, as it conveys the necessary degree of uncertainty to clinicians. Scans graded 0 to 1+ are considered to show no evidence of infarction. Early studies had suggested that localized uptake was characteristic of transmural infarction and diffuse uptake of subendocardial infarction. Although this may be a broad generalization, careful pathological studies have shown that this is not always the case. In contrast, the "doughnut" pattern, which is infrequently seen, is always associated with large transmural myocardial infarction [32].

The precise level set for positive and negative results influences the sensitivity (the percentage of patients with the disease in whom the test produces positive results) and the specificity (the percentage of patients without the disease in whom the test produces negative results). As discussed above, the interpretation of moderate diffuse PYP activity throughout the left ventricular region has proved most difficult. Berman et al. [31] studied 235 patients admitted to a coronary care unit. Of 81 patients with acute transmural infarction by electrocardiographic criteria, the results of the scan were positive in 76, equivocal in five and negative in none. Eighteen were judged to have a non-transmural infarct, and the results of the scan were positive in seven, equivocal in nine and negative in two. Of the remaining 126 patients without infarction, the results of the scan were negative in 87, equivocal in 35 and definitely positive in 4. In many patients a small diffuse increase in activity in the heart region

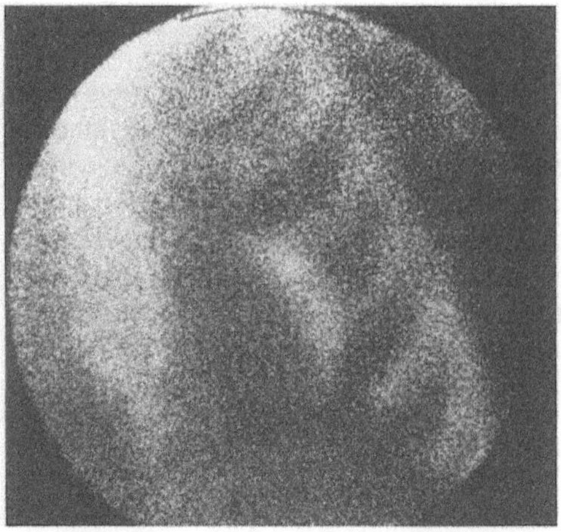

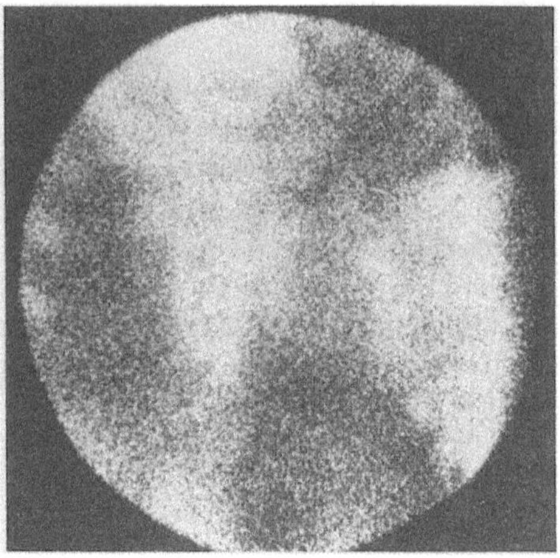

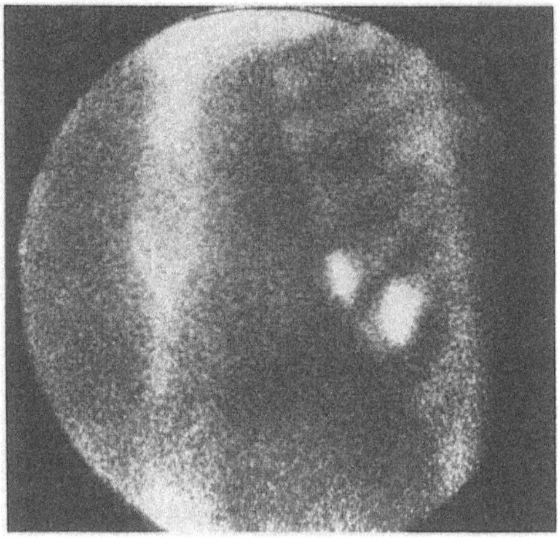

Fig. 3 *(upper left).* Lateral wall infarction

Fig. 4 *(upper right).* Extensive uptake of ^{99m}Tc PYP in skeletal muscle as well as myocardium in a patient who had required multiple defibrillation for repetitive ventricular fibrillation

Fig. 5 *(lower).* ^{99m}Tc PYP scintigram taken in a 48-year-old man admitted to our coronary care unit with atypical chest pain. No rib fracture was suspected until demonstrated by the scintigram. Radiological oblique views confirmed the rib fractures

may represent blood pool activity, and it is these patients we rescan 2 h later to determine whether there has been further clearance. Some equivocal results become clearly negative, but particularly in patients with unstable angina the diffuse appearance persists, a pattern noted by Donsky et al. [33] in 35% of patients with this clinical diagnosis. Whether this represents true but subclinical infarction remains controversial.

Any cause of myocardial necrosis will entail an uptake of ^{99m}Tc PYP, so that a scan may give positive results after cardioversion, cardiac tumour, cardiac trauma and dystrophic or metastatic cardiac calcification; findings may also be positive in some patients with left ventricular aneurysm, perhaps because of dystrophic cardiac calcification and continuing cell injury or because of the accentuated blood pool effect. Non-cardiac causes of apparently positive findings include bone, muscle or breast uptake because of bone fractures or neoplasms, muscle injury or cardioversion or inflammatory lesions of the breast (Figs. 4 and 5 [34].

4 The Role of Technetium-99m Pyrophosphate Scintigraphy

In the majority of patients diagnosis of myocardial infarction can easily be confirmed by electrocardiographic and serial cardiac enzyme changes, so that there is little need for ^{99m}Tc PYP scintigraphy in these patients [35]. Moreover, experience has shown that although some estimate of infarct size can be made in patients with anterior wall damage, assessment of infarct size in general is too unreliable for routine use. However, the ^{99m}Tc PYP scintigram provides unique information in clinical situations where interpretation of the electrocardiogram and enzyme changes is difficult.

4.1 Late Diagnosis

Late diagnosis occurs primarily when infarcts are suspected to have occurred some days before hospital admission or out-patient consultation. Evolutionary changes on the electrocardiogram are unlikely, and even changes in late-rising enzymes such as lactic dehydrogenase may be missed. In contrast, because the ^{99m}Tc PYP scan remains positive for 6 days or longer, this technique may prove helpful in the diagnosis of late suspected infarction. The finding of a strongly positive pyrophosphate scan result that reverts to negative 2–3 weeks later strongly supports the diagnosis of recent infarction.

In patients in whom the electrocardiogram can be misleading, such as those with left bundle-block or who have had previous infarctions, the diagnosis of further infarction is difficult. Even with a rise in cardiac enzymes, localization of the site of infarction may be impossible. As the site of infarction has considerable influence on prognosis, ^{99m}Tc PYP scintigraphy should be carried out to allow diagnosis and localization.

4.2 Myocardial Contusion

Myocardial contusion after blunt chest trauma, which can predispose to arrhythmias, produces non-specific electrocardiographic and enzymatic abnormalities, which are usually attributed to skeletal muscle trauma. Damage to the myocardium can be demonstrated by ^{99m}Tc PYP scintigraphy and can alert clinicians to the possibility of life-threatening arrhythmias [36].

4.3 *Unstable Angina*

Patients with anginal pain at rest that responds poorly to therapy (unstable angina) pose a particular clinical problem. These patients, by definition, do not show electrocardiographic and enzymatic evidence of myocardial infarction. However, approximately one-third of patients with this syndrome show low-grade positive ^{99m}Tc PYP myocardial scintigrams [33]. Poliner and colleagues [37] correlated scintigraphic, clinical and pathological findings in 52 patients studied by ^{99m}Tc PYP myocardial scintigraphy before death or surgical resection of the myocardium. Five of these cases were patients with unstable angina, and in all instances the positive ^{99m}Tc PYP scintigram was associated with evidence of multifocal irreversible myocardial damage, consisting of myocytolysis, coagulation necrosis and/or fibrosis. The histological age of lesions was compatible with acute injury corresponding to the time of injury. In these patients with unstable angina, small areas of necrosis may occur over a period of days, so that the total enzyme released into the bloodstream is small, but because PYP uptake continues for 6–7 days after infarction, the scan may detect this accumulated damage within that period.

4.4 *Right Ventricular Infarction*

It is also suggested that ^{99m}Tc PYP scintigraphy is specific for the diagnosis of right ventricular infarction. In patients with right ventricular infarction, accumulation of labelled PYP occurs in the inferior wall of the left ventricle and the free wall of the right ventricle. In some patients right ventricular infarction leads to systematic hypotension, with high venous pressure. Despite this high venous pressure it is appropriate to treat this group of patients with volume loading, so the diagnosis is important. However, disparity in function of the ventricles can be noted from radionuclide ventriculography, which may be more useful in the management of these patients than PYP imaging.

4.5 *Perioperative Infarction*

During cardiac surgery the heart is liable to myocardial cell damage, so that considerable effort has been expended in devising the best means of myocardial preservation during the period of circulatory arrest. The diagnosis of myocardial damage following cardiac surgery is, however, difficult. Non-specific electrocardiographic abnormalities frequently occur, and increases in serum enzymes are often noted in the absence of myocardial infarction. In contrast, a ^{99m}Tc PYP scan with positive results is indicative of acute infarction, provided the results of the pre-operative scan were negative and that the operative procedure did not involve excision of myocardial tissue. Our own experience is that patients with aortic stenosis are particularly at risk from myocardial damage during cardiac surgery, despite apparent cardioplegia. Presumably this condition relates to hypertrophy of the left ventricular muscle mass. Patients undergoing mitral valve replacement rarely show positive scintigraphic findings. In patients with aortic and mitral valve disease we have found that the findings are invariably negative pre-operatively, but in coronary artery disease pre-operative scintigraphy should be carried out to allow accurate diagnosis of perioperative infarction. We have noted that with improving myocardial preservation techniques the incidence of myocardial damage following coronary artery surgery has dropped from 10% to 2%. In patients in whom perioperative infarction has occurred, there is a reduction in left ventricular function after operation, indicating a loss of functioning myocardium which is often associated with a poor clinical outcome despite an apparently successful operation. In our institution ^{99m}Tc PYP scintigraphy has found its greatest role in the diagnosis of perioperative infarction.

5 Future Development

Image enhancement can be obtained by computer subtraction techniques, and the localization of the isotope in bone can be minimized by tomographic imaging. It is also likely that tomographic imaging will permit accurate localization and sizing of the damage to the myocardium. However, even if accurate localization and sizing of infarction were possible with ^{99m}Tc PYP scintigraphy, it would remain less than an ideal imaging agent. Its uptake relates too closely to myocardial blood flow, and the half-life of ^{99m}Tc is too long (6 h) to allow frequent repeated observations in the acute phase. Other infarct-avid radio-pharmaceuticals are being investigated [38]. Antimyosin antibodies show particular promise, as they localize in proportion to the amount of muscle cell injury, but labelling with ultra-short-half-life radio-nuclides has not yet been accomplished. An ideal agent would be one taken up equally by all the damaged myocardial cells. Positive results of scanning should be possible within 6 h of infarction, and the radiotracer itself should have a sufficiently short half-life to permit rescanning fairly frequently, so that therapeutic interventions aimed at limiting infarct size may be studied. However, such an imaging agent does not yet exist.

V Radio-Nuclide Explorations: Ventricular Function Studies

1 Introduction

The occurrence of acute myocardial ischaemia is invariably associated with impairment of left ventricular function [39]. Whether or not this is detected depends upon the sensitivity of the technique used to measure this parameter. Continuous monitoring of left ventricular pressure in patients with recurrent spontaneous episodes of myocardial ischaemia has shown elevation of the end-diastolic pressure which precedes the onset of electrocardiographic changes often by several minutes [40]. Furthermore, this rise in left ventricular end-diastolic pressure is associated with a fall in both contraction and relaxation peak rate of change of pressure, reflecting impairment of "contractility" of the ventricle. In other words, the ischaemic ventricle is in "acute failure", and this ventricular failure is an early manifestation which can be detected by a number of methods. The value of left ventricular pressure recording is obviously severely limited by its invasive nature. However, changes in left ventricular volume and regional contraction probably accompany the pressure changes, and recording these aspects of ventricular function will therefore probably provide useful diagnostic information. Contrast left ventriculography does not provide an adequate solution because of its invasive nature, its interference with cardiovascular physiology and the restriction of total contrast dose. Whilst echocardiography overcomes these problems, geometrical limitations preclude assessment of ventricular volume and impose some restriction on regional wall motion assessment. Many of the above-mentioned limitations can be overcome by radioisotopic methods of assessment of ventricular function.

2 Electrocardiogram-Gated Blood Pool Imaging

The ECG-gated blood pool imaging technique uses a scintillation camera to image the technetium-labelled cardiac blood pool [41]. Data are collected from several hundred cardiac cycles and those from corresponding time segments of the cardiac cycle are combined to produce a series of "frames" spanning one "averaged" cardiac cycle.

2.1 Blood Pool Labelling

Blood pool labelling can be achieved by withdrawing blood from the patient and labelling in vitro or, as is more commonly done, by labelling in vivo. This latter technique requires the intravenous injection of approximately 0.2 mg sodium (stannous) pyrophosphate per kilogram body weight, followed after an interval of approximately 30 min by 15–20 mCi technetium-99m as pertechnetate [42].

2.2 *Data Acquisition*

There are two basic modes of computerized data acquisition. In *list mode* the X, Y co-ordinates of each detected gamma event, together with the digitized ECG signal and 10-ms time markers, are stored on disc or magnetic tape in chronological order in the form of a continuous list. This is the more flexible method, as it allows any mode of reconstruction of the data into an averaged cardiac cycle and the simultaneous acquisition of other physiological signals. In *frame mode* the cardiac cycle is divided into time segments with reference to the R wave, and gamma events detected during each of these segments are positioned in a corresponding, memory-located matrix in such a way as to reproduce the spatial relationship of the detected events. In other words, a series of "images" spanning an averaged cardiac cycle is built up in the computer memory. The number of frames per cycle and the acquisition period must be preselected. This approach is far less flexible than list mode acquisition, but the software is less complicated and less data storage capacity is required. After frame mode acquisition the images can be displayed as soon as they are needed, but after list mode acquisition the images must first be created.

2.3 *Creation of Images from List Mode Data*

The first stage is to plot a histogram of the number of cardiac cycles of each given length and to calculate the modal cycle length [43]. Only those cycles whose length lies within an operator-selected window are used for image construction, the imaging-degrading effect of extrasystoles and marked heart rate variation can thus be minimized. Any number of frames per cycle can be selected, though it should be borne in mind that having many frames will mean fewer counts per frame and result in poor image quality. The duration of each frame is calculated as the modal cycle length divided by the number of frames required. Each cycle is then examined both forwards and backwards from each R wave (Fig. 1) and events in corresponding time segments of each cycle are located, most often, in a 64×64 matrix and summed over a selected acquisition period or total number of counts [43]. The result is a sequence of frames spanning an averaged cardiac cycle, including events during atrial systole (Fig. 2). Any error related to cycle length variation can be confined to one frame, which can be positioned in mid-diastole where volume change is minimal. The series of frames are viewed in cine format to facilitate the detection of regional abnormalities of wall motion.

2.4 *Clinical Application*

Blood pool imaging can be performed during supine bicycle exercise [44] or during other provocative tests such as the cold pressor test, hyperventilation and ergome-

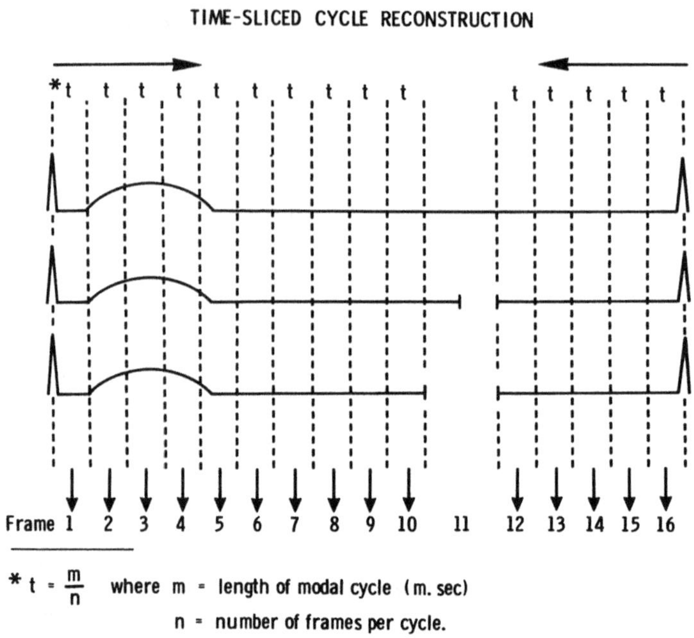

Fig. 1. Method of ECG-gated cycle reconstruction. All cycles of acceptable length are divided into *n* segments, where *t* = modal length/number of frames required. The cycle is thus divided progressing both forwards from the R wave and backwards from the next R wave. Corresponding segments from all cycles examined are summed to produce a series of images spanning one averaged cardiac cycle. This series includes events at end-diastole and the method enables the positioning of the frame containing errors due to cycle length variation in that part of the cycle where volume changes are minimal

trine injection [45]. Data acquisition must continue for at least 5 min, both during the basal state and after the onset of ECG change or chest pain.

The technique is useful for assessment of the resting state of the left ventricle, i.e. the detection of a dilated, hypokinetic ventricle (Fig. 3), of an extensive region of old infarction or of an aneurysm. Under these circumstances the period of data acquisition can be long in order to give good quality images. The detection of acute myocardial ischaemia is more difficult because of its transient nature. Imaging should span the whole period of detectable myocardial ischaemia and should therefore begin with, or after, the onset of ECG changes, where these occur, and finish before their resolution. Moreover, ischaemia must persist for several minutes because a steady state is required during the acquisition.

Using real time serial blood pool imaging at rest and on exercise, Borer et al. [44] were able to detect transient regional wall motion abnormalities during exercise in all 11 patients with significant coronary artery disease. These regional contraction abnormalities were associated with a fall in ejection fraction in ten patients, ranging between 7% and 47%. All 14 normals showed an increase in ejection fraction (mean ± SE = 23% ± 3%) and no regional wall motion abnormality. Several other workers have, more recently, demonstrated the high sensitivity of the technique in

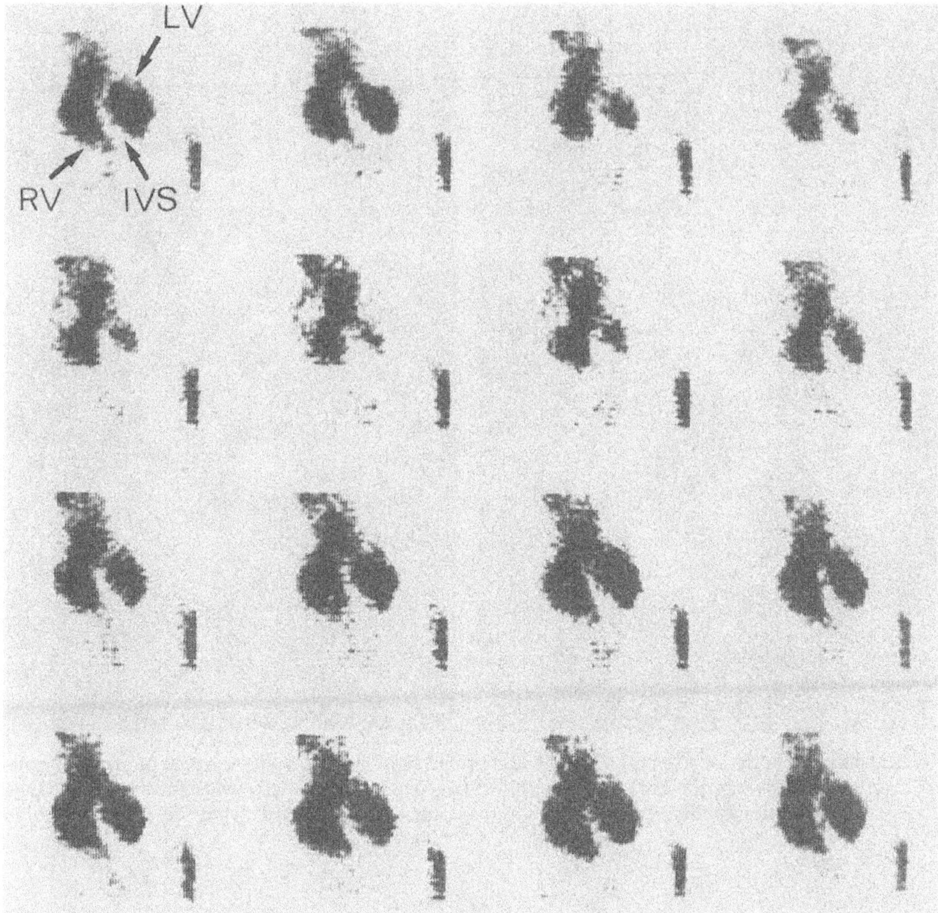

Fig. 2. A sequence of 16 frames, spanning an averaged cardiac cycle, of the ^{99m}Tc-labelled blood pool. *IVS:* interventricular septum; *RV:* right ventricle; *LV:* left ventricle. The size of the LV cavity falls during systole and returns towards the starting level as diastole progresses, completing the sequence

detecting the presence of significant coronary artery disease [46, 47]. The value of gated blood pool imaging in the detection of acute myocardial ischaemia has been compared to that of thallium-201 rest-exercise myocardial perfusion imaging. Elkayam et al. [48] found a sensitivity of 96%, 89% and 98% for the detection of significant coronary stenosis using ^{201}Tl imaging, gated blood pool imaging and the combined techniques respectively; the specificity of each method was 75%. Blood pool imaging was more sensitive for left anterior descending artery lesions, but ^{201}Tl scintigraphy was more specific and was more sensitive for right coronary artery lesions. Jengo et al. [49] found a sensitivity of 93% and 98% and a specificity of 94% and 100% for ^{201}Tl scintigraphy and gated blood pool imaging respectively in 42 patients with coronary artery disease and 16 normals.

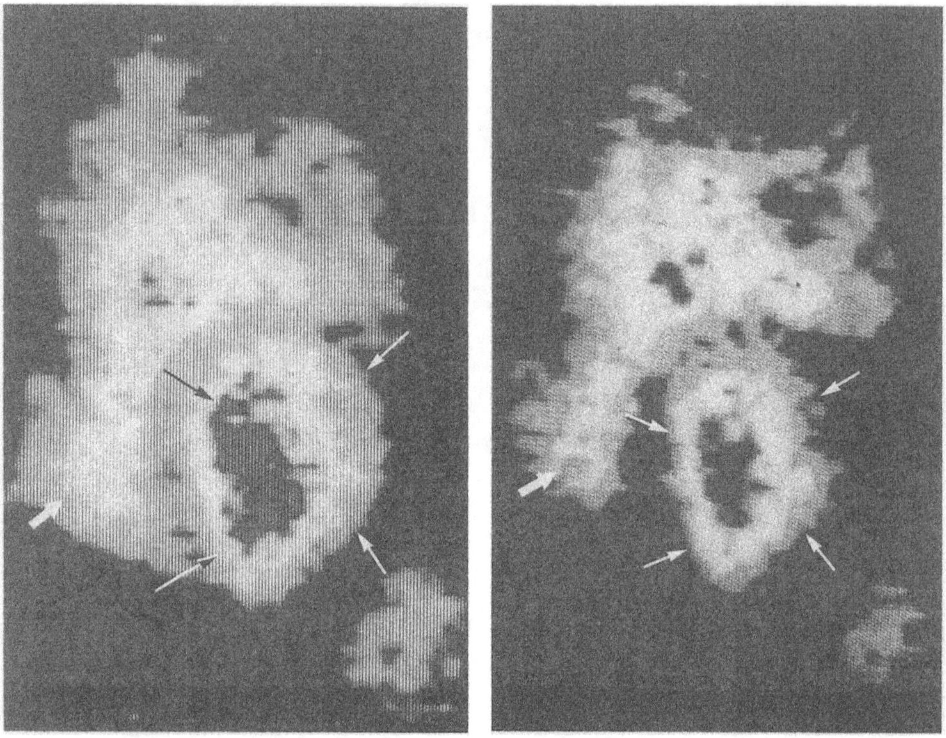

Fig. 3. On the *left* is shown the end-diastolic and on the *right* the end-systolic frame of an ECG-gated blood pool study of a patient with generalized hypokinesia of the left ventricle, clearly showing end-systolic dilatation of the left ventricle but good contraction of the right ventricle *(broad arrow)*

3 Continuous Precordial Counting

Because of the transient nature of attacks of myocardial ischaemia and the unpredictability of their occurrence, it would be desirable to monitor left ventricular function continuously from beat to beat. This is obviously not possible by imaging. However, changes in left ventricular volume accompany changes in regional left ventricular wall motion and can be assessed by counting the ^{99m}Tc-labelled blood pool activity over the left ventricle using a single scintillation probe [50]. This consists of a thallium-activated sodium iodide crystal 2 in. in diameter and 1½ in. thick with a 3½ in. long converging collimator (Fig. 4 upper). The probe is mounted on an arm which permits positioning freely over the chest (Fig. 4 lower) and control of two separate angular degrees of freedom. The beat-to-beat left ventricular time-activity curve is displayed in real time at 50-ms intervals on a cathode ray tube and the analogue output can be recorded on tape or on a strip chart recorder. The maximal count rate capacity of the system is 140000 counts/s. The positioning of the non-imaging probe requires orientation of the detector relative to the cardiac anatomy on the basis of a logically derived series of algorithms. Probe positions are determined

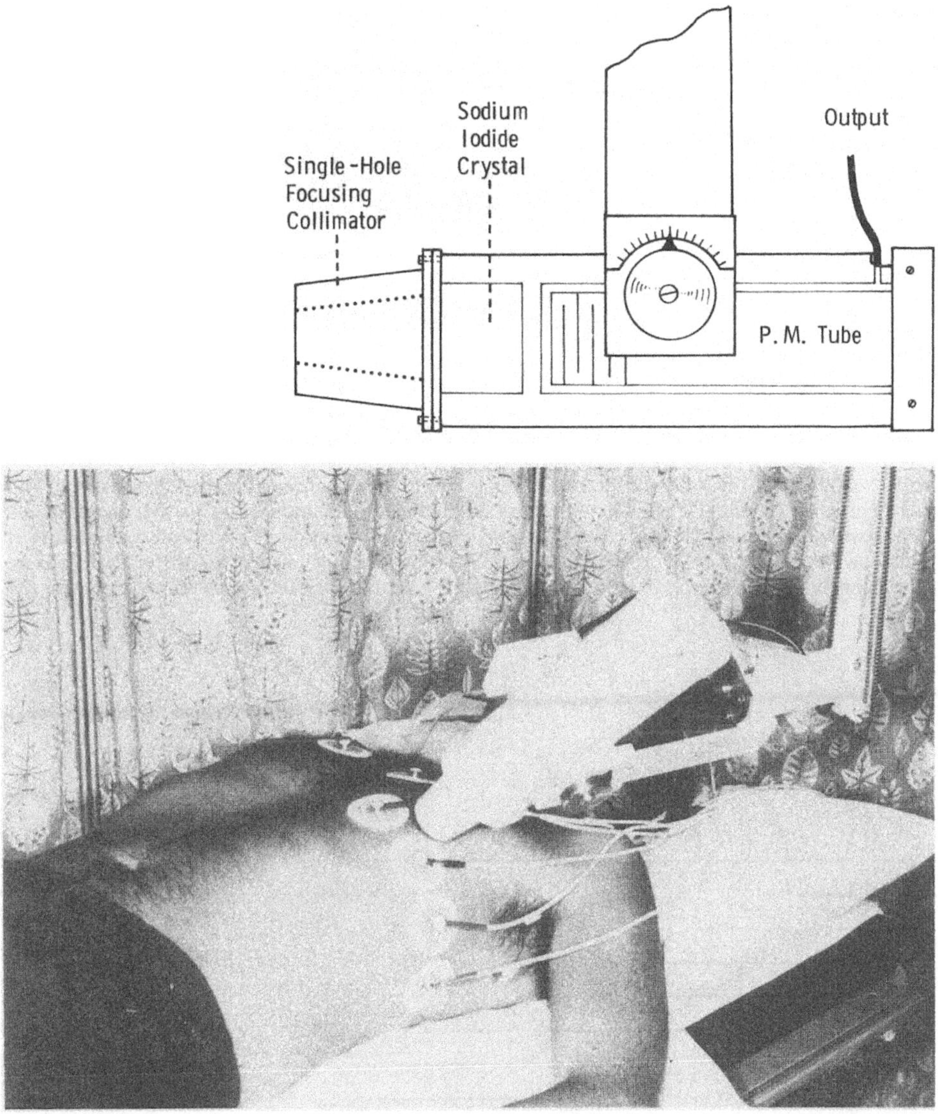

Fig. 4. *Upper:* Scintillation probe (Nuclear Stethoscope). It consists of a single-hole converging collimator, a thick thallium-activated sodium iodide crystal and a single photomultiplier *(P. M.)* tube. *Lower:* The scintillation probe is positioned over the left ventricle in the 40° left anterior oblique projection with 15° caudal angulation. Microprocessor-based algorithms facilitate fine adjustment of the instrument over the ventricle

empirically on the basis both of stroke counts (end-diastole minus end-systole) and of average counts (end-diastole plus end-systole divided by two) as recorded by the probe. The left ventricular region of interest is chosen as the position with the maximal ratio of stroke counts to average counts, taking into account also the shape of the volume curve. The background region of interest is chosen as a position imme-

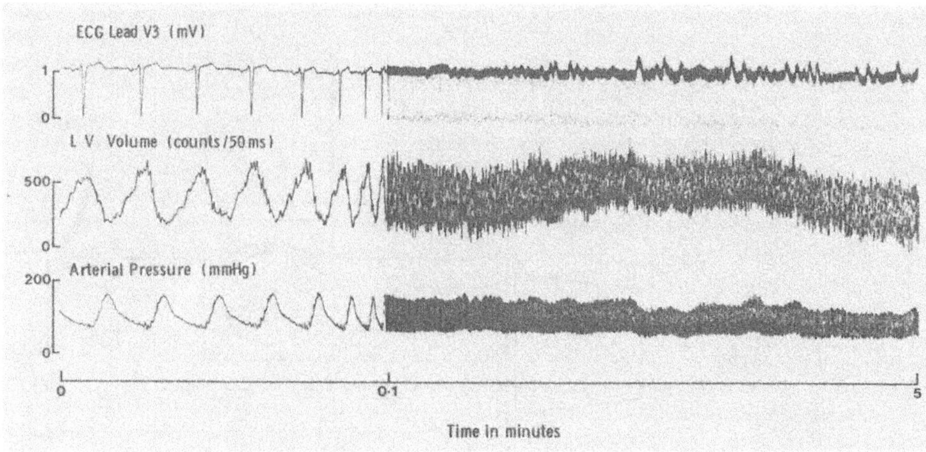

Fig. 5. A continuous recording of the ECG (V_3), left ventricular volume (Nuclear Stethoscope) and arterial pressure (brachial arterial cannula) during the basal state and during a spontaneous attack of myocardial ischaemia. There was a progressive increase in both end-systolic and end-diastolic volume, with a short plateau (approximately 2 min) followed by complete recovery. There was no significant change in the arterial pressure at the onset of the attack, which was entirely painless

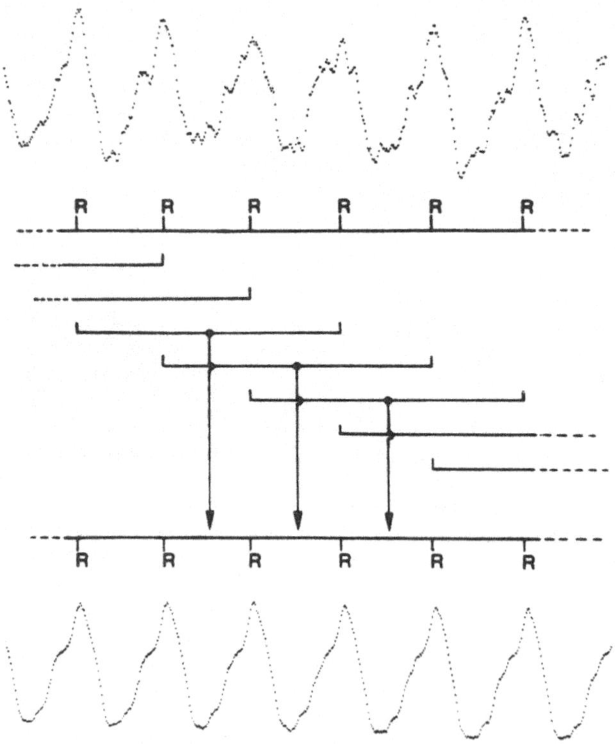

Fig. 6. Averaging of an input curve to produce an output curve: three cycles are used to produce each cycle of the output curve and the input curve is examined in a continuous, progressive manner. The corresponding time segment of each input cycle, synchronized by each R wave, is averaged

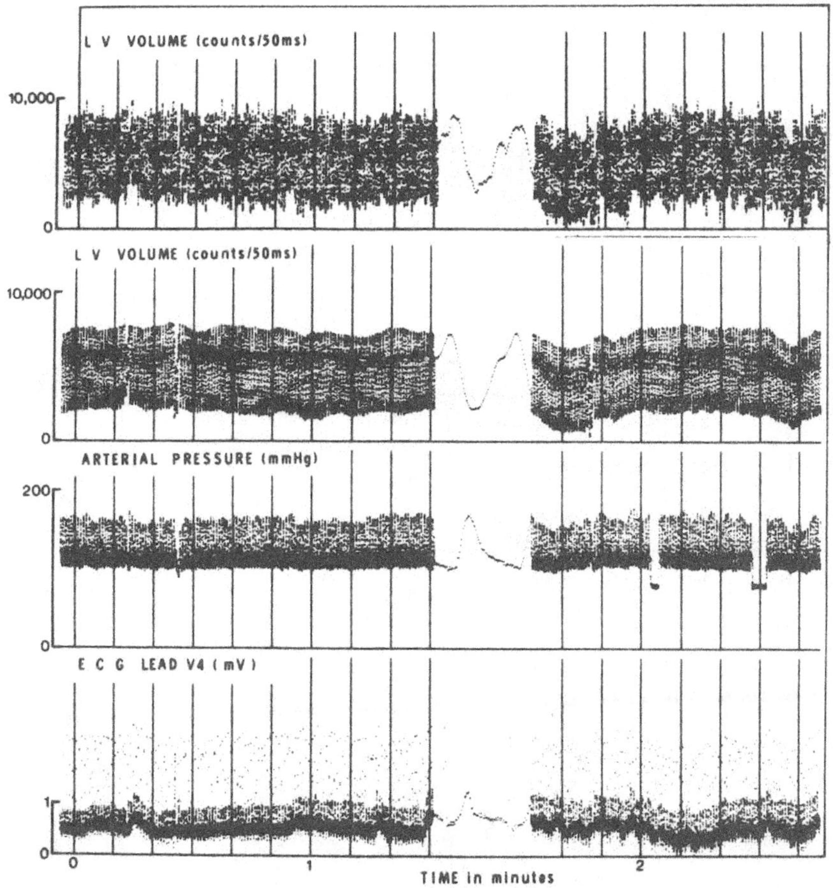

Fig. 7. The effect on the input curve *(top)* of averaging seven cycles. A continuous high-quality output curve is obtained, showing clearly the atrial contribution to diastolic left ventricular *(LV)* filling

diately anterolateral to the left ventricular region of interest, where stroke counts are minimal (no periodicity) and average counts first begin to decrease. The details of probe positioning and an assessment of beat-to-beat reproducibility of the technique have been published by Berger et al. [51].

After in vivo blood pool labelling (as for imaging) with 10 mCi ^{99m}Tc-pertechnetate, the patient lies supine, the 12 ECG leads are attached and the scintillation probe is positioned as above. Other analogue signals, such as arterial pressure, can be recorded simultaneously with the ECG and probe output on to analogue tape. The period of continuous recording may be extended for several hours with preservation of high-quality signals. Thus it is possible to detect spontaneous episodes of myocardial ischaemia in addition to those induced by exercise, cold pressor test, hyperventilation or ergometrine injection. Figure 5 shows the left ventricular volume signal recorded in the basal state and during an episode of spontaneous myocardial ischaemia. The background level of activity has been subtracted and therefore the peaks of the curve represent end-diastolic volume and the troughs represent end-

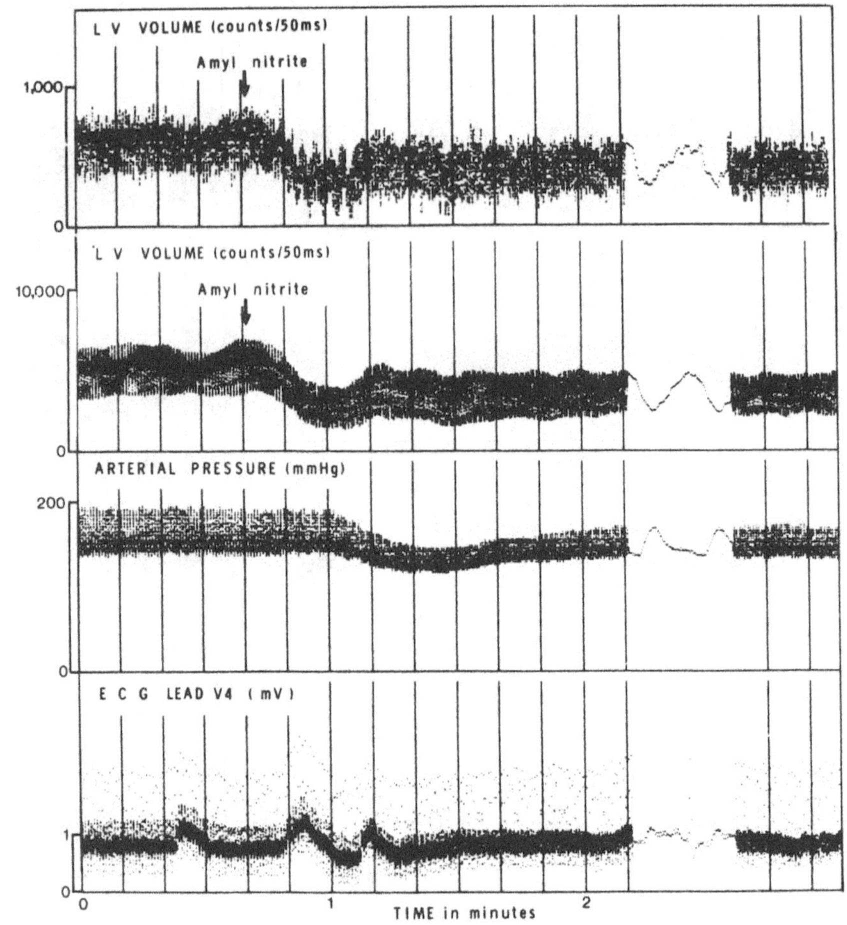

Fig. 8. The averaging process preserves the detection of the transient fall in left ventricular *(LV)* volume which is induced by amyl nitrite administered in this patient during acute myocardial ischaemia

systolic volume, the difference representing stroke volume. The data are replayed at high speed from tape to slow-moving paper in order to compress the time base. This facilitates the detection of transient changes in ventricle volume. End-diastolic and end-systolic dilatation of the left ventricle with reduction in stroke volume can be seen occurring during a spontaneous episode of acute transient myocardial ischaemia. The total duration of the attack is only 3 min, which is insufficient time for adequate ECG-gated imaging, particularly as the plateau of altered ventricular function is very brief. Left ventricular volume returns promptly to normal during the resolution phase.

The quality of the beat-to-beat curve can be substantially improved by ECG-gated cycle averaging [52], using just a few sequential cycles (e. g. seven) by the method depicted in Fig. 6. The figure illustrates three-cycle averaging; corresponding time segments of each cycle are averaged to produce the output curve. The input curve is examined in a progressive manner such that the output curve is also continuous. The effect of such averaging, using seven cardiac cycles, can be seen in Fig. 7. The quality of the curve is substantially improved and even allows the detection of the atrial contribution to diastolic filling. This averaging process does not impair the detection of a transient change in left ventricular volume, such as that induced by amyl nitrite (Fig. 8). Using this technique it has been demonstrated that ventricular dilatation with reduction in ejection fraction is an early manifestation of myocardial ischaemia [53]; it can be detected during asymptomatic attacks and during typical angina unaccompanied by diagnostic ECG changes.

4 Conclusion

An assessment of left ventricular function is of prime importance in the management of patients with suspected ischaemic heart disease. The basal condition of the ventricle can be assessed non-invasively by ECG-gated blood pool imaging and by echocardiography. Changes in left ventricular function during myocardial ischaemia can be assessed by blood pool imaging, if the episode is long, or by precordial counting. The detection of these transient changes in left ventricular function is of great diagnostic value.

References

1. Phelps ME, Hoffman EJ, Mullani NA et al. (1975) Application of annihilation coincidence detection to transaxial reconstruction tomography. J Nucl Med 16: 210
2. Phelps ME (1977) Emission computed tomography. Semin Nucl Med 7: 337
3. Ter-Pogossian MM, Raichle ME, Sobel BE (1980) Positron emission tomography. Sci Am 243: 170
4. Hoffman EJ, Huang SC, Phelps ME (1979) Quantitation in positron emission computed tomography. I. Effect of object size. J Comput Assis Tomogr 3: 299
5. Schelbert HR, Phelps ME, Hoffman EJ et al. (1979) Regional myocardial perfusion assessed with *N*-13 labelled ammonia and positron emission computerized axial tomography. Am J Cardiol 43: 209
6. Sobel BE, Weiss ES, Welch MJ et al. (1977) Detection of remote myocardial infarction in patients with positron emission transaxial tomography and intravenous ^{11}C-palmitate. Circulation 55: 853
7. Ratib O, Phelps ME, Huang SC, et al. (1982) Positron tomography with deoxyglucose for estimating local myocardial glucose metabolism. Clin Sci 23: 577
8. Selwyn AP, Allan RM, L'Abbate A et al. (1982) Relation between regional myocardial uptake of rubidium-82 and perfusion: absolute reduction of cation uptake in ischemia. Am J Cardiol 50: 112
9. Selwyn AP, Allan RM, Fox KM, et al. (1981) Prolonged myocardial ischemia in angina. Circulation 64 (Suppl IV): 83
10. Allan RM, Jones T, Rhodes C et al. (1981) Quantitation of myocardial perfusion in man using ^{15}O and positron tomography. Am J Cardiol 47: 481
11. Selwyn AP, Allan RM, Brady F (1981) Gallium-68 microspheres for in vivo quantitation of regional myocardial perfusion: experimental development. Clin Sci 62: 3
12. Allan RM, Pike V, Maseri A et al. (1981) Myocardial metabolism of ^{11}C-acetate: experimental and clinical studies. Circulation 64: 75
13. L'Abbate A, Biagini A, Michelassi G, Maseri A (1979) Myocardial kinetics of thallium and potassium in man. Circulation 60: 776

14. Love WD, Ishihara Y, Lyon LD, Smith RO (1968) Difference in the relationship between coronary blood flow and myocardial clearance of isotopes of potassium, rubidium and cesium. Am Heart J 76: 353
15. Maseri A, Parodi O, Severi S, Pesola A (1976) Transient transmural reduction of myocardial blood flow, demonstrated by thallium-201 scintigraphy, as a cause of variant angina. Circulation 54: 280
16. Uthurralt N, Davies GJ, Parodi O, Bencivelli W, Maseri A (1981) Comparative study of myocardial ischaemia during angina at rest and on exertion using thallium-201 scintigraphy. Am J Cardiol 48: 410
17. Parodi O, Uthurralt N, Severi S, Bencivelli W, Michelassi C, L'Abbate A, Maseri A (1981) Transient reduction of regional myocardial perfusion during angina at rest with ST segment depression or normalisation of negative T waves. Circulation 63: 1238
18. Wackers FJ Th, Busemann Sokole E, Samson G, Van der Schoot JB, Lie KI, Liem KL, Wellens HJJ (1976) Value and limitations of thallium-201 scintigraphy in the acute phase of myocardial infarction. N Engl J Med 95: 1
19. Wackers FJ Th, Van der Schoot JB, Busemann Sokole E, Samson G, Van Niftrik GJC, Lie KI, Durrer D, Wellens HJJ (1975) Non-invasive visualisation of acute myocardial infarction in man with thallium-201. Br Heart J 37: 741
20. Uthurralt N, Parodi O, Severi S, Davies GJ, Maseri A (1980) Thallium-201 scintigraphy for diagnosis of old myocardial infarction: comparison with electrocardiographic, ventriculographic and coronary arteriographic findings. Br Heart J 43: 527
21. Wynne J, Holman BL, Lesch M (1978) Myocardial scintigraphy by infarct-avid radiotracers. Prog Cardiovasc Dis 20: 243
22. Shen AC, Jennings RB (1972) Myocardial calcium and magnesium in acute ischaemic injury. Am J Pathol 67: 412
23. Bonte FJ, Parkey RW, Graham KD, Moore J, Stokely EM (1974) A new method of radionuclide imaging of myocardial infarcts. Radiology 110: 473
24. Buja ML, Parkey RW, Stokely EM, Bonte FJ, Willerson JT (1976) Pathophysiology of technetium 99m stannous pyrophosphate and thallium-201 scintigraphy of acute anterior myocardial infarcts in dogs. J Clin Invest 57: 1508
25. Dewanjee MK, Kahn PC (1977) Mechanism of localization of technetium 99m labelled pyrophosphate and tetracycline in infarcted myocardium. J Nucl Med 17: 639
26. Kronenberg M, Ettinger UR, Wilson GA, Schenk EA, Cohen J (1980) A comparison of radiotracer and biochemical methods for quantitation of experimental myocardial infarct weight: in vitro relationships. J Nucl Med 20: 224
27. Zaret LB, Dicola VC, Donabedian RK, Puri S, Wolfson S, Freedman GS, Cohen LS (1976) Dual radionuclide study of myocardial infarction. Relationships between myocardial uptake of potassium-43, technetium 99m stannous pyrophosphate, regional myocardial blood flow and creatine phosphokinase depletion. Circulation 53: 422
28. Buja ML, Tofe AJ, Kulkarni PV, Mukherjee A, Parkey RW, Francis MD, Bonte FJ, Willerson JT (1977) Sites and mechanisms of localization of technetium 99m phosphorus radiopharmaceuticals in acute myocardial infarcts and other tissues. J Clin Invest 60: 724
29. Willerson JT, Parkey RW, Bonte FJ, Meyer SL, Atkins JM, Stokely EM (1977) Technetium stannous pyrophosphate myocardial scintigrams in patients with chest pain of varying etiology. Circulation 51: 1046
30. Willerson JT, Parkey RW, Buja ML, Lewis SE, Bonte FJ (1979) Detection of acute myocardial infarcts using myocardial scintigraphy techniques. In: Parkey RW, Bonte JF, Buja ML, Willerson JT (eds), Clinical nuclear cardiology. Appleton, New York, p 141
31. Berman DS, Amsterdam EA, Hines HH, Selel AF, Bailey GJ, Denardo GL, Mason DT (1977) New approach to interpretation of technetium pyrophosphate scintigraphy in detection of acute myocardial infarction. Am J Cardiol 39: 341
32. Rude RE, Parkey RW, Bonte FJ, Lewis SE, Twieg D, Buja ML, Willerson JT (1979) Clinical implications of the technetium 99m stannous pyrophosphate myocardial scintigraphic "doughnut" pattern in patients with acute myocardial infarcts. Circulation 59: 721
33. Donsky MS, Curry GC, Parkey RW, Meyer SL, Bonte FJ, Willerson JT, Platt MR (1976) Unstable angina pectoris. Clinical, angiographic and myocardial scintigraphic observations. Br Heart J 38: 257

34. Willerson JT, Parkey RW, Bonte FJ (1981) The use of technetium 99m stannous pyrophosphate myocardial scintigraphy to establish the presence of myocardial infarction. In: Berwan DS, Mason DT (eds), Clinical nuclear cardiology. Grune and Stratton, New York, p 155
35. Bianco JA (1982) The saga of scintigraphy in acute myocardial infarction. J Nucl Med 22: 739
36. Go RT, Doty DB, Chiu CL, Christie J (1975) A new method of diagnosing myocardial contusion in man by radionuclide imaging. Radiology 116: 107
37. Poliner LR, Buja ML, Parkey RW, Bonte FJ, Willerson JT (1979) Clinicopathologic findings in 52 patients studied by technetium 99m stannous pyrophosphate myocardial scintigraphy. Circulation 59: 257
38. Khaw BA, Gold HK, Leinbach RC, Fallon JT, Strauss W, Pohost GM, Haver E (1978) Early imaging of experimental myocardial infarction by intracoronary administration of ^{131}I-labelled anticardiac myosin $(fab^1)_2$ fragments. Circulation 58: 1137
39. Guazzi M, Polese A, Fiorentini C, Magrini F, Olivari MT, Bartorelli C (1975) Left and right heart haemodynamics during spontaneous angina pectoris. Comparison between angina with S-T segment depression and angina with S-T segment elevation. Br Heart J 37: 401
40. Chierchia S, Brunelli C, Simonetti I, Lazzari M, Maseri A (1980) Sequence of events in angina at rest: primary reduction in coronary flow. Circulation 61: 759
41. Green MV, Ostrow HG, Douglas MA, Myers RW, Scott RN, Bailey JJ, Johnston GS (1975) High temporal resolution ECG gated scintigraphic angiocardiography. J Nucl Med 16: 95
42. Pavel DG, Zimmer AM, Patterson VN (1977) In-vivo labelling of red blood cells with ^{99m}Tc. A new approach to blood pool visualisation. J Nucl Med 18: 305
43. Davies GJ, Bencivelli W, Parodi O, Pisani P, Falchi E, L'Abbate A, Maseri A (1981) ECG gated blood pool imaging tailored to study transient changes in left ventricular contractility. In: Computers in cardiology. Conference, Williamsburg, Virginia, IEEE Computer Society, Los Angeles, p 295
44. Borer JS, Bacharach SL, Green MV, Kent KM, Epstein SE, Johnston GS (1977) Real-time radionuclide cineangiography in the non-invasive evaluation of global and regional left ventricular function at rest and during exercise in patients with coronary artery disease. N Engl J Med 296: 839
45. Wainwright RJ, Brennand-Roper DA, Cueni TA, Sowton E, Hilson AJW, Maisey MN (1979) Cold pressor test in detection of coronary heart disease and cardiomyopathy using technetium-99m gated blood pool imaging. Lancet II: 320
46. Newman GF, Rerych SK, Upton MT, Sabiston DC, Jones RH (1980) Comparison of electrocardiographic and left ventricular functional changes during exercise. Circulation 62: 1204
47. Jones RH, McEwan P, Newman GE, Port S, Rerych SK, Scholz PM, Upton MT, Peter CA, Austin EH, Leong KH, Gibbons RJ, Cobb FR, Coleman RE, Sabiston DC (1981) Accuracy of diagnosis of coronary artery disease by radionuclide measurement of left ventricular function during rest and exercise. Circulation 64: 586
48. Elkayam U, Weinstein M, Berman D, Maddahi J, Staniloff H, Freeman M, Waxman A, Swan HJC, Forrester J (1981) Stress thallium-201 myocardial scintigraphy and exercise technetium ventriculography in the detection and location of chronic coronary artery disease: comparison of sensitivity and specificity of these non-invasive tests alone and in combination. Am Heart J 101: 657
49. Jengo JA, Freeman R, Brizendine M, Mena I (1980) Detection of coronary artery disease: comparison of exercise stress radionuclide angiocardiography and thallium stress perfusion scanning. Am J Cardiol 46: 535
50. Wagner HN, Wake R, Nickoloff E, Natarajam TK (1976) The nuclear stethoscope: a simple device for generation of left ventricular volume curves. Am J Cardiol 38: 747
51. Berger H, Davies RA, Batsford WP, Hoffer PB, Gottschalk A, Zaret BL (1981) Beat to beat left ventricular performance assessed from the equilibrium cardiac blood pool using a computerized nuclear probe. Circulation 63: 133
52. Davies GJ, Bencivelli W, Morgan M, Pratt T, Chierchia S, Crea F, Maseri A: Monitoring left ventricular function to detect myocardial ischaemia. In: Computers in cardiology. Conference, Florence, Italy. IEEE Computer Society, Los Angeles, p 265
53. Davies GJ, Chierchia S, Myers M, Maseri A, Steiner RE (1981) Transient changes in left ventricular volume in acute myocardial ischaemia. Clin Sci 60: 13

Part II

X-Ray and Ultrasound Investigations

I Conventional Radiology

1 Methods

1.1 Choice of Techniques

The conventional radiological techniques used in the study of coronary artery disease have no particular specificity. Fluoroscopy and radiography should be employed as required, care being taken not to expose patients unnecessarily to radiation, especially if they are likely to receive high doses in the future during one or more coronary arteriographies. Conventional fluoroscopy should be abandoned entirely and replaced by television fluoroscopy image intensification. The choice of technique must be made judiciously. It is futile to look for coronary calcifications on standard plain films. Opacification of the oesophagus with barium is rarely useful. Performing radiography in four different projections is seldom worthwhile. In more than 90% of patients the standard frontal view is sufficient to enable observation of changes in the patient's radiological anatomy. An unusual or new technique may prove useful either for research purposes or to provide more information at a cost and radiation dose comparable to those of the traditional technique. An example of the former is the use of cineradiography or systematic video recording for improved detection of left ventricular contraction abnormalities and coronary calcifications [1, 2]. The latter case is illustrated by the process of integrated or ECG-gated interlaced radiography [2], an ECG-monitored system which controls the vertical movement of a lead grid with horizontal bars located between the X-ray source and the patient. A first exposure is made in end-diastole, then the grid is moved and a second exposure is made in end-systole. The heart border thus takes on a crenated appearance, with alternating systolic and diastolic segments. This technique is the modern version of kymography.

1.2 Contribution of Conventional Radiographic Projections

The frontal postero-anterior projection allows measurement of the cardiothoracic ratio and detection of left ventricular or left atrial dilatation and of pulmonary vascularization anomalies, most often due to left ventricular insufficiency. It is important to take the customary precautions: to have the frontal plane of the subject parallel to the film; to await apnoea at the end of a deep inspiration; to make sure that the X-ray source is at least 2 m from the film; and to use a short time exposure ($\leqslant$ 0.03 s), a high voltage and a filter which softens the contrast between the mediastinum and the lungs.

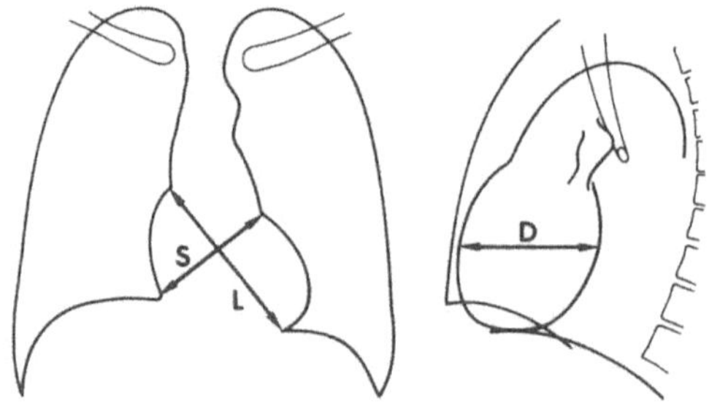

Fig. 1. Determination of the relative cardiac volume $=(L \times S \times D \times K)/\mathrm{BSA}$. *L:* long axis of the heart; *S:* short axis; *D:* the greatest anteroposterior diameter; *BSA*: body surface area; *K*: constant related to the X-ray focus-film distance

The lateral projection is seldom truly useful. It is indicated (with a barium-filled oesophagus) in the case of suspected left atrial dilatation or to search for an aneurysm of the inferior wall, but the results are generally disappointing. This transverse view is necessary when estimated left ventricular volume is to be measured (Fig. 1).

The right anterior oblique (RAO) projection is ideal for the assessment of left atrial size when the oesophagus is filled with barium paste. The left anterior oblique (LAO) projection provides the best view of the lateral left ventricular wall, supplementing the frontal view in an assessment of left ventricular dilatation.

In the particular case of acute myocardial infarction, thoracic radiography is very often performed under difficult conditions: equipment must be transported to the patient's bed; the patient is wholly or partially recumbent; wires, electrodes and catheters must be used for monitoring; there is insufficient inspiration; there is magnification of the image; etc. These difficulties have to be handled as well as possible, for the examination is very useful in assessing the patient's clinical and haemodynamic state [3].

1.3 Contribution of Television Fluoroscopy

The study of left ventricular contraction requires a frontal projection for viewing the anterolateral wall and the apex, and 45°–60° LAO projection for the lateral wall. The inferior or diaphragmatic wall is more or less hidden by the diaphragm according to the patient's morphological type, RAO projection being best for observing it if the fatty LPD epicardial groove is sufficiently visible.

The search for coronary artery calcifications is difficult, disappointing and misleading in conventional radiographies but is greatly facilitated by observation of cardiac dynamics on the television screen or, better yet, on a cine film. The operator must pick out the radiotransparent fatty lines of the atrioventricular and interventricular grooves against which the coronary calcifications stand out. The ideal projections are slight LAO for the left coronary common trunk, 45°–60° for the bifurcation of the left anterior descending artery (LAD) and the circumflex (Cx), transverse for the mid and distal LAD, and 30° RAO and transverse for the right coronary artery (RCA) (Fig. 2). The vertical orientation and the rapid motion of the RCA facilitate its identification. The patient should be examined in apnoea, at the end of a deep inspiration, so as to immobilize the extracardiac calcifications.

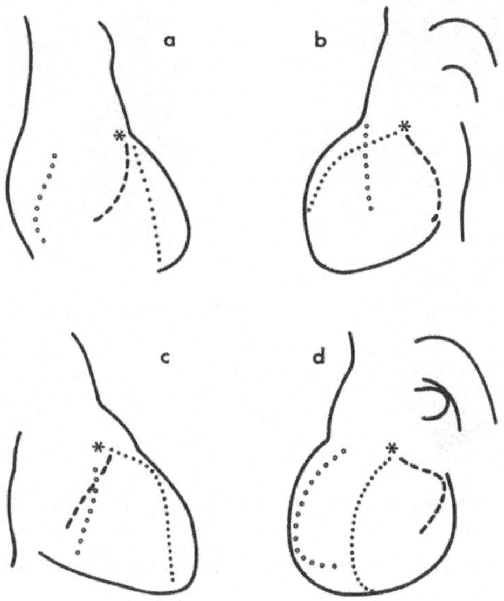

Fig. 2 a–d. The best projections for detecting coronary calcifications in the classic projections; **a** frontal, **b** transverse, **c** right anterior oblique, **d** left anterior oblique

2 Results

2.1 Deformations of the Cardiac Silhouette

Deformations of the cardiac silhouette depend essentially on left ventricular dilatation and occasionally on left atrial dilatation. The discovery of a cardiomegaly in coronary artery disease is rare and almost always indicates a certain degree of left ventricular failure. In a consecutive series of 207 patients it was observed only 16 times [3]. Very large cardiomegalies are found mainly when the coronary artery disease causes no pain syndrome and mimics a congestive-type primary myocardiopathy. Such circumstances are exceptional. A heart of normal size is found in one case out of four of moderate left ventricular insufficiency [4]. The most common abnormalities of the cardiac outline are ventricular aneurysms. Any bulge-like projection that breaks the continuity of the left ventricular outline of the anterior wall and the apex in RAO or frontal projection, or of the lateral wall in LAO projection, may be an aneurysm. In fact, a left ventricle that is simply dilated always retains its regular convex outline. Large aneurysms on the anterior wall produce a very marked bulge of the left border, which is either convex or angular, with a quadrilateral form or a *coeur en sabot* contour, and which may sometimes make contact with the left lateral thoracic wall (Figs. 3 and 4). The visualization of aneurysms of the septal and inferior walls requires angiography, since traditional radiological techniques cannot detect them, which is also true for many anterior or lateral aneurysms if they are not of sufficient size. When ECG changes suggest the presence of a ventricular aneurysm not confirmed by traditional radiography, left ventriculography should be performed in all cases. The fluoroscopic observation of systolic expansion of a left ventricular wall is not a proof of aneurysm, as it occurs in all cases of akinesis subsequent to myocardial infarction. The fibrous tissue of the infarcts and aneurysms can become calcified (Fig. 5). These calcifications are usually fine and

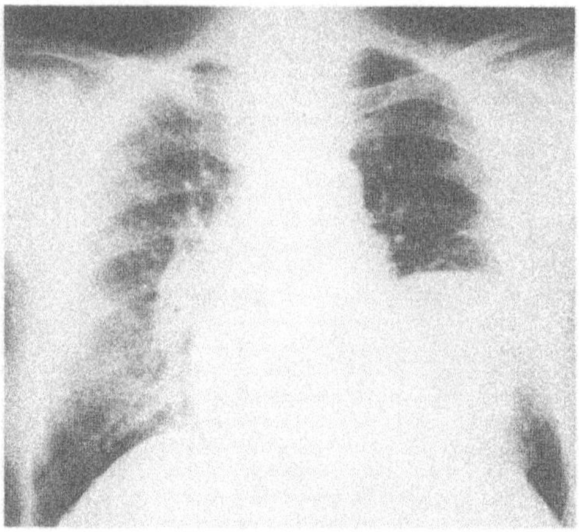

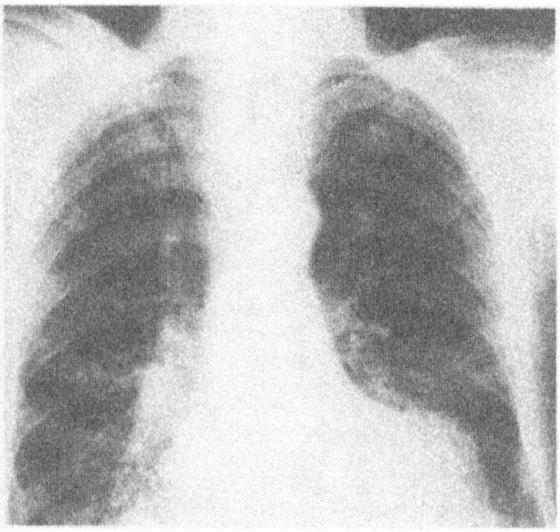

Fig. 3 *(left)*. Left ventricular aneurysm. Frontal view: an angulated shape resembling the *coeur en sabot*

Fig. 4 *(right)*. Left ventricular aneurysm. Frontal view: a classic rounded shape

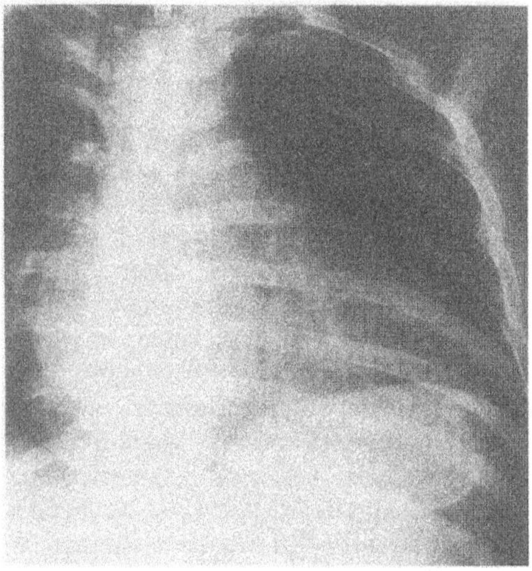

Fig. 5. Subepicardial calcification of an old antero-apical myocardial infarct. A tangential projection of the calcification is needed to enable good visualization

regular, superficial and parallel to the cardiac outline, and visible in the projection in which the X-ray strikes them at an angle (Fig. 6). When not clearly superficial, they indicate calcification of an intraventricular thrombus. They are easy to distinguish from pericardial calcifications, which are located preferentially along the atrioventricular and interventricular grooves and are more spread out and irregular.

Left atrial dilatation appears either when left ventricular function is quite altered and there is increased filling pressure, or when there is mitral regurgitation due to fibrosis or ischaemic dysfunction of a papillary muscle. The double atrial contour on the right border of the outline is more common than the left appendage bulging on the left border.

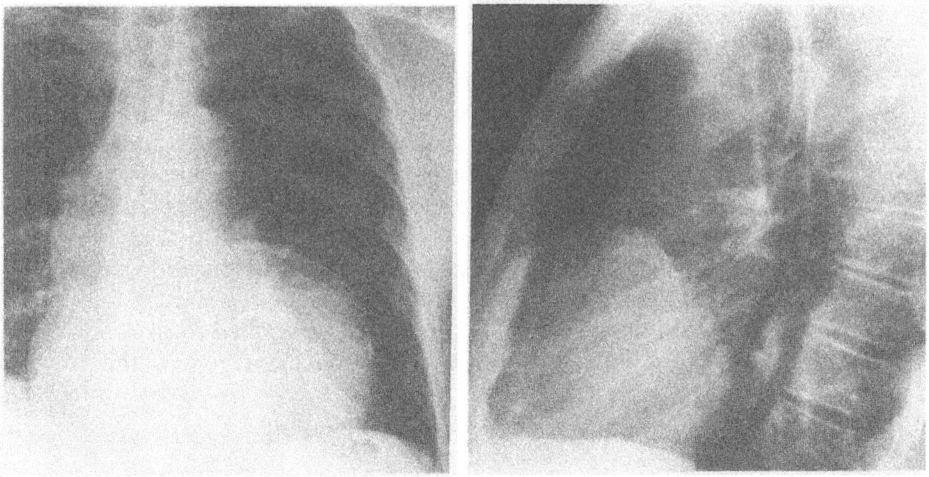

Fig. 6. Frontal *(left)* and *(right)* lateral views of a large anterolateral left ventricular aneurysm well delineated by thin, extensive, eggshell-like calcification

2.2 Pulmonary Vascularization Abnormalities

The radiological signs of pulmonary venous hypertension and of pulmonary oedema are mainly found in the acute phase of myocardial infarction with left ventricular failure, but also in cases of acute mitral regurgitation due to rupture of chordae tendineae or of the head of a papillary muscle resulting from ischaemia with or without signs of myocardial infarction. It is known that pulmonary radiological signs reflect a rise in capillary pressure [5], with the following developments:

- distention of the pulmonary veins and increase in the arterial flow of the upper lobes;
- appearance of interstitial oedema with Kerley's lines and perivascular blur; and
- alveolar oedema indicating capillary pressure greater than 25 mmHg.

More than 50% of patients with acute myocardial infarction present one or more radiological signs of congestive cardiac insufficiency, and the clinical signs often appear later than the radiological signs [6]. In general, the severity of the pulmonary radiological signs is in good agreement with the degree of left ventricular failure and the prognosis for the patient, and the improvement of the radiological image is a good indication of the clinical improvement of the patient's condition following treatment [6, 7]. However, thoracic radiography often loses its predictive value in cases of cardiogenic shock [7]. According to Kostuk, there is a significant correlation between the estimated left ventricular volume indicated by the thoracic film in the first 3 days after infarction and the chances of short- or middle-term survival [6]. When the estimated left ventricular volume is normal, the mortality rate is 4% in the 1st month and 8% in the next 10 months. For the same periods these rates rise to 26% and 24% respectively when left ventricular volume is abnormal.

2.3 *Analysis of Left Ventricular Kinetics*

The study of left ventricular walls by fluoroscopy is of very limited value in that the septal and inferior walls are not taken into consideration and that this non-quantitative method ordinarily provides no information additional to that obtained by standard radiography and the ECG. It should be recalled that any postinfarction akinetic sequela, and not just aneurysms, may be subject to systolic expansion. For valid assessment of left ventricular wall contraction anomalies, especially segmentary hypokineses, it is absolutely necessary to observe the kinetics of the endocardial outline of the ventricle and then to have recourse to angiography. Among the simple methods involving low radiation doses for the patient, intergated chest X-ray is recommended, as it permits good detection of the abnormal movements of the left ventricular free wall [2].

2.4 *Searching for Coronary Arterial Calcifications*

The search for coronary artery calcifications is carried out using an image intensifier viewed directly on the television screen or by video recording or cine film (Fig. 7). Opinion is divided as to its usefulness. Bartel [8] and then Saltiel [1] have shown that the discovery of coronary calcifications is highly significative of severe coronary stenoses in patients presenting an anginal syndrome. Aldrich [9] has demonstrated that the association of calcifications and of a positive exercise test is 96% predictive of coronary artery disease. Crochet's study [10] devoted to 200 coronary arteriography patients confirms and supplements earlier studies [1, 8, 11–14]. When the calcifications affect the three main vessels, these show significant stenosis in 82% of cases. The site of the calcification is of importance. The LAD is the most frequently calcified artery (91%), then the RCA (60%) and finally the Cx (33.5%). The sensitivity or predictive value of a stenosis relative to the presence of a calcification is 93.5% for the LAD, 72.4% for the RCA and 47.5% for the Cx. The specificity or

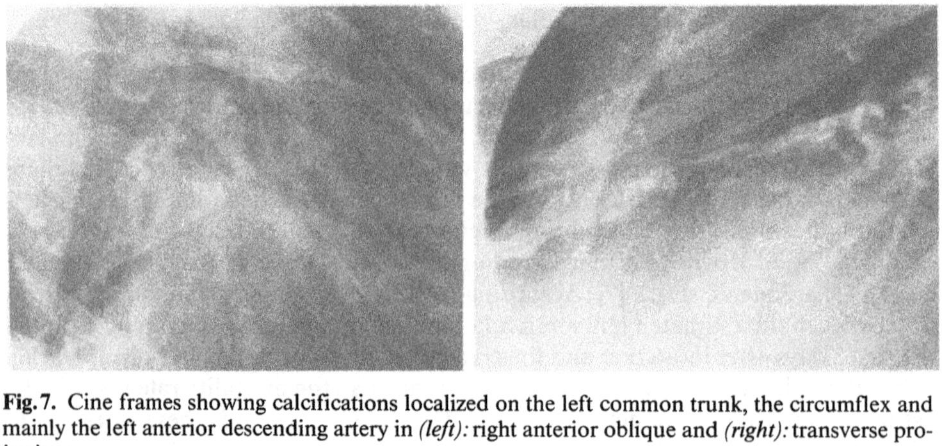

Fig. 7. Cine frames showing calcifications localized on the left common trunk, the circumflex and mainly the left anterior descending artery in *(left):* right anterior oblique and *(right):* transverse projections

predictive value of a calcification relative to the presence of a stenosis is 26.6% for the LAD, 76.1% for the RCA and 78.6% for the Cx. Thus the LAD is often calcified independently of the presence of significant stenoses. On the other hand, the Cx is rarely calcified, but a calcification in this artery is strongly predictive of severe stenosis. The site and the extent of calcifications allow the quality of the "downstream arterial bed" to be estimated approximately. A calcification of the Cx, whether proximal or distal, indicates a severely involved distal artery in more than 50% of cases. For the LAD and the RCA, the distal arterial lumen is inadequate in 80% of cases if the calcifications have a distal site. The analysis of coronary calcifications thus provides approximate but valuable information concerning the severity and localization of stenoses as well as the quality of the distal portions of the coronary arteries. However, it should be noted that the detection of coronary calcifications is only of real value in young subjects and in the absence of decisive proof favouring the diagnosis of coronary artery disease.

References

1. Saltiel J, Crochet D, Petitier H: Apport de la cinéfluorographie dans la maladie coronarienne. Enc Méd Chir Radiodiagnostic 1: 32270 A 40
2. Dinsmore RE, Wernikoff RE, Miller SW, Pohost GM, Block PC, Potsaid MS (1979) The evaluation of left ventricular free wall asynergy due to coronary artery disease: the use of an interlaced ECG-gated radiography system. AJR 132: 909
3. Aintablian A, Hamby RL, Garsman J (1976) Correlation of heart size with clinical and hemodynamic findings in patients with coronary artery disease. Am Heart J 91: 21
4. Stein PD, Lewison H, Potts KH (1974) Cardiac size and left ventricular performance. JAMA 229: 1614
5. Milne ENC (1973) Correlations of physiologic findings with chest roentgenology. Radiol Clin North Am 11: 17
6. Kostuk W, Barr JW, Simon AL, Ross J (1973) Correlations between the chest film and hemodynamics in acute myocardial infarction. Circulation 48: 624
7. Cascade PN, Kantrowitz A, Wajszczuk WJ, Rubenfire M (1976) The chest X-ray in acute left ventricular power failure: an aid to determining prognosis of patients supported by intraaortic balloon pumping. AJR 126: 1147
8. Bartel AG, Chen JT, Peter RH, Behar VS, Lester RG (1974) The significance of coronary calcifications detected by fluoroscopy. A report of 360 patients. Circulation 49: 1247
9. Aldrich RF, Brensike JF, Battaglini JW, Richardson JM, Loh IK, Stone NJ, Passamani ER, Ackerstein H, Seningen R, Borer JS, Levy RI, Epstein SE (1979) Coronary calcification in the detection of coronary artery disease and comparison with electrocardiographic exercise testing. Circulation 59: 1113
10. Crochet D, Lavenant F, Krause D, Wanlin P, Bizais Y, Delumeau J, Petitier H (1981) Intérêt de l'étude des calcifications dans le bilan de la maladie artérielle coronaire athéromateuse. J Radiol 62: 221
11. Hamby RI, Tabrah F, Wisoff BG, Harstein ML (1974) Coronary artery calcification: clinical implications and angiographic correlates. Am Heart J 87: 565
12. Langou RA, Huang EK, Kelley MJ, Cohen LS (1980) Predictive accuracy of coronary artery calcification and abnormal exercise test for coronary disease in asymptomatic men. Circulation 62: 1196
13. Margolis JR, Chen JTT, Yihong Kong, Peter RH, Behar VS, Kisslo JA (1980) The diagnostic and prognostic significance of coronary artery calcification. Radiology 137: 609
14. Oliver MF (1970) The diagnostic value of detecting coronary calcifications. Circulation 42: 981

II Angiographic Explorations: Techniques

1 Introduction

The name of Mason Sones is inseparably associated with the concept of selective coronary arteriography. Thanks to his work, the examination has become a routine part of cardiological exploration. Sones' achievement is to have created a veritable doctrine of the selective examination of the coronary arteries. His method is based on the introduction of the catheter probe into the brachial artery by arteriotomy and on the recording of the images by radio-cinematography. The first examinations performed by the pioneers of the method used the direct view of the image intensifier output screen. Beginning in 1958, technical advances proceeded apace. Improvements in the chemical structures of contrast media reduced the rate of ventricular fibrillations. The gradual replacement of cradles by different systems of stands with arms rotating around the patient, the increased resolution power of image intensifiers, and the perfecting of axial oblique, sagittal oblique and double-oblique (craniocaudal and caudocranial) projections made detection of stenotic lesions more reliable. The association of coronary arteriography with other procedures (pharmacological tests, exercise tests, atrial stimulation with measurement of the products of cardiac metabolic degradation in the coronary sinus, injection of various radio-nuclides into the coronary arteries) led to a better understanding of the physiology of myocardial ischaemia. It may be added that examination of the coronary arteries is necessarily accompanied by left ventriculography to explore the muscle side of myocardial ischaemia.

Although the role of coronary arteriography in the diagnostic assessment of myocardial ischaemia is currently contested when compared with non-invasive techniques, it still remains the reference method and is indispensable to pre-operative evaluation of lesions.

2 Diagnostic Use of Radiographic Methods in Coronary Disease

Coronary angiography, which is in effect a technique combining left ventriculography and coronary arteriography, plays a dominant role among the imaging methods used to diagnose coronary affections. At the present time, no other technique can replace it for identifying a congenital or acquired coronary lesion, measuring a coronary artery stenosis, assessing the results of aortocoronary bypass surgery, detecting mitral regurgitation or determining the size of a ventricular aneurysm. The coronary and ventricular operability of a patient cannot be judged without reference to this technique.

Table 1. Indications for coronary arteriography

Coronary artery disease
Angina posing a particular socioprofessional risk
Disabling stable angina (Canadian classes 2–4[a])
Unstable angina: prolonged, accelerated or variant
Threat of extension of the infarct
Postinfarction residual angina
Residual angina after heart surgery
Heart failure after aortocoronary bypass
Infarction with complications: septal rupture, mitral regurgitation, aneurysm
Valvular disease (pre-operative assessment)
Patient over 54 years of age
Patient with angina or coronary calcifications
Acute mitral regurgitation
Hypertensive or diabetic patient
Cardiomyopathies
Patient with angina
Congestive cardiomyopathies (systematically for all cases)
Congenital cardiopathies
Congenital coronary anomalies
Tetralogy of Fallot
Complex cases of transposition or malposition
Various diseases
Cardiac traumatisms
Cardiac tumours
Idiopathic ventricular tachycardia

[a] Campeau L (1976) Grading of angina pectoris. Circulation 54: 522

Coronary arteriography thus remains the reference method. Its privileged position is due mainly to the quality of the radiographic image. All the non-invasive examinations run up against the difficulty of obtaining a sufficient degree of resolution, but only the radiographic image provides a resolution of 0.1 mm, a superiority it will probably retain for many years. Unfortunately, this method is not free from complications, since it requires hospitalization of the patient, is relatively expensive and entails exposure to X-rays. For these reasons, the indications for coronary arteriography (see Table 1) should be specific and well respected. In Sect. 1 of Part I the necessity of making a clear distinction between the techniques which detect coronary artery obstruction and those which detect myocardial ischaemia was indicated. The latter are applied before coronary arteriography whenever clinical signs and the ECG at rest are not sufficient to show that there is disabling coronary artery disease. It would be a mistake to perform coronary arteriography before obtaining an echocardiogram in a patient presenting atypical thoracic pains in connection with mitral valve prolapse. On the other hand, it would be unreasonable to call for other examinations than coronary arteriography in a patient suffering from typical unstable angina with permanent depression of the ST segment in the anterior precordial leads.

Since 1959, coronary arteriography has been perfected and enriched by complementary tests. In association with catheterization of the coronary sinus, it permits study of myocardial metabolism at rest, during exertion and under atrial pacing. Various pharmacological tests can be used to assess the reversibility of left ventricular segmental contraction anomalies and to make coronary artery spasm appear or disappear. Coronary arteriography has thus become a very complete physiopathological method of evaluating coronary artery disease.

This technique is now a therapeutic tool, thanks to Andreas Grüntzig, who developed coronary transluminal angioplasty, and to Peter Rentrop, who performed the first arterial recanalization by fibrinolysis in cases of acute myocardial infarction. Today, the progress being made in computerized angiographic imaging poses questions about the evolution of coronary arteriography. In the near future, the new technology should permit a reduction in cost and in the patient's radiation dose, although it will not be possible to abandon the selective arterial approach. It is to be hoped that in the more distant future coronary arteriography will become a non-invasive method requiring only injections of contrast medium into the vena cava system.

3 Material

The material used during coronary arteriography is in part very similar to that used in any cardiac catheterization. However, there are a few peculiarities with respect to the radiological material and catheter probes. For the brachial approach, the operator needs the usual surgical equipment. Conventional instruments are used for incision of the skin, blunt dissection of the artery, isolation and incision of the vessel and suture of the arterial wall and of the skin. Fogarthy catheters are available in case of arterial obstruction by clotting, which is an exceptional occurrence. For the femoral approach, the operator makes use of the classic material of Seldinger or that of Désilets-Hoffman, adapted to the arterial route by means of an antireflux valve system.

The cardiorespiratory intensive care material is not specific to the catheterization laboratory: defibrillator, bipolar electrode catheter for pacing, equipment needed for artificial ventilation, and the ordinary drugs for cardiac intensive care. The monitoring equipment must be sufficient to assure constant surveillance of the electrocardiogram and of the arterial pressure at the distal end of the catheter. In a well-equipped unit it is now possible to monitor and record simultaneously two or three electrocardiographic leads and two or three different pressure curves, and the most modern installations are computerized.

The radiological equipment must satisfy very demanding criteria, for it must produce excellent images of small vessels which are barely visible (approximately 0.1 mm in size) and sometimes characterized by extremely rapid motion. An image intensifier that has an input field with electronic zoom (varying between 15 und 23 or 17 and 25 cm) is chosen by most operators. The accompanying image recorder is a 35-mm cine camera, whose superiority is attested not only by the rapidity with which it may be used but also by the fact that it is the only instrument providing continuous televised and video-taped monitoring of arterial opacification. In addition, the cine film provides a dynamic study which offers valuable information in some special situations: spasms, myocardial bridge, collateral circulation and inter-

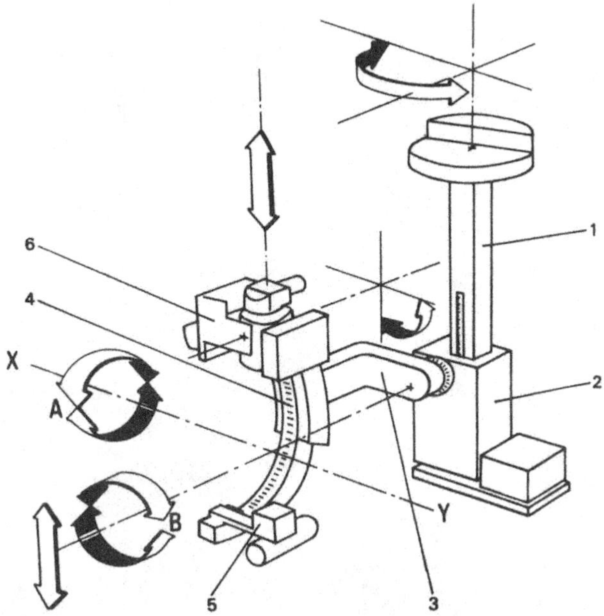

Fig. 1. Stand permitting examination in isocentric and double-oblique projections. *XY:* long axis of the patient; *A:* rotation of the C arm to provide the classic oblique projections; *B:* rotation of the L arm to provide caudocranial or craniocaudal oblique projections; *1:* floor-to-ceiling column; *2:* lift (not absolutely necessary if the vertical movement of the table is motor-controlled); *3:* L arm; *4:* C arm; *5:* X-ray tube; *6:* fixture for the image intensifier. Two stands of this type can be combined to form an isocentric biplane system (by courtesy of Siemens)

coronary anastomoses. A relatively slow filming speed (25 frames per second) is sufficient for coronary arteriography, whereas ventriculography is normally performed at a speed of 50 frames per second, and even of 100 frames per second when left ventricular contraction is to be thoroughly analysed. Video tape recording is necessarily combined with the filming. It offers the operator the possibility of instantaneous play-back of the filmed sequence and thus of choosing the most satisfactory projections for diagnostic purposes. A camera providing a 70×70 or 100×100 mm format, at two to six frames per second, can be a useful addition because the still image has a better quality than that of cine film and is thus appreciated by surgeons in the operating-room.

Most of the stands currently in use have motorized arms allowing rapid rotation of the tube and image intensifier around the patient and in most cases providing double-oblique (craniocaudal or caudocranial) projections (Figs. 1 and 2). Cradles have practically been abandoned. Their sole advantage was that they offered the operator better protection from radiation as a result of their removable lead screens.

Various studies have been devoted to the effects of contrast media on the myocardium [1–5]. Recent products with low osmolarity (around 600 mosmol/kg H_2O), which have a dimeric ionic structure or a non-ionic structure, are being increasingly used. These new molecules (ioxaglic acid, iopamidol, metrizamide) disturb myocardial electrophysiology less, reducing the frequency of arrhythmias, and can

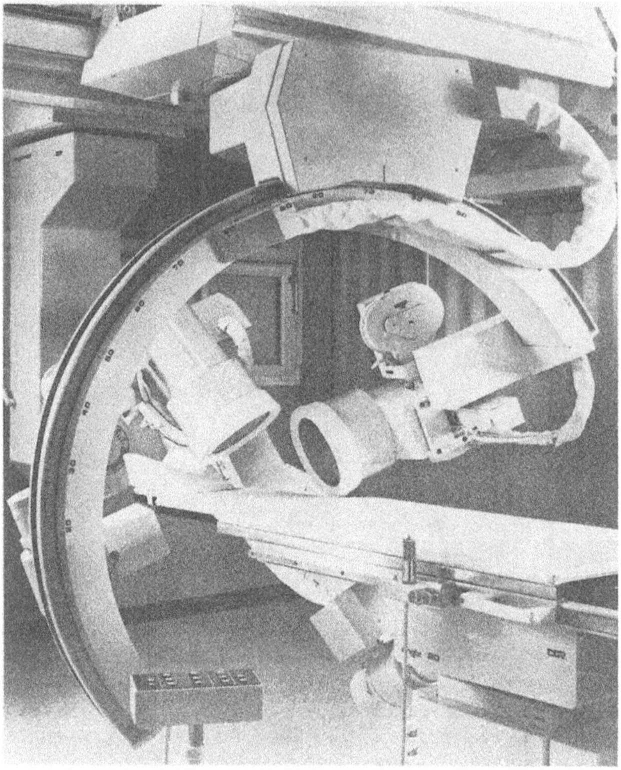

Fig. 2. Isocentric biplane stand with an L arm for the classic oblique projections and a C arm for caudocranial and craniocaudal projections (by courtesy of Compagnie Generale de Radiologie)

be used in much greater amounts (up to 6 ml/kg body wt.) than the more classic products.

It is important to give consideration to the qualities of the catheters used: a smooth and non-thrombogenic surface, sufficient flexibility to avoid traumatisms, sufficient rigidity for the catheter to have a certain degree of "memory" and to respond to axial rotation at the hub end. Sones catheters are made of Dacron, are 80–120 cm in length and have a calibre of between 6 F and 8 F. Of the different models available, the most popular is model 5421-8F-USCI (Fig. 3). This catheter was designed as a single instrument to be used for catheterization of the left ventricle as well as of both coronary arteries, and even of aorta to coronary venous bypasses. To catheterize the coronary arteries, the catheter must be buckled against the aortic valves so that it moves up along the aorta wall and its distal end is directed towards the corresponding coronary ostium. When it is necessary to use the humeral route because of an iliofemoral arteriopathy, operators unfamiliar with the Sones technique may find it preferable to use Amplatz's preshaped brachiocoronary catheters. There are three main types of percutaneous catheter introduced by the femoral artery route: those of Judkins, Amplatz and Bourassa (Fig. 4). These catheters are preshaped differently for the left ventricle, the right coronary artery and the left coronary artery (Fig. 5). The coronary catheters normally have only one distal opening. For an untrained operator, the catheterization of vessels is often easier

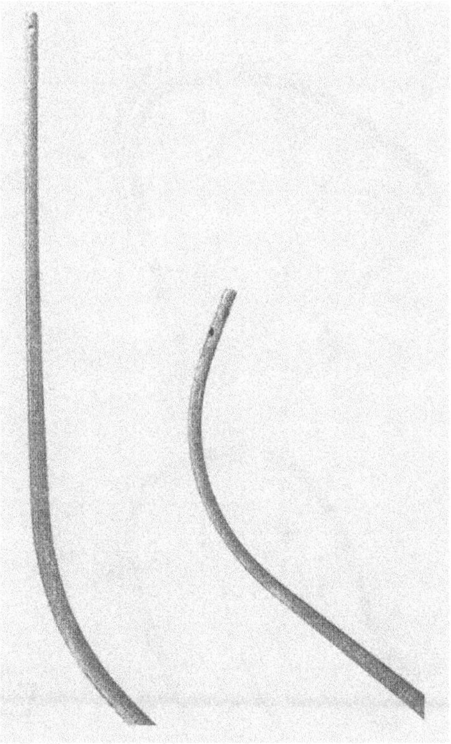

Fig. 3. Sones catheters

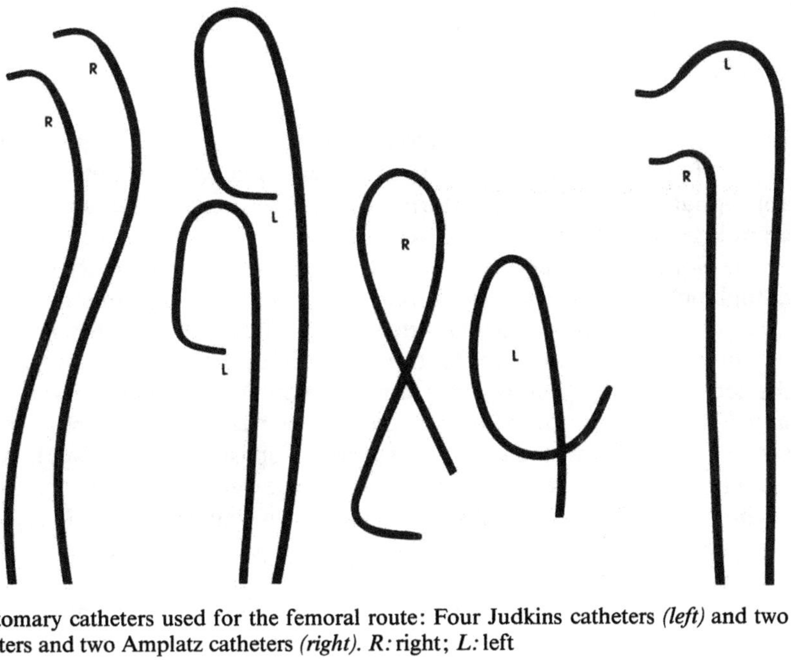

Fig. 4. The customary catheters used for the femoral route: Four Judkins catheters *(left)* and two Bourassa catheters and two Amplatz catheters *(right)*. *R:* right; *L:* left

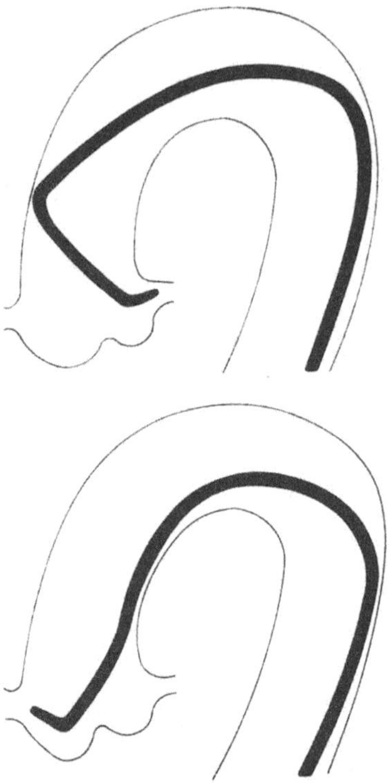

Fig. 5. The Judkins catheters are preshaped to facilitate catheterization of the coronary arteries

with these models than with those of Sones, yet it is certainly more dangerous, especially when there is an ostial or para-ostial stenosis of the coronary arteries.

4 Mode of Operation

Some coronary angiographic factors, such as the approach route and the catheterization of the vessels, are specific to each technique, whereas others, such as the most appropriate projections, monitoring during the examination and pharmacoangiographic tests, are common to all techniques.

The Sones technique is the oldest method used in coronary arteriography, although not the most common. It requires some experience or surgical observation, given the approach by brachial arteriotomy. Those who practise it routinely attribute the following advantages to it: use of a single catheter; the possibility, and even the necessity, of performing the examination under anticoagulants; a greater facility in negotiating an aortic stenosis and in catheterizing both coronary arteries successively and rapidly in the case of a suspected spasm; and the fact this technique is ideal in the case of arterial obstruction in the lower limbs. However, catheterization of the coronary arteries is often much more difficult than with Judkins' technique, and projections between 60° left anterior oblique (LAO) and transverse are not always easy to carry out.

The Judkins technique (and Bourassa's variant of it) almost always uses the femoral route, and exceptionally the axillary route. As a general rule, catheterization of the coronary ostia is easier than by the brachial route. The main drawback is the need to change catheters three times. However, the use of Désilets-Hoffman sheaths adapted to the arterial passage has considerably facilitated the changing of the catheters, providing an appreciable saving of time and a reduction in arterial traumatism. The very great advantage of this method is the total freedom with which the C or U arm can be rotated around the thorax of the patient; the operator can choose at will any single- or double-oblique projection he desires.

Whatever method is chosen, left intraventricular pressure is first recorded and ventriculography is performed in 30°–40° right anterior oblique (RAO) projection by injection of 30–45 ml contrast medium at a rate of 10–15 ml/s. If necessary, ventriculography can be performed a second time in LAO projection. The ideal arrangement is to use a biplane stand. Angiography constitutes a test of volume overload, so that it is always of interest to check the change in left ventricular end-diastolic pressure 2 min after ventriculography. The opacification of the left ventricle is sometimes repeated to assess the effect of a drug, usually nitroglycerin. The second phase of the operation consists in performing successive and multiple selective injections according to the different projections of the two coronary arteries. Ordinarily, the left coronary artery is explored before the right in order to know at the outset if coronary circulation is left preponderant. In all cases, it is wise to use a semi-selective injection and a limited dose of contrast medium to test the reactivity of each coronary artery and to search for a possible ostial or para-ostial stenosis, especially a severe stenosis of the left main coronary trunk. The operator must withdraw the catheter and never inject contrast medium when the pressure drops or when the contour of the curve takes on a ventricular pattern. Between injections he must wait until the electrocardiogram has returned to its initial aspect and any pain has subsided. A minimum 2-min waiting period must strictly be observed between two coronary injections, even when the examination runs its course easily and without incident.

For an experienced operator, it is ideal to know both the preceding techniques and to choose whichever is the better one in terms of the clinical state of the patient or the difficulty of an approach route. In the case of arteriopathy of the lower limbs and in aged subjects (over 70), the humeral approach is to be chosen without hesitation. In a young manual worker, for example, the femoral route is preferable. Local complications are more frequent with the Sones technique, but the risk of cardiac complications or cerebral embolism is certainly lower. The situation is just the opposite with the Judkins technique.

5 Radiological Projections

For the right coronary artery, the basic projections (Fig. 6) are 45° LAO and 30° RAO. Additional useful projections are the transverse, which reveals the initial part and the second vertical segment of the right coronary artery, and the 30° LAO, either standard or with caudocranial angulation, which shows remarkably well the region of the crux and the diaphragmatic arteries that perfuse the inferior wall of the left ventricle (Fig. 7).

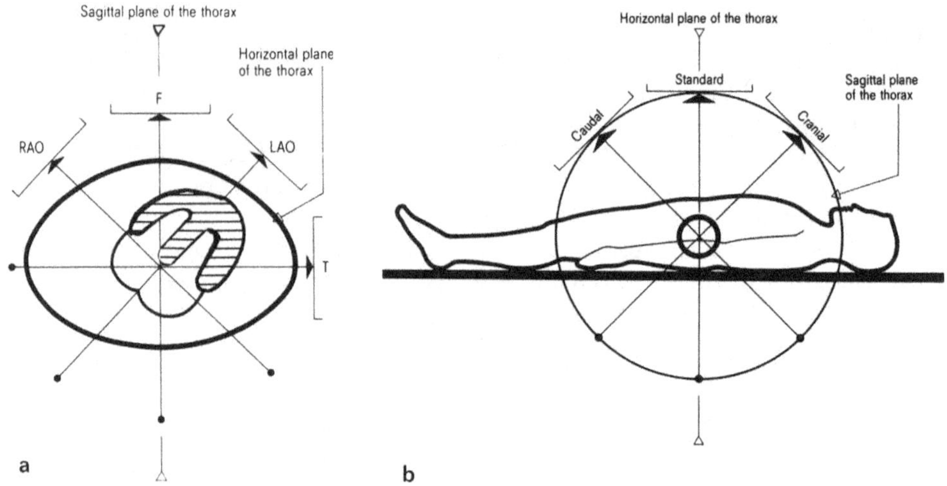

Fig. 6 a, b. Principles and diagrams of double-oblique projections. **a** standard oblique projections; **b** caudocranial and craniocaudal oblique projections. *LAO:* left anterior oblique; *RAO:* right anterior oblique; *F:* frontal; *T:* transverse

For the left coronary artery the basic projections are 30° RAO and 45° LAO with a 20°–25° caudocranial angulation. The former allows good analysis of the circumflex artery and its left marginal branches and of the mid and distal parts of the left anterior descending artery (Fig.8). The latter is very useful in the study of the initial part of the left anterior descending artery and of its diagonal branches (Fig. 9). Two other projections may also be regarded as basic: 60° LAO, which provides additional information about the proximal part of the circumflex artery; and, even more so, the transverse, which reveals the entire left anterior descending artery and its septal branches very clearly. Among the other projections there are two of capital importance: the frontal or slightly RAO projection with craniocaudal angulation of the incident beam, which provides an optimal view of the bifurcation between the left anterior descending artery and the circumflex artery; and the 25° LAO projection with 20° caudocranial angulation which gives an ideal view of the left coronary main trunk (Fig. 10). Some operators, as a measure of maximum security, always begin coronary arteriography with this projection.

During an examination the operator can, of course, modify a customary projection by 15°–20° in one direction or the other to obtain better analysis of an arterial segment, to bring into view a stenosis partially hidden by an adjacent artery or to adapt the viewing angle to a peculiar anatomical configuration.

6 Monitoring of Cardiac Parameters

During coronary arteriography in any type of patient there must be strict monitoring of the electrocardiogram and of aortic pressure. In very high risk patients with a very reduced systemic flow, some authors suggest performance of coronary arteriography under aortic counterpulsation. Such circulatory assistance is recom-

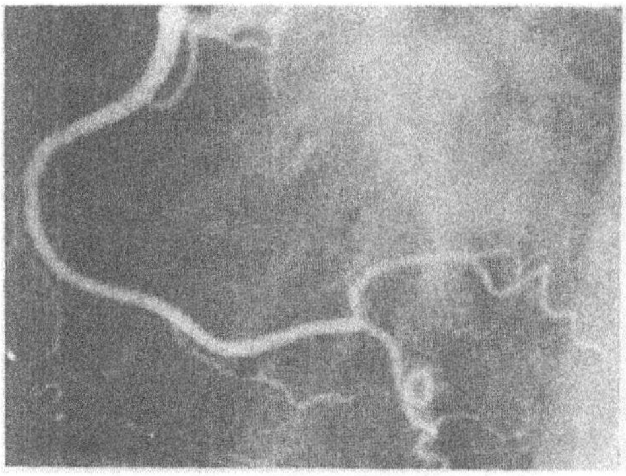
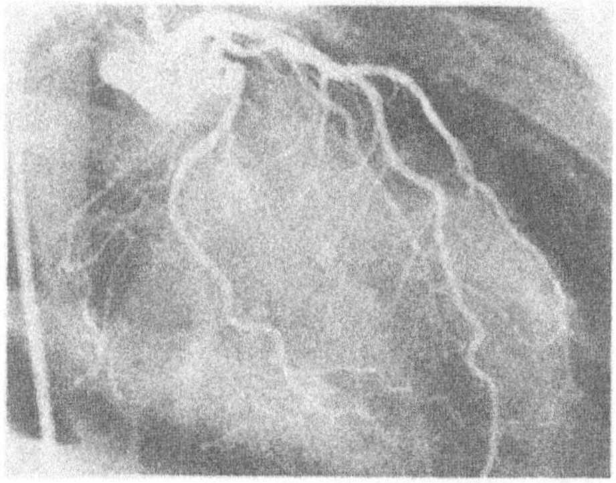
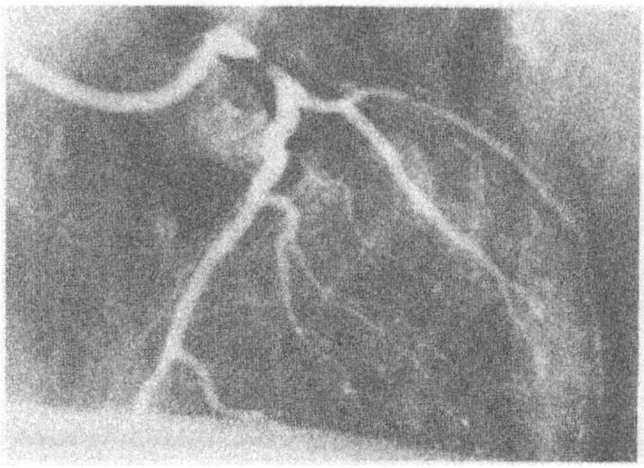
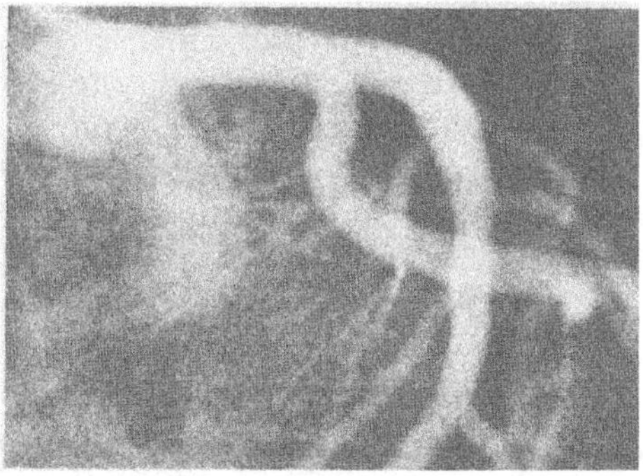

Fig. 7 *(upper left).* View of the right coronary artery in 30° left anterior oblique and 20° caudocranial double-oblique projection. This projection is of interest for examination of the diaphragmatic branches to the inferior wall of the left ventricle

Fig. 8 *(upper right).* View of the left coronary artery (LCA) in 30° right anterior oblique projection. The main drawback to this basic projection is that the first diagonal branches are often superimposed on the proximal segment of the left anterior descending artery. In this patient the LCA perfuses the totally obstructed right coronary artery by means of an anastomotic left Kugel artery

Fig. 9 *(lower left).* View of the left coronary artery in 45° left anterior oblique and 25° caudocranial double-oblique projection, which is mainly useful for analysis of the origin of the diagonal branches of the left anterior descending artery

Fig. 10 *(lower right).* View of the left coronary artery in 25° left anterior oblique and 20° caudocranial double-oblique projection, providing an unobstructed image of the left coronary main trunk

mended mainly when there are mechanical complications of the infarct (septal rupture, mitral regurgitation). Particularly vigilant monitoring during the hours following coronary arteriography is recommended in the following cases: left ventricular insufficiency, cardiomyopathy with cardiac failure, unstable angina, recent infarction, and aortic stenosis associated with coronary artery disease. Patients who present significant clinical or electrocardiographic alterations during the examination, as well as those who have very severe myocardial or arterial lesions, should benefit from several hours of hospitalization in the intensive care unit after coronary arteriography.

7 Pharmacological Tests

In recent years, the information provided by coronary arteriography has been supplemented by the use of pharmacological tests.

7.1 Coronary Arteries

The dilatation of the coronary arteries is currently induced by means of nitroglycerin. It is used sublingually, intravenously or intracoronarily. Slow administration of an infusion containing 4 mg nitroglycerin in 100 ml saline or glucose isotonic solution should be carried out under very strict and constant monitoring of arterial pressure. The infusion is stopped if systolic pressure drops below 90–80 mmHg. The intracoronary injection of nitroglycerin in a 0.1–0.3 mg dose requires the same precautions. The resulting vasodilatation provides better visualization of atheromatous plaques, stenoses and anastomotic reinjections because of the improved transstenotic gradient under the effect of the vasodilator. Nitroglycerin is also indicated when there is suspicion that a proximal stenosis, or less often a distal stenosis, is induced by a spastic mechanism. Such a possibility must be considered whenever a stenosis is regular and well centred, and nitroglycerin must be administered as a matter of urgency should there be any alteration in the ST segment of the electrocardiogram, anginal pain or, a fortiori, ventricular rhythm disturbances or hypotension. Nifedipine is another drug which can induce coronary arterial dilatation [6].

Stimulation of coronary vasoconstriction has been proposed as a means of inducing spasm in some patients afflicted with spontaneous angina, particularly Prinzmetal's angina, whose arteries are healthy or have only slight lesions [7–11]. Among the applicable tests, the most common one uses derivatives of rye ergot: ergonovine or methylergometrine maleates. Most authors recommend performing this test in stages, starting with the injection of an intravenous bolus of 0.1 mg of the diluted product. The patient's clinical and electrocardiographic state is then monitored during the next 5 min, the electrocardiogram being taken using three peripheral leads (D1, D2, D3) and two or three precordial leads. In the absence of reaction, a control coronary opacification is performed before administration of a second 0.1-mg bolus. The procedure can be repeated to a maximum total dose of 0.4 mg. When a spasm is induced, it must be suppressed as soon as it has been observed and filmed. A 0.1–0.3 mg dose of intracoronary nitroglycerin is ordinarily very effective in eliminating the spasm. Some serious complications have been reported following such spasm stimulation tests [8, 9, 11–13], with the result that some authors limit their use to patients whose coronary network is angiographically normal. Other authors employ it systematically in cases of spontaneous angina, even when there are siginificant atheromatous lesions [14]. Among the other pharmacological tests proposed for use during coronary arteriography, the following may be cited: intravenous administration of alkaline solute (bicarbonate of soda or TRIS buffer), voluntary hyperventilation and the cold pressor test requiring prolonged immersion of the hands in iced water; all are means of inducing coronary vasoconstriction [15, 16].

7.2 Left Ventricle

Pharmacological tests are also useful in analysing left ventricular contraction. The nitroglycerin test consists in repeating left ventriculography 5 min after sublingual absorption of nitroglycerin. This drug induces a lowering of left ventricular end-diastolic pressure and of intramyocardial tension, thus favouring improved contraction of an ischaemic wall segment. Atrial pacing and bicycle or handgrip exercise tests have also been used to study the behaviour of the left ventricle when submitted to an increase in cardiac demand and work-load. The controlled inducement of ventricular extrasystolic beats during left ventriculography allows assessment of the adaptation possibilities of one or more segments of ventricular wall to intensification of contractility and to an increase in preload. According to the conditions in which they are used, these tests have one of two objectives:

1. To verify that a wall segment which is apparently normal during initial ventriculography retains its contractile functions during the test
2. To try to determine whether a segment hypokinetic during initial ventriculography can increase the amplitude of its contraction during the test, which would suggest that the abnormality is not due to myocardial fibrosis or to scar tissue but is consequent to an ischaemia possibly reversible by myocardial revascularization.

8 Accidents and Risks of Coronary Arteriography

The main complications of coronary arteriography have been analysed in large serial studies [17–23]. These co-operative studies (Table 2) have shown that the risks attending the examination increase significantly when operators do not perform a

Table 2. Type and percentage of complications following coronary arteriography

	Adams 1979 Co-operative Study [17]		Davis 1979 Co-operative Study [18]			Judkins 1976 [19]		Montreal Heart Institute 1976 [20]	Lyons Cardiology Hospital 1975 [22]
Method	Sones	Judkins	Sones	Judkins	Total	Without heparin	With heparin	Bourassa	Sones
No. of patients	43080	45999	1187	6328	7553	7000	880	5251	670
Deaths (%)	0.12	0.16	0.51	0.14	0.2	0.07	0	0.23	0.1
Myocardial infarction (%)	0.15	0.20	0.42	0.22	0.25	0.12	0	0.09	0.4
Serious arrhythmia (%)	0.70	0.82			0.63			0.48	0.5
Cerebral embolism (%)	0.08	0.09	0.08	0.005	0.02	0.13	0	0.13	0
Arterial thrombosis (%)	1.13	0.23	1.85	0.24	0.49	0.3	0.11	0.68	2

sufficient number of examinations per year. A team carrying out less than 200 explorations per year records four times as many complications as a team during 700 per year. The rate of complications is still significantly related to the following factors: non-heparinized material, stenosis of the left main coronary trunk, para-ostial stenosis, triple-vessel disease, unstable angina, cardiac insufficiency and arterial hypertension [17–21, 23–25]. Rhythm disturbances and myocardial infarction, which were initially complications specific to coronary arteriography as compared with other types of cardiac exploration, have become exceptional. It has now been clearly established that the risks of coronary arteriography are directly related to the training and experience of the operators and to obedience to the safety rules formulated by the most experienced authors: Sones, Judkins, Bourassa and Gensini. Judkins' observation is apt: the work of a coronary arteriography unit may be considered very good if the mortality rate is less than 0.1%, and bad and needing revision if the rate is over 0.3% [24]. Complications are more frequent in unstable angina than in stable angina because the coronary and left ventricular lesions are more severe [23].

The patient and operator radiation dose due to direct and scattered radiation is theoretically less intense during coronary arteriography than during exploration of valve disease. With a trained operator, the mean duration of fluoroscopy should be easily under 10 min, unless there is an associated aortic stenosis [26–29]. The radiation dose received by the operator is greater when the stand has a rotating arm than when the patient is in a cradle [26]. In classic catheterization, there is as much radiation from the fluoroscopic examination as from the radio-cinematography. In coronary arteriography, the radio-cinematography contributes more to the radiation dose. It is therefore advisable to film the coronary arteries at a rather low speed (25 frames per second). The doses of radiation received during the examination by an operator wearing a protective lead apron can be estimated at the following levels: 25 mR for the eyes, 15 mR for the hands and 5 mR for the gonads [26–29]. The doses received by the paramedical personnel vary greatly according to the source of statistics. They should be insignificant and even nil if the operator refrains from using fluoroscopy when a technician or nurse comes near the examination table and if the generator control panel and the cardiac monitoring equipment are located out of the room or behind efficient protective screens. The patient's gonads receive higher doses with Judkins' method than with that of Sones, and such doses are greater for women (approximately 35 mR per examination). The dose of radiation received by a patient during a complete examination can total 25–30 R [29].

References

1. Crochet D, Petitier H, De Laguerenne J, Wanlin P (1979) Modifications de la performance ventriculaire gauche induites par la coronarographie avec un nouvel opacifiant à faible osmolarité. Ann Radiol 22: 313
2. Higgins CB, Schmidt W (1978) Direct and reflex myocardial effects of intracoronary administered contrast materials in the anesthetized and conscious dog: comparison of standard and newer contrast materials. Invest Radiol 13: 205
3. Yamazaki H, Banka VS, Bodenheimer MM, Hattori S, Agarwall JB, Helfant RH (1981) Differ-

ential effects of Renografin 76 on the ischemic and non-ischemic myocardium. Am J Cardiol 47: 597

4. Higgins CB, Gerber KH (1982) Regional myocardial hemodynamic and metabolic effects of ionic and nonionic contrast media in the normal and ischemic state. In: Amiel M (ed) Contrast media in radiology. Springer, Berlin Heidelberg New York, p 84
5. Petitier H, Crochet D, Wanlin P, De Laguerenne J, Krause D (1982) Changes in left ventricular preload and afterload induced by coronary angiography: influence of contrast medium osmolality. In: Amiel M (ed) Contrast media in radiology. Springer, Berlin Heidelberg New York, p 92
6. Kaltenbach M, Schultz W, Kober G (1979) Effects of nifedipine after intravenous and intracoronary administration. Am J Cardiol 44: 832
7. Higgins CB, Wexler L, Silverman JF, Hayden WG, Anderson WL, Schroeder JH (1976) Spontaneously and pharmacologically provoked coronary arterial spasm in Prinzmetal variant angina. Radiology 119: 521
8. Curry RC, Pepine CJ, Sabom MB, Feldman RL, Christie LG, Conti CR (1977) Effects of ergonovine in patients with and without coronary artery disease. Circulation 56: 803
9. Heupler FA, Proudfit WL, Razavi M, Shirley EK, Greenstreet R, Sheldon WC (1978) The ergonovine maleate provocative test for coronary artery spasm. Am J Cardiol 41: 631
10. Schroeder JS, Bolen JL, Quint RA, Clark DA, Hayden WG, Higgins CB, Wexler L (1977) Provocation of coronary spasm with ergonovine maleate. New test with results in 57 patients undergoing coronary arteriography. Am J Cardiol 40: 487
11. Bertrand ME, Rousseau MF, Lablanche JM, Warembourg H Jr, Carre AG, Lekieffre JP (1979) La détection du spasme des artères coronaires par le test à la méthylergomètrine. Technique, résultats, indications. Arch Mal Coeur 72: 123
12. Nelson C, Nowak B, Childs H, Weinrauch L, Forwand S (1977) Provocative testing for coronary arterial spasm: rationale, risk, and clinical illustrations. Am J Cardiol 41: 624
13. Chérrier F (1981) Test de provocation à l'ergomètrine, risques et accidents. Etude coopérative française. In: Bertrand ME (ed) Coronary arterial spasm. Laboratoires Dausse, Paris
14. Bertrand ME, Lablanche JM, Tilmant PY, Thieuleux FA, Delforge MR, Carre AG, Asseman P, Berzin B, Libersa C, Laurent JM (1982) Frequency of provoked coronary arterial spasm in 1089 consecutive patients undergoing coronary arteriography. Circulation 65: 1299
15. Yasue H, Nagao M, Omote S, Takizawa A, Miwa K, Tanaka S (1978) Coronary arterial spasm and Prinzmetal's variant form of angina induced by hyperventilation and Tris-buffer infusion. Circulation 58: 56
16. Raizner AE, Chahine RA, Ishimori T, Verani MS, Zacca N, Nasiruddin J, Miller RR, Luchi RJ (1980) Provocation of coronary artery spasm by the cold pressor test: hemodynamic, arteriographic and quantitative angiographic observation. Circulation 62: 925
17. Adams DF, Abrams HL (1979) Complications of coronary arteriography: a follow-up report. Cardiovasc Radiol 2: 89
18. Davis K, Kennedy JW, Kemp HG Jr, Judkins MP, Gosselin AJ, Killip T (1979) Complications of coronary arteriography from the collaborative study of coronary artery surgery (CASS). Circulation 59: 1105
19. Gander MP, Judkins MP (1976) Advances in coronary arteriography using the Judkins technique. In: Lichtlen PR (ed) Coronary angiography and angina pectoris. Thieme, Stuttgart, p 26
20. Bourassa MG, Lesperance J (1976) New advances with the Bourassa technique of coronary arteriography. In: Lichtlen PR (ed) Coronary angiography and angina pectoris. Thieme, Stuttgart, p 31
21. Bourassa MG, Noble J (1976) Complication rate of coronary arteriography. A review of 5,250 cases studied by percutaneous femoral technique. Circulation 53: 106
22. Age C, Clermont A, Dalloz C, Amiel M (1975) Etude rétrospective des accidents de la coronarographie. Lyon Medical 233: 29
23. Delaye J (1980) Le risque de la coronarographie dans l'angor instable. Etude coopérative française. Arch Mal Coeur 73: 211
24. Judkins MP, Gander MP (1974) Prevention of complications of coronary arteriography. Circulation 49: 599
25. Lipton MJ, Pfeifer JF, Murphy ML, Hultgren HN (1977) Dangers of left main coronary artery lesions: angiographic technique and evaluation. Invest Radiol 12: 447

26. Amiel M, Sobotka F, Philippon L (1977) Irradiation du médecin, du patient et du personnel paramédical dans les explorations cardiaques et vasculaires. J Radiol 58: 534
27. Balter S, Sones FM Jr, Brancato R (1978) Radiation exposure to the operator performing cardiac angiography with U arm systems. Circulation 58: 925
28. Begg FR, Hans LF (1975) Radiation exposure to the angiographer during coronary arteriography using U arm image amplifier. Cathet Cardiovasc Diagn 1: 261
29. Rueter FG (1978) Physician and patient exposure during cardiac catheterization. Circulation 58: 134

III Angiographic Explorations: Normal Results

1 Left Ventricle and Left Ventricular Function

1.1 Radiological Anatomy

The left ventricle (LV) can be compared to two partially amalgamated and connected cones representing the filling and ejection chambers (Fig. 1), with a common point towards the front and two adjoining bases towards the spine. The input orifice of the filling chamber and the output orifice of the ejection chamber are connected by the intervalvular trigone, a fibrous formation joining together the mitral septal leaflet and the posterior and left aortic semi-lunar valves (Fig. 2). A cross-sectional view of the LV, perpendicular to its longitudinal axis (Fig. 3), shows a septal wall and three free walls which seem to form a single regularly convex wall successively anterior, lateral and inferior. The practice of left ventriculography in right anterior oblique (RAO) and left anterior oblique (LAO) projections has led to the adoption of a suitable terminology to designate the LV walls: anterior and inferior clearly visible in RAO projection, lateral and septal in LAO projection (Figs. 4 and 5). These

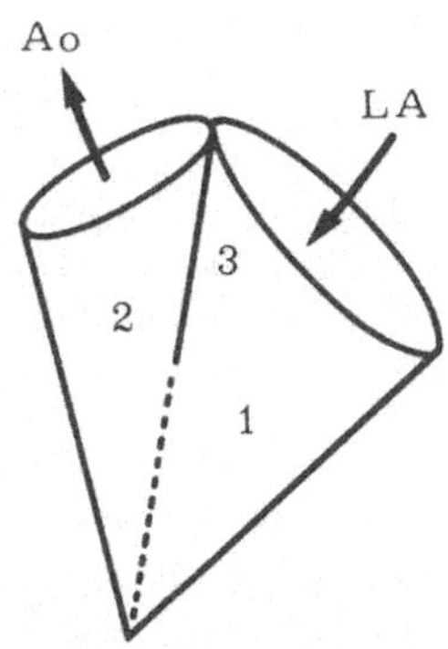

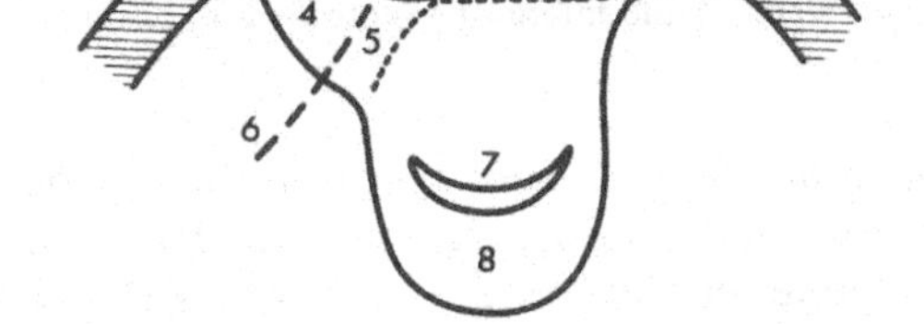

Fig. 1 *(left)*. Schematic left anterior oblique view of the left ventricle. The cone-shaped inlet *(1)* and outlet *(2)* chambers are divided by the septal leaflet *(3)*. *Ao:* aorta; *LA:* left atrium

Fig. 2 *(right)*. The aortoventricular membrane (McAlpine [34]) *RCA:* right coronary artery; *LCO:* left coronary ostium; *L, R, P:* left, right and posterior aortic sinuses; *1:* left anterior fibrous trigone; *2:* right anterior fibrous trigone; *3:* intervalvular trigone; *4:* ventricular membranous septum; *5:* atrial membranous septum; *6:* septal leaflet of the tricuspid valve; *7:* septal (anterior) leaflet of the mitral valve; *8:* lateral (posterior) leaflet of the mitral valve

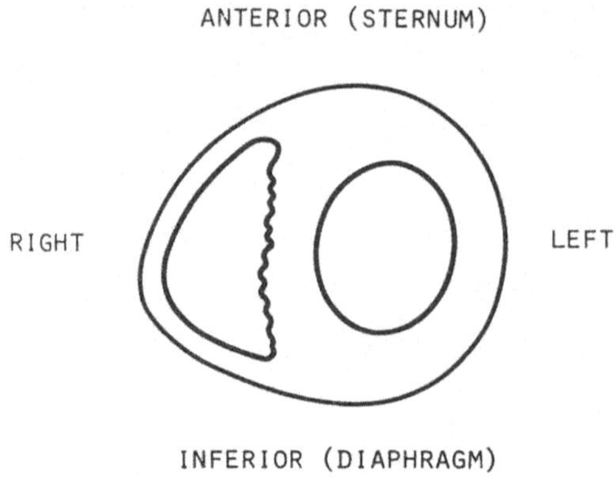

Fig. 3. Cross-section of the two ventricles at right angles to the left ventricular long axis: a plea for identification of four left ventricular walls

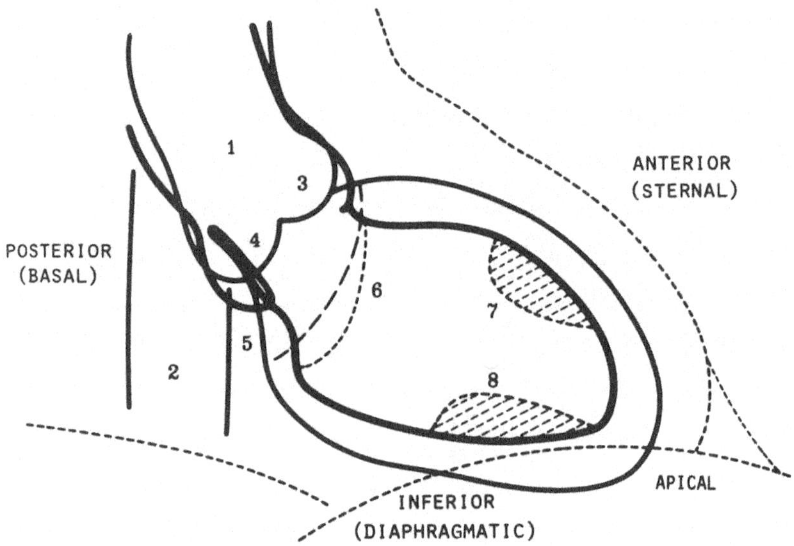

Fig. 4. Thirty-degree right anterior oblique view of the left ventricle. *1:* ascending aorta; *2:* descending aorta; *3, 4:* right coronary and posterior non-coronary Valsalva sinuses; *5:* atrial side of the mitral septal leaflet; *6:* attachment line of the posterolateral leaflet on the mitral annulus; *7, 8:* anterior (anterolateral) and inferior (posteromedial) papillary muscles

anatomic features correspond to the functional distribution of coronary vascularization. In the most common case, that of right-preponderant coronary circulation, the anterior wall of the LV is vascularized by the left anterior descending artery (LAD) and its branches, the lateral wall by the circumflex (Cx) and its branches, the inferior wall by the distal branches of the right coronary artery (RCA), and the septal wall by the septal branches arising from the LAD and the posterior descending artery (PDA). The general orientation of the LV is rather difficult to define, considering the spiral form of the interventricular septum. Relative to the basic thoracic planes, the mean LV longitudinal axis forms a 40° angle with the frontal plane, a 60° angle with the sagittal plane and a 60° angle with the horizontal plane in a well-

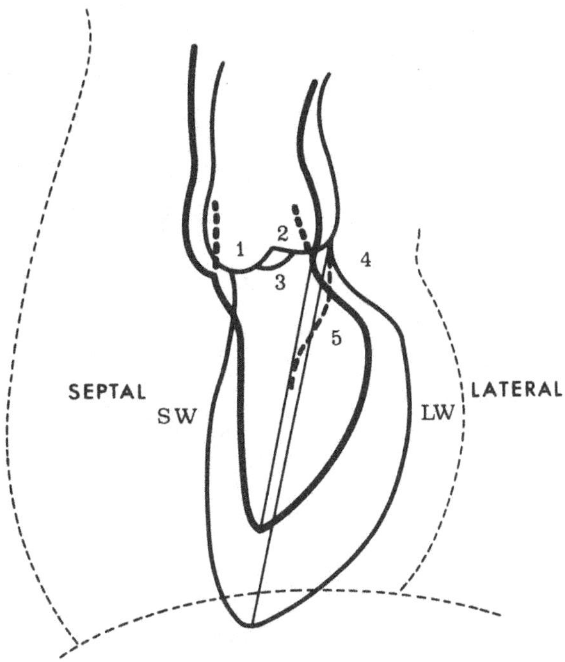

Fig. 5. Forty-five degree left anterior oblique view of the left ventricle (asthenic-vertical type). *SW:* septal wall; *LW:* lateral wall; *1, 2, 3:* right coronary, left coronary, posterior non-coronary Valsalva sinuses; *4:* left atrium; *5:* septal leaflet of the mitral valve

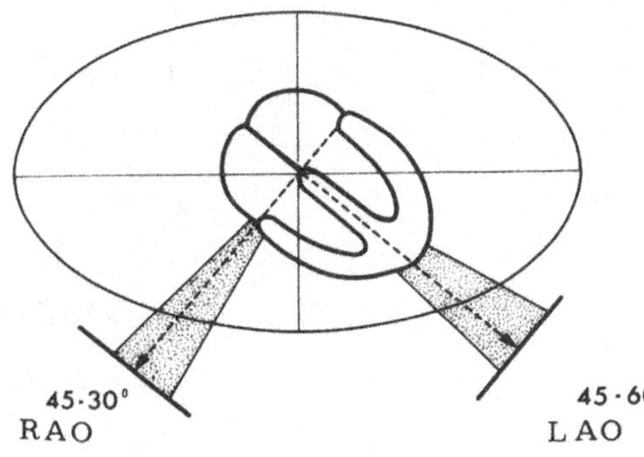

Fig. 6. The two basic projections for left ventriculography and coronary arteriography: superior view of a horizontal thoracic cross-section. *RAO:* right anterior oblique; *LAO:* left anterior oblique

proportioned sthenic person. This orientation explains why the LV is viewed obliquely in the classic anteroposterior and lateral projections of the thorax. To obtain a better view of the LV, it is preferable to radiograph it in 30°–40° RAO, which places the plane of the interventricular septum and the long axis of the LV parallel to the image recorder (image intensifier or film), and in 45–60° LAO projection, which places the septal plane perpendicular to the recorder (Figs. 6 and 7). The best projection for studying the septum and the lateral wall comprises a double angulation (LAO and caudocranial), so that the septal plane remains perpendicular to the film, whereas the long axis of the ventricle is parallel to the film (Fig. 8).

When the LV contour is described according to the different projections, it is customary to regard the diastolic image as the basis for determining systolic modifications.

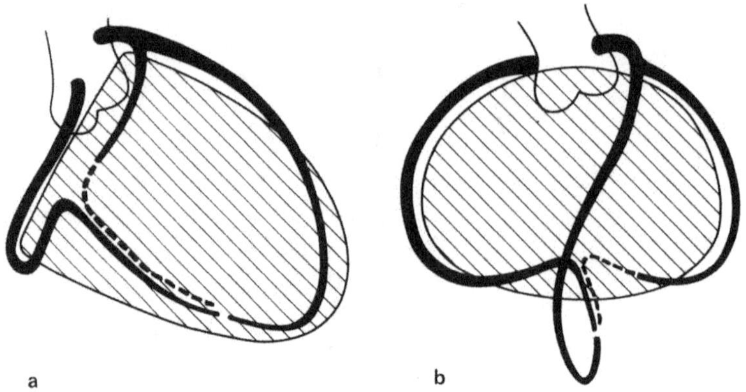

a b

Fig. 7 a, b. The two basic projections for analysis of the coronary arterial network. **a** right anterior oblique projection of the interventricular septal plane; **b** left anterior oblique projection of the plane of the atrioventricular orifices

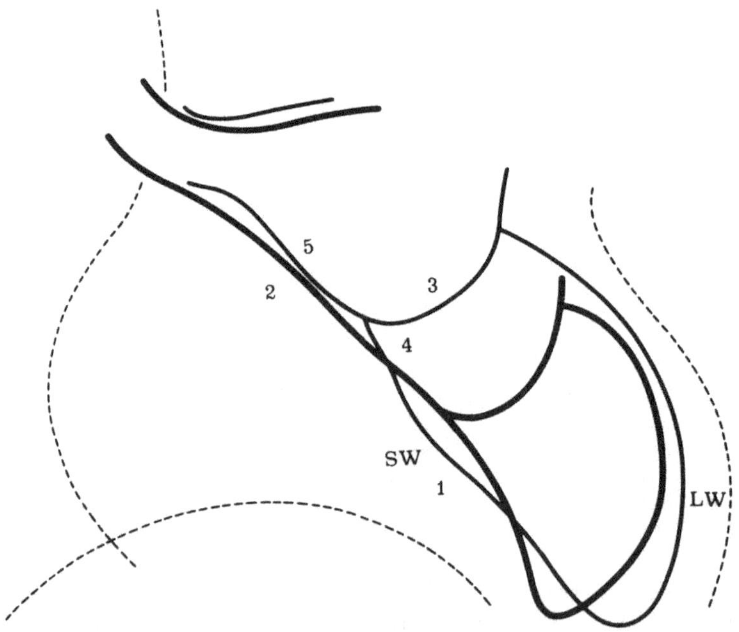

Fig. 8. Thirty-five-degree left anterior oblique and 25° caudocranial projection of left atrium and left ventricle. Superimposition of end-diastolic and end-systolic drawings. *SW, LW,* septal and lateral walls; *1:* interventricular septum; *2:* interatrial septum; *3:* diastolic position of mitral valve; *4, 5:* diastolic position of membranous septum and foramen ovale

The 30°–40° RAO projection is fundamental, as it provides information on the contractile quality of the anterior and inferior (posterodiaphragmatic) walls and on the functioning of the mitral and aortic valves. The ventricular chamber is visible in its greatest dimension and may consistently be compared to an ellipsoid (Fig. 9). Relative to the horizontal plane, the longitudinal axis of the LV is tilted 30° and the

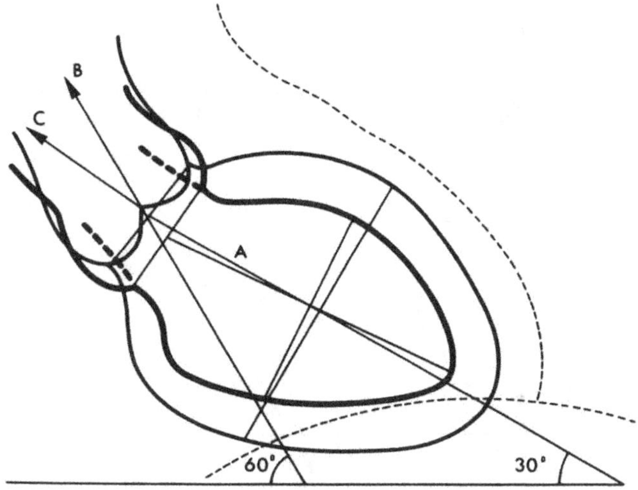

Fig. 9. Thirty-degree right anterior oblique projection of the left ventricle. Representation of ventricular *(A)*, aortic *(B)* and ejection chamber *(C)* axes

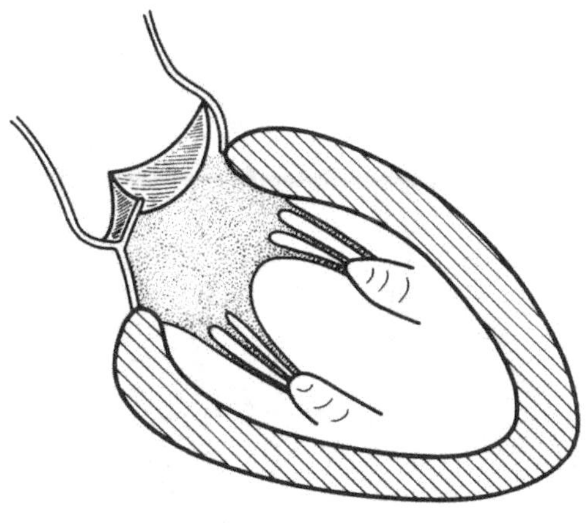

Fig. 10. Left ventricular oblique vertical section passing through the mitro-aortic junction, parallel to the major ventricular axis (McAlpine [34])

long axis of the ascending aorta 60°. The anterior free wall of the LV corresponds to the convex anterosuperior border of the cavity, which extends from the junction point of the two coronary aortic semi-lunar valves to the apex. The inferior wall corresponds to the lower border of the cavity, extending from the apex to the apparent junction point of the non-coronary posterior aortic semi-lunar valve with the mitral valve. The anterior two-thirds of this inferior border is nearly horizontal, while the posterior third forms the "heel" of the ventricle (fulcrum), being convex posteriorly and inferiorly in its lower part and concave in its upper part. This subaortic segment of the inferior border corresponds to the atrial side of the inferior part of the mitral valve (Fig. 10). The membranous leaflets of the mitral valve are parallel to the film and thus not visible. The insertion line of the small mitral valve, corresponding to the left half of the mitral ring, is clearly visualized in systole and when accentuated by contrast material as a wide and regularly curving convex line opposite to the apex. The outlines of the papillary muscles are ordinarily invisible in diastole, but

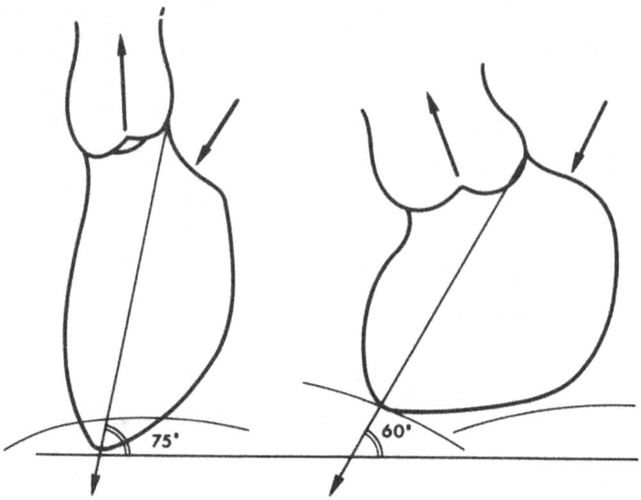

Fig. 11. Left anterior oblique projection of the left ventricle. Variable direction of the main axes related to anatomic configuration: asthenic-vertical type on the *left*, pyknic-horizontal type on the *right*

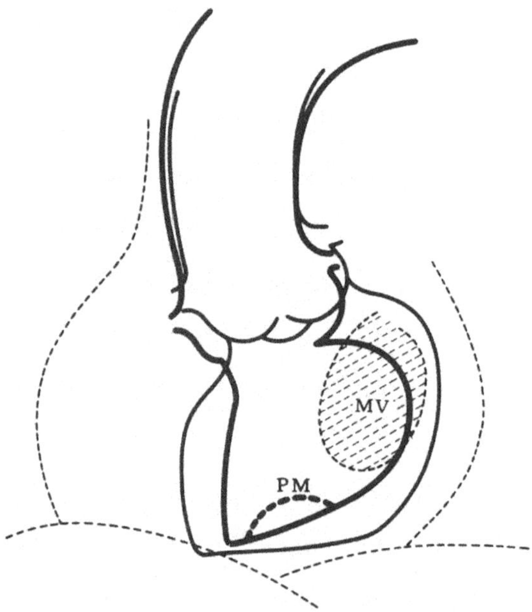

Fig. 12. Left anterior oblique view of the left ventricle (horizontal type): ventricular end-diastolic and end-systolic silhouettes. Projection of opening mitral valve *(oMV)* and inferior (posterior) papillary muscle *(PM)*

are intermittently visible in systole in the form of two protruding radiolucent spaces in the apical third of the cavity.

The LAO projection should be 45° for a vertical heart and 60° for a horizontal heart. The ventricular cavity presents an irregular oval shape (Figs. 11 and 12), with an external border corresponding mainly to the projection of the lateral wall, and a smoother internal border corresponding to the septal wall. The upper part of the external border marks the atrial limit of the mitral ring. The septum has a double curvature: concave towards the centre of the ventricle for the lower two-thirds and con-

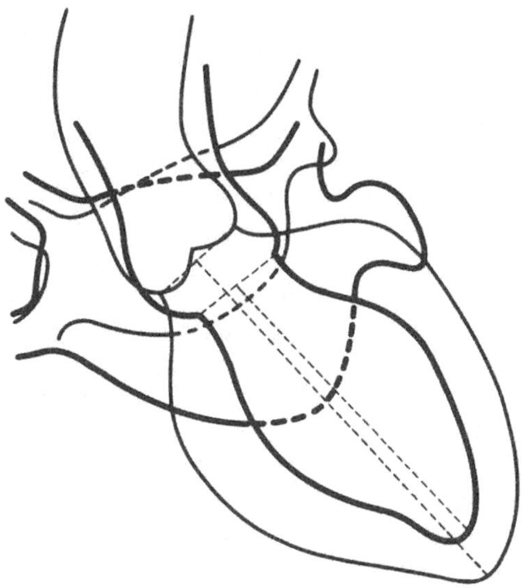

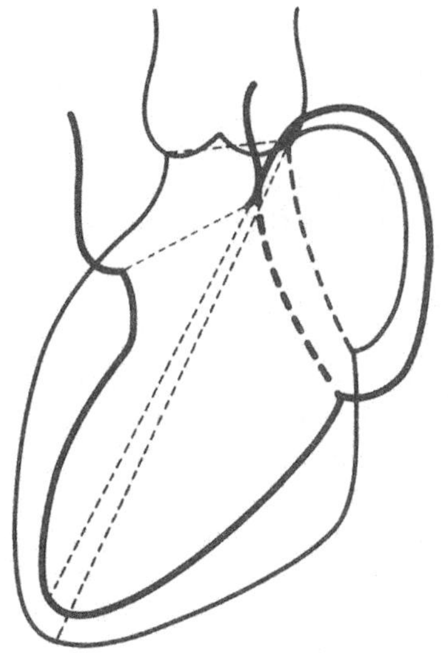

Fig. 13 *(left)*. Frontal projection of left cardiac chambers. Position of the orifices and main axes at the end of ventricular diastole and systole

Fig. 14 *(right)*. Lateral projection of left cardiac chambers. Ventricular end-diastolic and end-systolic position of the orifices and main axes (same individual as in Fig. 13, from biplanar cine film)

vex for the upper third. The immediately subaortic segment of the internal border corresponds to the membranous septum. The aortic orifice forms the upper limits of the cavity. The mitral valve is visible in diastole in the form of a rounded radiolucent area, more or less clearly defined, situated in the concavity of the upper part of the lateral border (Fig. 12). The septal leaflet of the mitral valve becomes more clearly visible as the projection angle is increased (60° or more). The posterolateral leaflet is not ordinarily visible. When a caudocranial angulation of the X-ray beam is associated with the LAO projection, the long axis of the LV becomes parallel to the film plane and the double septal curvature is straightened out, thus providing better viewing of the entire length of the septum as well as of the aortomitral junction.

Frontal postero-anterior and transverse projections (Figs. 13 and 14) are ordinarily of little interest in coronary artery disease. From an angiographic point of view, it might be said that the frontal projection is a poor RAO view and the lateral projection a poor LAO view. The main value of the transverse projection is to allow good analysis of the septal leaflet of the mitral valve.

1.2 Normal Kinetics

Left ventricular volume reaches its maximum value at the end of diastole. During systole the volume diminishes gradually, so that it may be assumed, in the absence of demonstration, that the heart muscle contracts around its geometrical centre or its centre of mass. The best-adapted and most popular geometrical model of the LV is that of an ellipsoid with a thick wall corresponding to the myocardium. During the isovolumic phase of contraction, the outer ventricular surface tends to become more spherical, with a discrete shortening of the longitudinal axis and a discrete lengthening of the transverse axis [1]. At the same time, the ventricular cavity itself shows practically no deformation. The decrease in ventricular volume occurs during the ejection phase. Minimum volume is reached at the end of systole. During systole, the external ventricular envelope shows very little deformation. Analysis of kinetics is thus concerned essentially with deformations of the endocardial outline, and possibly with modifications of wall thickness. During diastole, the various diameters of the LV increase as a result of ventricular filling. At the end of diastole atrial contraction ensures the completion of ventricular filling, which precedes mitral closure. The movement of the orifices and the axial modifications of the LV during the cardiac cycle are rather complex because of the multidirectional arrangement of the myocardial fibres which become inserted into the periorificial fibrous trigones. Analysis is facilitated by comparing the orthogonal projections in biplanar radio-cinema and by studying patients with prosthetic valves. During systole, the aortic orifice moves downwards and forwards (translation) and tilts slightly, so that its upper side faces more to the front and right. The mitral orifice moves in the direction of the apex (translation), and its anterior side faces more downwards and to the left. The apex moves closer to the base, which is due in part to its obliteration when the apical part of the anterior wall approaches the inferior wall. The longitudinal axis of the LV tilts slightly around its centre (Fig. 9), and its midpoint makes a translation of 1–6 cm towards the base. The tilting of the long axis is of the order of 10°. The translation of the orifices is not greater than 10–15 mm. Finally, study of the prosthetic valves shows that the mitral and aortic orifices are also subject to a slight rotation around their longitudinal axes.

1.3 Analysis of Wall Contraction

Study of the wall kinetics of the LV chamber is of considerable interest because of the frequency of contraction abnormalities induced by myocardial ischaemia. To analyse the kinetics correctly, the outline of the LV, its main symmetrical axis and its geometrical centre or centre of mass must be clearly defined, so that myocardial movements between end-systole and end-diastole can be validly compared. In RAO projection the symmetrical axis ordinarily used passes through the middle of the aortic orifice to the apex or through the mitro-aortic junction to the apex. With a computer it is possible to define a mean axis starting from the apex and intersecting the base at any point, so that the area of ventricular outline divides into two equal parts. Analysis of LV movement, in the simplest hypothesis (analysis of two frames per cycle), consists in superimposing the end-systolic and end-diastolic outlines. Several frames (up to 25 or 50, for example) may be analysed during one cycle, but this is usually done only for research purposes. One of the great problems in analysis of LV contraction is connected with the choice of the correction technique for changes in axis and for translations of the aortic orifice and the apex (Fig. 15). Obtaining thoracic immobility of the patient during apnoea is the best means of overcoming this difficulty. Some authors have used natural landmarks, such as the spine

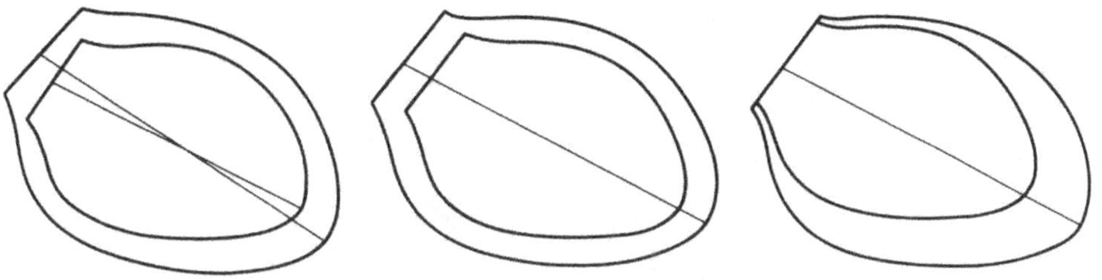

Fig. 15. Various possibilities for superimposition of end-diastolic and end-systolic silhouettes

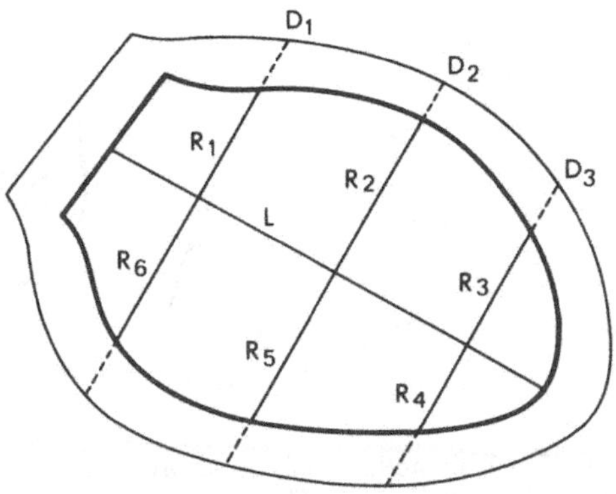

Fig. 16. Analysis of the segmental wall motion: quadrisection of the long axis *(L)* by perpendicular transverse basal *(D1)*, medial *(D2)* and apical *(D3)* axes. Each transverse axis is divided into two hemiaxes: anterobasal *(R1)*, anteromedial *(R2)*, antero-apical *(R3)*, infero-apical *(R4)*, inferomedial *(R5)*, inferobasal *(R6)*

and the ribs [2], or a catheter placed in the coronary sinus [3], or external markers affixed to the image intensifier screen [4]. The superimposition of the aortic orifices [4, 5] is not adequate because it exaggerates apical and inferobasal kinetics. Brower's comparative studies [6] demonstrate the importance of realigning the longitudinal axis and/or the apex during the cardiac cycle.

The quantitative analysis of wall motion rests on the principle of the division of the endocardial outline, using either transverse axes perpendicular to the longitudinal axis (Figs. 16 and 17a) or lines radiating from the centre of the ventricle (Fig. 17b). The methods used today are varied, but they all derive from the propositions made by the following authors: Herman [7] and Leighton [2] for the principle of transverse hemiaxes; Scampardonis [8] and Rickards [9] for the principle of radial hemiaxes.

Wall motion is measured by the percentage of systolic shortening of the axes or hemiaxes. A negative value indicates a dyskinesis with systolic expansion of a wall segment (percentage of elongation). Figure 16 expresses the principle of these methods schematically for a limited calculation based on end-systolic and end-diastolic images of a cardiac cycle. Tables 1 and 2 give the results obtained by various authors. It may be noted that the motion of the inferior wall is less than that of the anterior wall, and that the shortening of the longitudinal axis is less than that of the transverse axes. These methods become very efficient when computers are used to produce the tracing of the axes, increasing their number at will and allowing study of many frames during the same cycle (Fig. 18). Dividing up the ventricular image

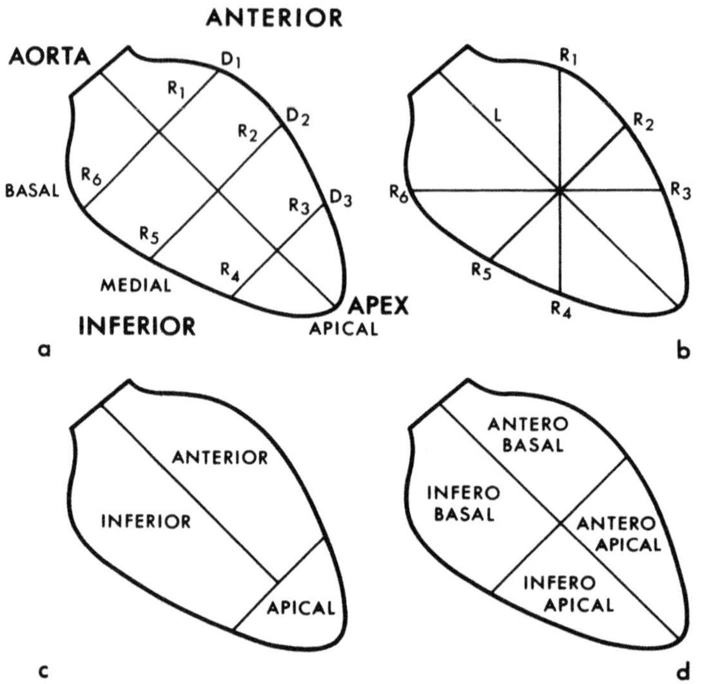

Fig. 17. a Wall motion analysis according to the reference method of Herman [7]. Quadrisection of the longitudinal axis *L*. The transverse axes *(D1, D2, D3)* evaluate basal, medial or apical whole-left-ventricular contraction. The transverse hemiaxes *(R1–R6)* attempt to analyse a more localized segmental motion dependent on the anterior or the inferior wall. **b** Wall motion analysis according to the reference method of Scampardonis [8]: six radial hemiaxes, with a 45° angle between each pair, are used to evaluate segmental wall motion. **c, d** Wall motion analysis by means of the percentage of change in area between end-diastolic and end-systolic silhouettes. The left ventricle is divided into three or four areas

Table 1. Wall motion analysis: mean values of percentage axis shortening. The transverse axes (*D*1, *D*2, *D*3) evaluate basal, medial or apical whole-left-ventricular contraction

Author	*D*1	*D*2	*D*3
Leighton [2]	53	52	57
Nakhjavan [12]	39.4	45.4	57.9

Table 2. Wall motion analysis: mean values of percentage axis shortening

Author	*R*1	*R*6	*R*2	*R*5	*R*3	*R*4	*L*
Bertrand [13]	47	30	39	33	38	39	23
Carroll [14]	51.3	39.3	46.6	44.1	50.0	48.5	
Scampardonis [8][a]	48.9	28.4	58.0	50.8	56.9	52.7	24.8
Sniderman [3][b]	42	45	40	62	45	70	

[a] Radial method; [b] superimposed aortic orifices

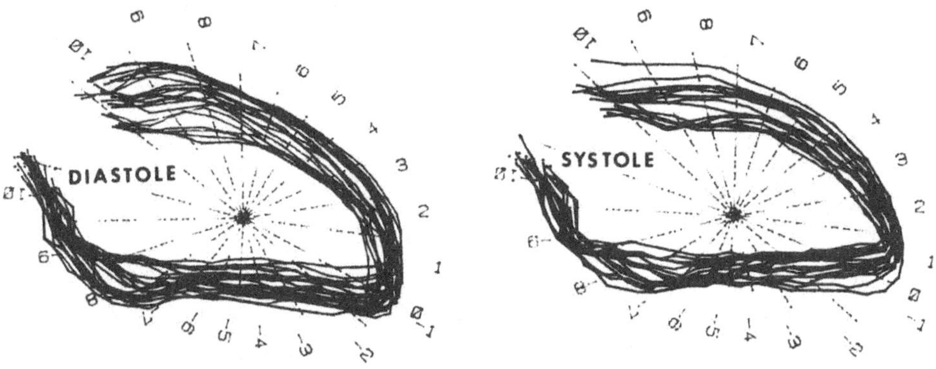

Fig. 18. Superimposition of the endocardial contours in multiframe analysis of left ventriculography

into areas (Fig. 17 c, d) has been proposed [10, 11], but seems no better as a method. Analysis of segmentary contraction provides results comparable to those obtained with measurement of the ejection fraction in assessment of LV function [12].

1.4 Volumes and Function Indexes

The methods for measuring LV end-diastolic and end-systolic volumes are based on the principle of calculating a volume from its planar image as projected on one or two planes. The ellipsoid is the geometrical model with which the LV is generally identified. Theoretically, the most exact methods are those using simultaneous biplanar filming of the LV, with application of Simpson's rule to the geometrical reconstruction of the LV. These methods have been developed by Chapman [15] and Besse [16] and are especially useful in cases involving very deformed ventricles (aneurysm, obstructive myocardiopathy). However, single-plane methods are used far more often: Greene's method [17], Snow's method [18] and especially Dodge's area-length method [19], which has certainly been most universally adopted. These methods have been tested on ventricular casts, compared with conventional methods of measuring cardiac output and systolic ejection volume, and then corrected by regression equations suitable to each and to the radiological projections used. When the image magnification factor is correctly measured [16, 20], these methods are absolutely reliable in routine practice. Figure 19 provides a schematic representation of the principles and computation formulae for the three main methods. Table 3 gives the results obtained by various authors with different methods. The volume values are indexed per square meter of body surface area.

Left ventricular ejection fraction remains one of the best indices of LV function and even of contractility, and is the one most often used in routine practice. In the absence of mitral regurgitation or of interventricular communication, it expresses the percentage of end-diastolic volume ejected into the aorta during each systole: ejection fraction = (end-diastolic volume − end-systolic volume)/end-diastolic volume. Its normal value as determined by various authors is given in Table 3.

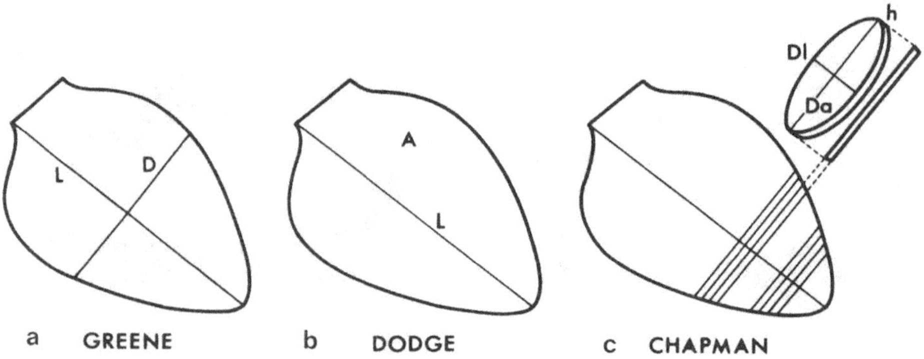

Fig. 19a–c. Diagrams and formulae for the three main methods of measuring left ventricular volumes *(V)*. Representation of the ventricular outline in 30° right anterior oblique projection. **a** Axes method (Greene): *Single-plane:* $V=\frac{4}{3}\pi\frac{D}{2}\cdot\frac{D}{2}\cdot\frac{L}{2}=\frac{\pi D^2 L}{6}$ The antero-inferior transverse axis *D* is assumed to be equal to the septolateral transverse axis *D*. *Biplanar:* $V=\frac{4}{3}\pi\frac{Da}{2}\cdot\frac{Dl}{2}\cdot\frac{L}{2}$ The antero-inferior *Da* and septolateral *Dl* transverse axes are measured according to the corresponding projections: postero-anterior or right anterior oblique on one plane, transverse or left anterior oblique on the other plane. **b** Area-length method (Dodge): this method is applicable to a single-plane or biplane system. The transverse axis *D* is calculated from the planimetred area *A* of the left ventricular outline: $V=\frac{\pi D^2 L}{6}$ where $D=\frac{4A}{\pi L}$. **c** Method of summing the slices of the left ventricle (Chapman): the volume of each ventricle slice is equal to $\Delta V=\pi h\cdot\frac{d}{2}\cdot\frac{d'}{2}$.

In order to obtain true left ventricular volume, the theoretical volume provided by the above formulae is corrected for image magnification, and a regression equation specific to each method is applied, taking the selected projection(s) into account. These regression equations are derived from calculations using left ventricular casts.

Table 3. Left Ventricular volumes (ml/m^2 body surface area) and ejection fraction (EF)

Author	Method	No. of Patients	EDV	ESV	SV	EF
Amiel [21]	RAO SinglePlane	10	60 ±12	16 ± 3	(44)	0.63
Arvidsson [22]	Arvidsson biplanar	16	57.3	14.6	(42.7)	0.74
Besse [16]	Chapman modified biplanar	39	99 ±22	35 ±11	(64)	0.63±0.03
Brun [23]	Simpson biplanar	8	72.3±13	26.9± 7.4	(45.4)	0.62±0.03
Falsetti [24]	RAO single-plane	5	104	31	(73)	0.70
Hermann [25]	Dodge modified biplanar	6	71 ±8	30 ±4	(41)	0.63±0.02
Kennedy [26]	Dodge biplanar	16	70 ±20	24 ±10	45 ±13	0.67±0.08
Petitier [27]	RAO Dodge single-plane	25	77.4±23.2	27.2± 9.0	50.2±15.9	0.64±0.06
Wynne [28]	Dodge biplanar	17	72 ±15	20 ± 8	51 ± 8	0.72±0.08

SV: value of stroke volume calculated from the values of end-diastolic volume (EDV) and end-systolic volume (ESV) given by the authors; *RAO:* right anterior oblique view

It is easy, if the image magnification factor is known, to measure the thickness of the LV anterior free wall on the basis of the tracings of internal and external ventricle outline in 30° RAO projection. If possible, this measurement is taken on the LV equatorial transverse axis. Myocardial mass is most often computed in end-diastole only, according to the method of Rackley [29], by assuming that the ventricular chamber is totally surrounded by cardiac muscle, even in the mitro-aortic region, and that the wall is of equal thickness at all points. The calculation principle is simple: external LV volume – internal LV volume = LV wall volume; LV wall volume × specific weight of the myocardium = myocardial mass. The normal values of wall thickness and myocardial mass indexed per square meter of body surface area are indicated in Table 4. The amplitude and thickness variation rate of the wall during the cardiac cycle are also valid indices of LV function. According to Ritman [32], the rate of systolic thickening is a sensitive index of myocardial ischaemia.

The equatorial mean fibre-shortening velocity (VCF) gives the shortening velocity of fibres in the plane perpendicular to the midpoint of the longitudinal axis of the LV [33]. Measurement of the transverse axis or minor axis *M* at end-diastole (EDM) and end-systole (ESM) and of systolic ejection time (SET) enables computation of mean VCF according to the formula: mean VCF = (EDM – ESM) / (EDM × SET). Mean VCF is expressed in circumferences per second. The normal value is of the order of 1.30–1.40. It is possible to base the computation of mean VCF on several transverse axes as well as to study variations in instantaneous VCF by frame-by-frame analysis during systole in order to determine the peak VCF, that is, the maximum value of instantaneous VCF.

This brief review of the methods of studying LV function is derived solely from angiographic and cine-angiographic techniques. It is perhaps unnecessary to mention that the use of cut film has been abandoned in this field. The methods described are those used in everyday routine. However, it should be noted that today there is a proliferation of sophisticated methods for computing LV function indices. This is the result of computer assistance, providing rapid calculation as well as the possibility of digitizing images and of recording ventricular outlines and pressure curves rapidly by means of graph pens. These various indices are the result of simultaneous study of pressure und flow parameters, on the one hand, and of those of volume and dimensions on the other. Their elaboration is based on mechanical notions of stress, strain and compliance which are beyond the scope of our approach, which is limited to diagnostic imaging.

Table 4. End-diastolic anterior wall thickness (mm) and left ventricular (LV) mass (g/m2 body surface area)

Author	No. of patients	Wall Thickness	LV mass
Kennedy [26]	22	10.9 ± 2.0	92 ± 16
Kreulen [30]	7		91.5 ± 2.7
Besse [16]	39	7 ± 1.8	78 ± 15
Petitier [27]	23	9.40 ± 2.0	
Amiel [21]	10	9.40 ± 1.3	
Mirsky [31]	10	9 ± 0.05	

2 Coronary Arteries and Veins

Myocardial vascularization is provided by the RCA and the left coronary artery (LCA). The LCA originates as a short stem which almost immediately bifurcates into two main branches: the LAD and the Cx. In functional terms, it is customary to speak of three main coronary trunks, the RCA, the LAD and the Cx, in that each of these trunks actually plays an important role in the nutritional and metabolic support of the LV, the essential component of the heart pump whose deterioration jeopardizes the chances of survival.

2.1 Origin, Calibre and Preponderance of the Coronary Arteries

The coronary arteries depart from the root of the ascending aorta in the upper region of the right and left sinuses of Valsalva (Fig. 20). Usually, the left ostium is at the same level or a little above the ring marking the transition between the dilated area of the sinus and the aorta itself. The right ostium, however, is found above the ring in only 1% or 2% of cases. The precise studies of McAlpine show that in the great majority of cases the right orifice lies in the arc between 335° and 355°, relative to aortic circumference, and the left orifice between 110° and 130° (Fig. 21). This configuration indicates why only an LAO projection in coronary arteriography allows the first part of the two coronary arteries to be free from all aortic superimposition. The LCA orifice is higher than that of the RCA because of the slant of the aortic orifice plane (Fig. 20). The RCA takes off at a right angle from the aorta, whereas the left main coronary trunk (LMCT) forms a wide (approximately 60°) angle with the aorta, opening downwards and to the front. As a rule, there is only a single left coronary ostium, if exception is made for the apparent separate origins of the LAD and the Cx due to the extreme shortness of the LMCT, which is sometimes nearly non-existent. However, it is fairly common to observe two right coronary orifices separated by 1 or 2 mm, one corresponding to the RCA itself and the other to the right conus artery. This configuration is evident in nearly 50% of subjects.

According to McAlpine [34], the coronary orifices are oval and are wider than they are high (RCA orifice 3.7 and 2.4 mm, and LCA orifice 4.7 and 3.2 mm). Studies in vivo [35, 36] show that the calibre of the LCA is greater than that of the

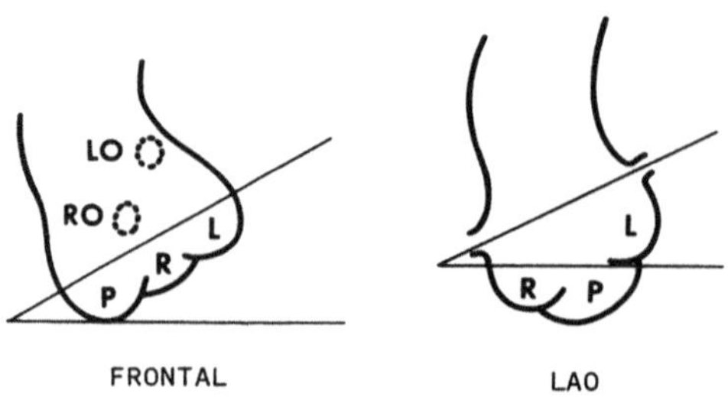

Fig. 20. Orientation of the planes of the aortic orifice and coronary ostia. *LO, RO:* left and right coronary ostia; *L, R, P:* left coronary, right coronary and posterior non-coronary aortic sinuses; *LAO:* left anterior oblique

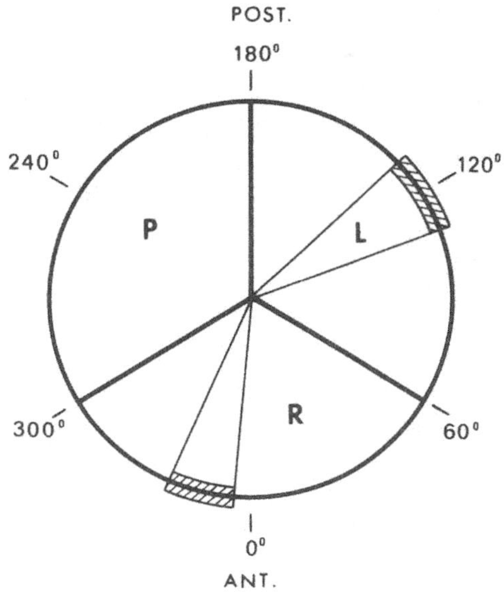

Fig. 21. The usual location of the coronary orifices on the aortic circumference in the horizontal plane (McAlpine [34]). *L, R, P:* left coronary, right coronary and posterior non-coronary aortic sinuses

Table 5. Calibre (mm) of the coronary arteries

	MacAlpin [35]	Vieweg [36]
Left main trunk	4	4.7–5.2
Proximal LAD	3.4	3.9
Distal LAD	2	2.4
Circumflex artery	3	3.2–4
Diagonal branch	2	
Marginal branch	2.5	
Proximal RCA	3.2	2.7–4.1
Distal RCA	2.7	2.9–3.4

LAD: left anterior descending artery; *RCA:* right coronary artery

RCA in 83% of cases, and that this preponderance is more frequent in men than in women. The mean values of the calibre of the main branches are given in Table 5. The ratio of the coronary area (24 mm^2) to the body surface area (1.84 m^2) is 13.1 [36]. With respect to coronary preponderance, three types of coronary circulation are possible: preponderant RCA, preponderant LCA and balanced coronary distribution. In the case of preponderant RCA (Fig. 22), the RCA runs from its point of origin along the right atrioventricular sulcus to the crux or anatomic cross of the heart, skirting the tricuspid ring. The artery divides into two main branches: the PDA and the retroventricular artery. The former advances along the posterior interventricular sulcus, and the latter continues the course of the RCA along the left atrioventricular sulcus, towards the left border of the LV, giving off branches to its diaphragmatic wall.

The first part of the LCA runs towards the left, then forwards, and divides into two main branches behind the pulmonary artery and below the left atrial appendage. The LAD continues the curvilinear course of the common trunk. It passes

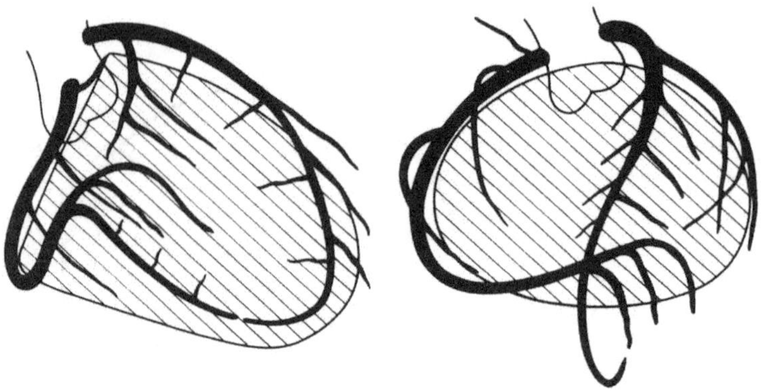

Fig. 22. Right-predominant coronary artery system

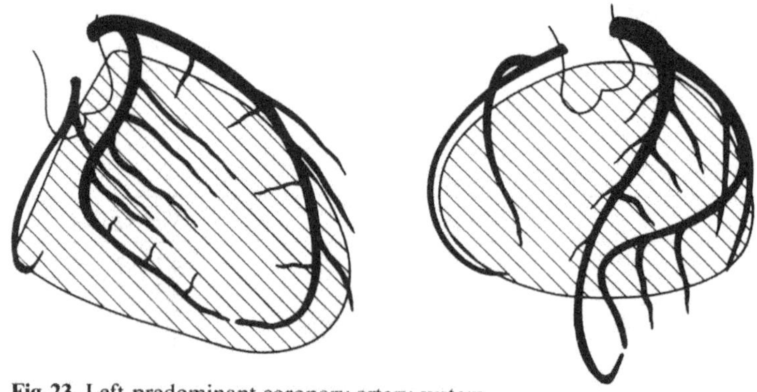

Fig. 23. Left-predominant coronary artery system

along the left side of the pulmonary artery at the level of its valvular orifice and then courses towards the anterior interventricular sulcus, which it follows as far as the apex. During its course it gives off branches mainly to the interventricular septum and to the anterior wall of the LV. The Cx takes off at a right angle from the LMCT and runs downwards and to the left. It courses along the left atrioventricular sulcus, skirting the mitral ring, and terminates at some point in this groove before reaching the crux. During its course it gives off branches mainly to the lateral wall of the LV.

In the case of a preponderant LCA (Fig. 23) the RCA does not go beyond the crux and is said to be hypotrophic. The LCA is characterized by a well-developed Cx, the mirror image to some extent of a preponderant RCA. This artery runs along the entire length of the left atrioventricular sulcus to the crux and is continued by the PDA. The arteries to the diaphragmatic wall of the LV originate from the lower part of the Cx.

When the coronary distribution is balanced (Fig. 24), the RCA gives off the PDA but no branch to the diaphragmatic wall of the LV. The LCA provides the branches to the diaphragmatic wall of the LV and sometimes a second PDA.

To sum up, the network is right preponderant when the RCA provides the PDA and vascularizes the diaphragmatic wall of the LV (80% of cases); it is left prepon-

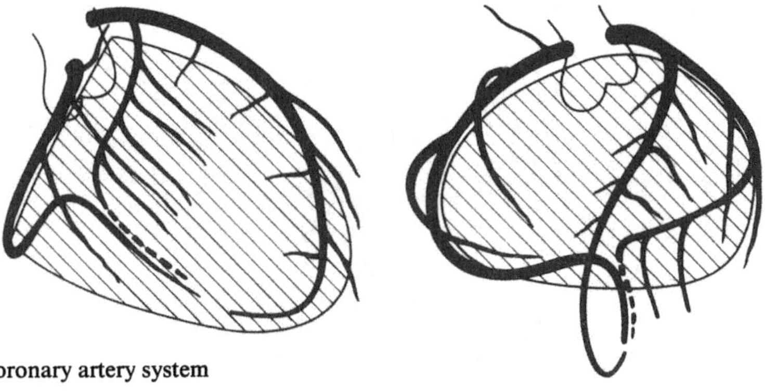

Fig. 24. Balanced coronary artery system

Table 6. Terminology applied to the branches of the coronary arteries (adapted from O'Reilly [37])

Left coronary artery
- Branches of the left anterior descending artery (LAD) to the anterior and anterolateral wall of the left ventricle (LV): diagonal branches, anterolateral branches, left ventricular (LV) branches, left muscular branches
- Ramus medianus between the LAD and the circumflex (Cx) in the case of trifurcation of the left coronary main trunk: median branch, first branch to LV
- Branches of the Cx to the "posterolateral" (diaphragmatic) wall of the LV: posterolateral branches, muscular branches, posterior branches to the LV, marginal branches, and median Cx branches
- Branches of the Cx to the lateral wall of the LV: obtuse marginal branch, left marginal and left border artery for the largest of its branches; lateral branches, lateral Cx and left marginal branches for the others
- Continuation of the Cx in the left atrioventricular sulcus: atrioventricular branch, second portion Cx and distal Cx

Right coronary artery
- Branches to anterior and diaphragmatic wall of the right ventricle (RV): right ventricular branches, marginal branches, muscular branches, and branches to RV
- Largest branch to RV: acute marginal branch, right marginal branch, right border artery and dominating branch to RV
- Branches originating distal to the posterior descending artery, supplying posterior LV wall: posterolateral branches, LV posterior branches, branches to back of LV, branches to LV.

Authors consulted: Abrams, Di Guglielmo, Gensini, James, Judkins, Levin, Paulin, Sewell, Sones and Wilson

derant when the LCA provides the PDA and vascularizes the diaphragmatic wall of the LV (10%–12% of cases); and it is balanced when the RCA provides the PDA and the LCA gives off the branches to the diaphragmatic wall of the LV (8%–10% of cases).

2.2 *Nomenclature and Segmentation of the Coronary Arteries*

A varying terminology is used by anatomists. O'Reilly [37] has compiled the different denominations currently in use to designate the main branches of the coronary

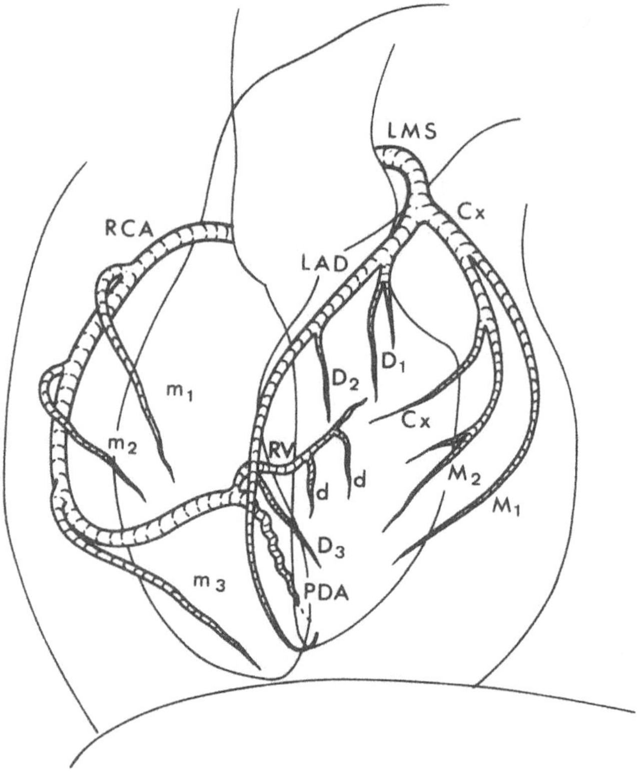

Fig. 25. Basic left anterior oblique view of the coronary arteries. *RCA:* right coronary artery; *LMS:* left main stem; *LAD:* left anterior descending artery; *Cx:* circumflex; m_1, m_2, m_3: right marginal branches; D_1, D_2, D_3: diagonal branches; *RV:* retroventricular artery; *d:* diaphragmatic branches; *PDA*, posterior descending artery; M_1, M_2: left marginal branches

network (see Table 6). The nomenclature presented here is indebted to a study by the Société Française de Cardiologie [13].

The LCA (Figs. 25–30) has a LMCT extending from the ostium to the point of origin of the Cx. The LAD gives off anterior septal arteries and arteries referred to as diagonal arteries which vascularize the anterior wall of the LV. All these arteries are numbered and identified in order of origin, for example first, second, third septal artery or diagonal artery. When one of these arteries is preponderant, it is said to be main (for example, main second diagonal artery). The LAD is proximal until the origin of the first septal artery, middle between the first septal and the second diagonal arteries, and distal beyond that. In the absence of these indicators, the artery is divided into thirds labelled proximal, middle and distal parts. The non-preponderant Cx provides the lateral wall of the LV with left marginal arteries numbered in order of origin (first, second etc.), the most important being identified as main but retaining its order number (for example, main second marginal artery). The Cx is proximal until the origin of the main marginal artery and distal beyond that point. In the absence of this indication, it is divided into two equal proximal and distal parts.

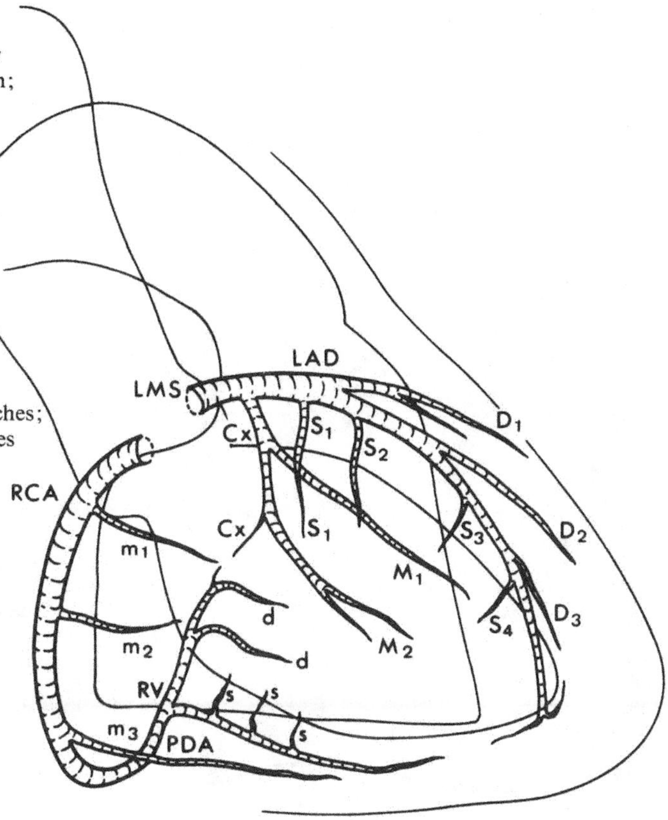

Fig. 26. Basic right anterior oblique view of the coronary arteries. *LMS:* left main stem; *RCA:* right coronary artery; m_1, m_2, m_3: right marginal branches; *RV:* retroventricular artery; *PDA:* posterior descending artery; *LAD:* left anterior descending artery; *Cx:* circumflex; *d:* diaphragmatic branches; *s:* inferior septal branches; S_1, S_2, S_3, S_4: anterior septal branches; M_1, M_2: left marginal branches; D_1, D_2, D_3: diagonal branches

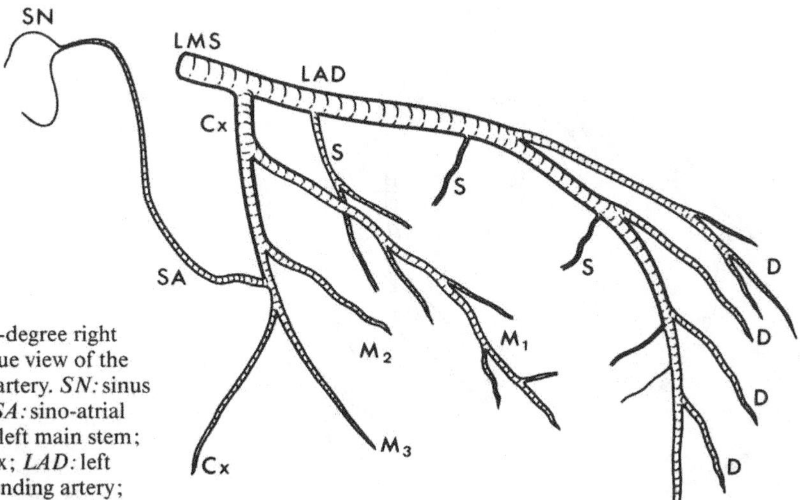

Fig. 27. Thirty-degree right anterior oblique view of the left coronary artery. *SN:* sinus node artery; *SA:* sino-atrial artery; *LMS:* left main stem; *Cx:* circumflex; *LAD:* left anterior descending artery; *S:* anterior septal branches; M_1, M_2, M_3: left marginal branches; *D:* diagonal branches

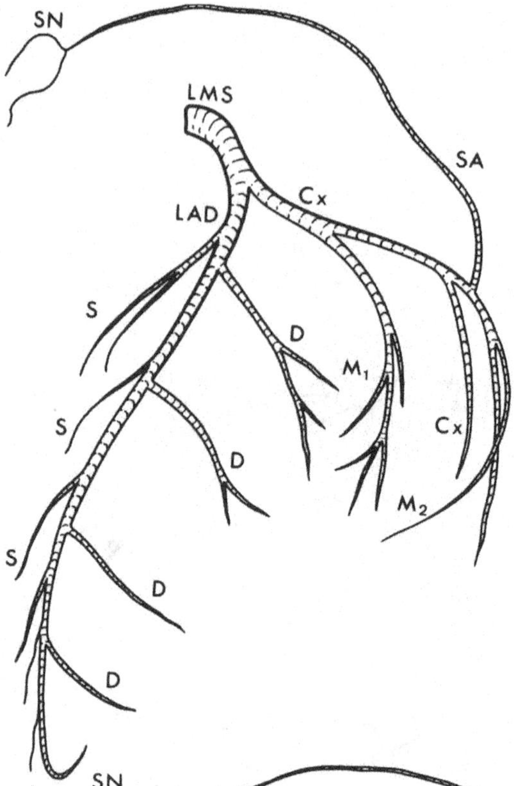

Fig. 28: Forty-five-degree left anterior oblique view of the left coronary artery. *SN:* sinus node artery; *LMS:* left main stem; *LAD:* left anterior descending artery; *S:* anterior septal branches; *Cx:* circumflex; *D:* diagonal branches; M_1, M_2: left marginal branches; *SA:* sino-atrial artery

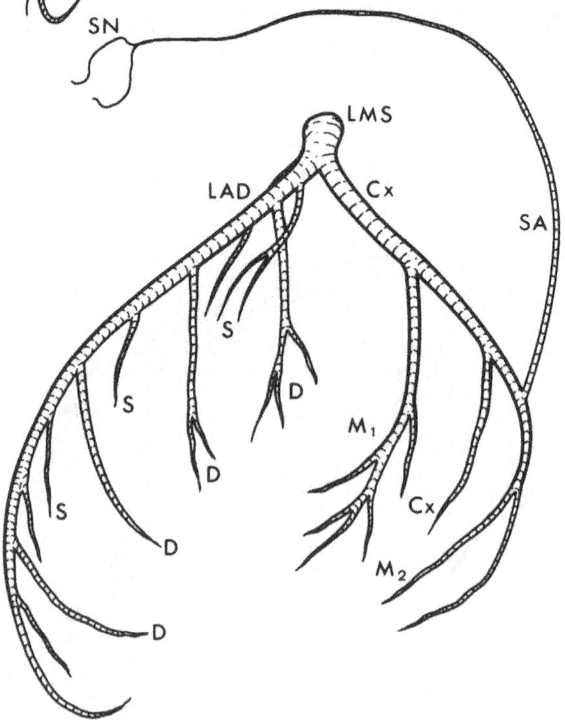

Fig. 29. Sixty-degree left anterior oblique view of the left coronary artery. *SN:* sinus node artery; *LAD:* left anterior descending artery; *S:* anterior septal branches; *D:* diagonal branches; *LMS:* left main stem; *Cx:* circumflex; M_1, M_2: left marginal branches; *SA:* sino-atrial artery

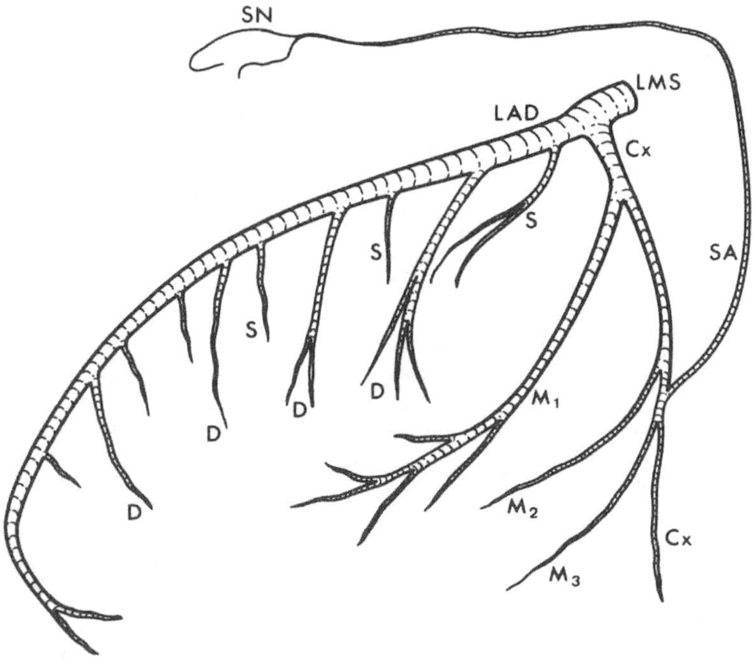

Fig. 30. Transverse view of the left coronary artery. *SN:* sinus node artery; *LAD:* left anterior descending artery; *S:* anterior septal branches; *D:* diagonal branches; *LMS:* left main stem; *Cx:* circumflex M_1, M_1, M_3: left marginal branches; *SA:* sino-atrial artery

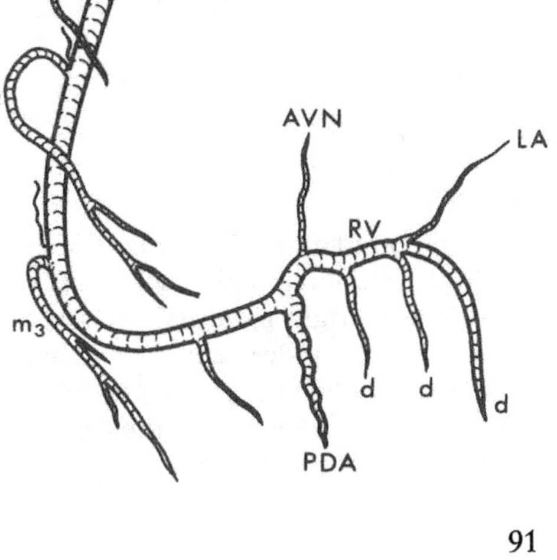

Fig. 31. Forty-five-degree left anterior oblique view of the right coronary artery. *CA:* conus artery; m_1, m_2, m_3: right marginal branches; *SN:* sinus node artery; *LA:* left atrial branch; *AVN:* atrioventricular node artery; *PDA:* posterior descending artery; *RV:* retroventricular artery; *d:* diaphragmatic branches

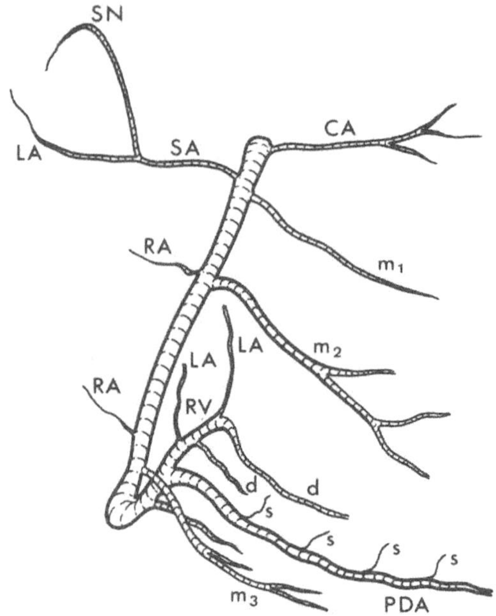

Fig. 32. Thirty-degree right anterior oblique view of the right coronary artery. *SN:* sinus node artery; *LA:* left atrial branch; *SA:* sino-atrial artery; *RA:* right atrial branch; *LA:* left atrial branch; *RV:* retroventricular artery; *d:* diaphragmatic branches; *s:* inferior septal branches; m_1, m_2, m_3: right marginal branches; *PDA:* posterior

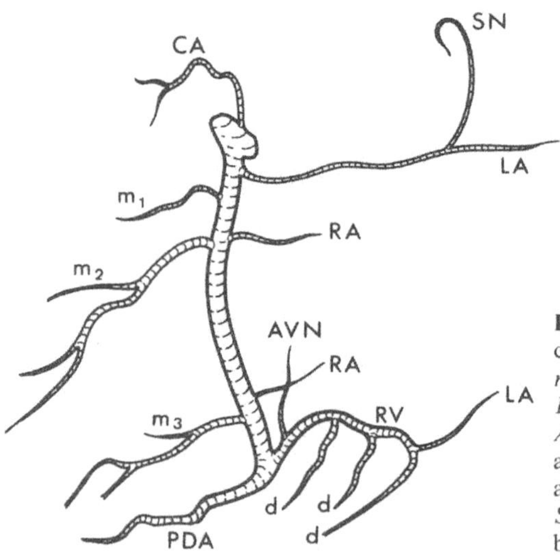

Fig. 33. Transverse view of the right coronary artery. *CA:* conus artery; m_1, m_2, m_3: right marginal branches; *PDA:* posterior descending artery; *AVN:* atrioventricular node artery; *RA:* right atrial branch; *RV:* retroventricular artery; *d:* diaphragmatic branches; *SN:* sinus node artery; *LA:* left atrial branch

The preponderant RCA (Figs. 25, 26, 31–33) provides branches to the free wall and to the diaphragmatic wall of the right ventricle, which are referred to as right ventricular or right marginal arteries and numbered by order of origin. If one is preponderant, it is designated as main but keeps its number. The PDA gives off septal branches called inferior septal arteries. Beyond the crux and the point of origin of the PDA, the extension of the RCA in the left atrioventricular sulcus is referred to as the retroventricular artery, whose branches to the diaphragmatic wall of the LV are called diaphragmatic arteries and are numbered by order of origin. The part of the RCA from the ostium to the crux, referred to as the circumflex part, is C-shaped. It is divided into three segments: proximal, middle and distal, or numbers 1, 2 and 3. Both in balanced distribution (Fig. 24) and in left preponderance (Fig. 23), the diaphragmatic arteries to the inferior wall of the LV originate from the distal Cx.

This nomenclature has the advantage of dispensing with certain ambiguous terms such as right or left border artery, muscular artery, posterolateral artery and circumflex lateral artery. Each artery, regardless of anatomical variation, has a designation relative to its purpose: diagonal for the anterior wall of the LV, left marginal for the lateral wall of the LV, diaphragmatic for the diaphragmatic or inferior wall of the LV, right marginal for the anterior and the diaphragmatic walls of the RV. The use of this nomenclature for several years has allowed us to establish an easily understood language for physicians and surgeons, no matter what anatomical variation is encountered in the collateral branches of the three main trunks.

2.3 A Reminder About the Physiology of Coronary Circulation

Coronary circulation makes use of an extremely rich intramyocardial capillary network comprising approximately 4000 capillaries/mm^3 in a normal heart. The density of this capillary network is greater in the subendocardial layer. Each capillary has a precapillary sphincter. Coronary blood flow is expressed by the equation $Q = p/R$, where Q is coronary blood flow, p the gradient between mean aortic pressure and mean right atrial pressure, that is 80 and 2 mmHg respectively under normal conditions, and R the resistance opposed to coronary flow. The resistance components are varied: intrinsic resistance due to vasomotor tone and extrinsic resistance related to LV end-diastolic pressure, but also to systolic intramyocardial tension, which is greater in the subendocardial region than in the subepicardial region. Blood circulation in the coronary network occurs essentially during diastole. As coronary output is proportional to p, the flow increases when diastolic time is longer and decreases when LV end-diastolic pressure rises (LV insufficiency) or when aortic diastolic pressure drops (aortic insufficiency or cardiogenic shock). The diastolic flow contributes to about 75% of total left coronary flow and to only 50% of total right coronary flow. Coronary flow is equivalent to 5% of cardiac output, hence 250 ml/min or about 100 ml/min per 100 g myocardium. Average coronary circulation time is about 4 s. In simple terms, it may be said that coronary circulation depends on three main types of regulation:

1. Metabolic: hypoxia and adenosine induce coronary vasodilatation
2. Nervous: sympathetic fibres are vasoconstrictive and parasympathetic fibres are vasodilative
3. Auto-regulation: an initial vasoconstriction is quickly offset by a vasodilatation.

2.4 Angiographic Anatomy

2.4.1 Left Coronary Artery (Figs. 25–30)

The course of the LMCT is initially transverse, moving towards the left and slightly to the rear behind the pulmonary artery, so that this portion of the left trunk may be best studied in 20° LAO and 20° caudocranial projection. Its length is variable: practically non-existent if the origins of the LAD and the Cx are side by side (10% of cases); short if 5 mm or less (25% of cases); intermediary if 6–20 mm (60% of cases); and very long if more than 20 mm (5% of cases). The LMCT bifurcates into two terminal branches, the LAD and the Cx, the resulting angle varying between 30° and 90° but being most often around 80°. In 10% of cases the LMCT trifurcates into the LAD, the Cx and a diagonal artery sometimes referred to as the bisecting artery. In exceptional cases there is quadrifurcation, with a left marginal artery or the first septal artery taking off at the same point as the other three vessels. As a rule, the LMCT does not give off collaterals, though in rare instances it provides the first artery of the right ventricle, that is the left conus artery, which ordinarily originates from the LAD.

The LAD continues in the direction originally taken by the left trunk and skirts the pulmonary artery before running along the anterior interventricular sulcus towards the apex. Thus it follows a very elongated S-shaped course, clearly visible in 45° LAO and 20° craniocaudal projection. It terminates in two recurrent branches, one going towards the left border and the other towards the right border, so that in frontal and RAO projections there is a characteristic anchor image. The length of the artery is variable. According to Di Guglielmo, it terminates at the apex in 24% of cases, continues in the posterior interventricular sulcus in 68% of cases and ends before the apex in 8% of cases. It is double in 4% of cases. The LAD is sometimes intramyocardial during part of its course, most often during the first third. In 45° LAO projection, the LAD slants downwards to the right almost in the middle of the heart shadow. In 30° LAO and 25° caudocranial projection, the entire proximal portion of the LAD is clearly visible. Beyond this initial part, the lateral projection best reveals the LAD, whose first segment is nearly horizontal, whereas the second bends gradually downwards.

The collateral branches of the LAD are, in the most common order of origin, the first diagonal, the first septal, the first right ventricular artery, the second and third septals, the second diagonal, and then in varying number other septal and diagonal branches. The number of septal arteries which may be discerned on a coronary arteriogram normally ranges between four and seven. They arise at a right angle from the lower side of the LAD and enter directly into the septum. They are long, supplying the upper two-thirds of the interventricular septum, and are easy to pick out on lateral and RAO projections. The first septal artery is generally small, the second often being the largest. The first septal artery may originate from the RCA, and the first diagonal artery may also give off septal arteries. The diagonal arteries depart at acute angles from the left side of the LAD. In 30° RAO projection, they appear above and partly behind the LAD, which is more or less superimposed on them. In 45°–60° LAO projection, the diagonal arteries are visible midway between the LAD and the Cx. In 30°–45° LAO and 20° caudocranial projection, the diagonal arteries appear on the left side of the LAD and may be easily distinguished from the septal arteries which are on the right side of the LAD. The bifurcation angles between the LAD and the diagonal arteries are clearly apparent in this projection. The number of diagonal arteries angiographically visible ranges from two to seven. There are usually two diagonal branches with significant calibre, the first and second or the second and third. The branches to the right ventricle are rarely visible angiographically. In transverse and 60–75° LAO projection, they course forwards towards the sternum and above the LAD.

The Cx is a relatively short branch in most subjects, since right-preponderant circulation is virtually the rule (80%). In 30° RAO projection, it takes off perpendicularly from the LMCT and moves downwards and a little to the rear, standing out in contrast to the radiolucency of the fatty left atrioventricular sulcus. It provides between one and three left marginal branches, which take off anteriorly towards the apex of the LV to vascularize its lateral wall. In LAO projection, the course of the Cx bends inwards, with its concavity facing the centre of the cardiac mass. At the origin of the artery there is often superimposition of the Cx and its marginal collateral branches. The Cx provides a terminal left marginal artery in 20% of cases, and in the ohter 80% it ends by a very thin distal Cx which gives out either before reaching the diaphragmatic wall of the LV (30%) or before reaching the crux (70%). The lateral projection is preferable to the LAO to separate the marginal arteries from the Cx.

The collateral branches of the Cx are relatively numerous. Generally, there are three left marginal arteries to the lateral wall of the LV. Often there is a preponderant or single large marginal artery which continues the course of the proximal Cx and slants across the entire lateral wall of the LV (obtuse marginal), giving off secondary branches. The Cx also provides atrial arteries, often three in number: superior, for the roof of the left atrium; middle, for its lateral wall; and inferior, for its lower wall. The first two are almost always present, but the third exists in only 80% of cases. In 30%–40% of subjects, the superior (or sometimes the middle) left atrial artery extends along the upper wall of the right atrium as far as the orifice of the superior vena cava to provide the sino-atrial node artery. The left Kugel artery takes off either directly from the Cx or from the left superior atrial artery. It runs in the plane of the mitral orifice towards the upper part of the interatrial septum, where it descends to join the atrioventricular node artery at the crux. It may anastomose with the right Kugel artery. These arteries are angiographically visible only in pathological conditions. In 20% of cases the left inferior atrial artery is provided by the RCA.

2.4.2 Right Coronary Artery (Figs. 25, 26, 31–33)

In 45°–60° LAO projection, the RCA is clearly visualized in its circumflex part, whereas in RAO projection the first and third segments of this artery are seen according to their main axes, which are parallel to the X-ray beam. When the RCA is preponderant (80% of the population), it divides at the level of the crux into its two terminal branches: the PDA and the retroventricular artery. The latter ends at the junction of the diaphragmatic and lateral walls of the LV (16%) or between the crux and this junction (64%). When the LCA is preponderant (10% of the population), the RCA divides early into two or three thin branches which give out before the crux, either on the free wall of the right ventricle (2%) or its diaphragmatic wall (8%). In cases of balanced distribution, the RCA has a single terminal branch, the PDA. At the level of the crux, beyond the origin of the PDA, the RCA or the retroventricular artery generally forms an upward convex curve similar to an inverted U.

There are numerous collateral branches of the RCA. The right conus artery may have its own ostium (40%) or take off during the first millimeters of the vessel (60%). In RAO projection, it heads forwards and upwards. It joins a homologous artery coming from the LCA to form the anastomotic ring of Vieussens in front of the pulmonary conus arteriosus or right ventricular infundibulum. In the same projection, the right marginal arteries take off perpendicularly from the front side of the RCA and run forwards. In 90% of cases there are only two or three right marginal arteries, the second being the largest. Sometimes a very long marginal artery, originating early, slants across the entire free wall of the right ventricle until the apex. The right marginal arteries supply the anterior free wall and the diaphragmatic wall of the right ventricle. The right atrial arteries may be superior, middle or inferior, as in the case of the homologous left ones. The right superior atrial artery is the most frequent. In RAO projection it runs to the rear and upwards, vascularizing the upper wall of the right atrium and, in 60% of subjects, providing the artery for the sinus node, which is then justly referred to as the sino-atrial node artery. The middle atrial artery is present in 80% of subjects and the inferior atrial artery in 60%. The last important atrial branch provided by the RCA in 85% of subjects is the atrioventricular node artery, which arises from the inverted U-shaped RCA segment at the level of the crux and ascends perpendicularly towards the interatrial septum.

The course of the PDA in the posterior interventricular sulcus is more or less long. Sometimes it takes off from the RCA before the crux and slants across the diaphragmatic wall of the right ventricle to reach the posterior interventricular sulcus in its middle part. In rare instances there are two PDAs, both coming from the RCA or both from the LCA or one from each coronary artery. In 30°–50° RAO projection, the PDA is seen laterally along all its length. It gives off inferior septal branches to the lower part of the interventricular septum, and also provides a few branches to the diaphragmatic wall of the right ventricle as well as the LV. The retroventricular artery and the diaphragmatic arteries (between one and five) that it provides to the inferior wall of the LV are quite clearly exposed in 30°–40° LAO and 15°–20° caudocranial projection. In RAO projection they are more or less superimposed on the PDA.

2.4.3 Vascularization of Nodes and the Conduction System

The sinus node ordinarily receives a single artery coming either from the RCA (60%–70% of cases) by intermediary of the right superior atrial artery (nine times out of ten) or from the LCA (30%–40% of cases) by intermediary of the left superior or middle atrial artery. In exceptional cases, the sinus node receives a branch from both coronary arteries. The vascularization of the atrioventricular node is provided by the atrioventricular node artery, originating from the RCA in 85% of cases and from the LCA in 15%, depending on which of the coronary arteries reaches the crux. The vascularization of the bundle if His is rich and not angiographically specific; it is effected by the atrioventricular node artery and by the first anterior and inferior septal arteries originating from the LAD and PDA.

2.4.4 Interconnecting Anastomoses

Anastomotic vessels are invisible in vivo if the coronary arteries are normal; they are only visualized when there are severe arterial stenoses. They vary considerably in number from one individual to another. Apparently for genetic reasons, certain subjects have more anastomotic potential. Selective coronary angiography makes it possible to reveal anastomoses with a calibre equal to or greater than 200 μm. Some attain a calibre of more than 1 mm. These anastomoses are intramyocardial or subepicardial, and homo- or intercoronary. Inter- and heterocoronary anastomoses connecting branches of different arteries are more frequent (60%) than homocoronary anastomoses connecting segments of the same artery.

2.5 Coronary Veins (Figs. 34 and 35)

The venous blood of the myocardium is collected by two groups of cardiac veins: deep intramyocardial veins and superficial epicardial veins. The former comprise the small heart veins, which empty directly into the right atrium, and the Thebesian veins, which open into the four heart cavities. The latter include mainly the anterior interventricular vein or great cardiac vein, which is continued in the left atrioventricular sulcus by the coronary sinus that receives on its anterior side the posterior vein of the LV, the posterior interventricular vein and, finally, the small cardiac vein coming from the right ventricle. In the normal subject, only the superficial venous system is visible with coronary arteriography, appearing about 4 s after the beginning of arterial opacification. During left coronary arteriography, the terminal segment of the great cardiac vein and the coronary sinus are generally well opacified.

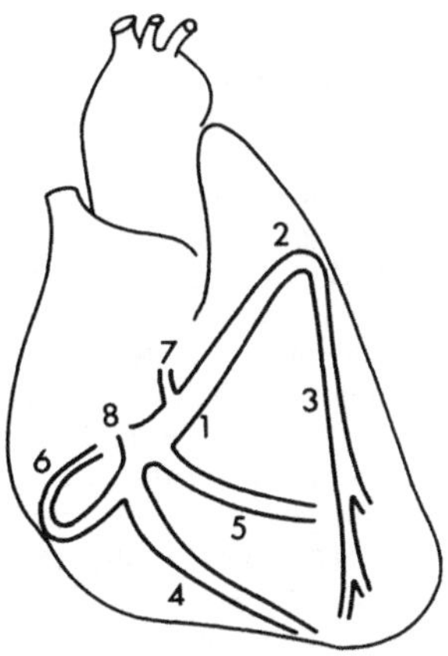

Fig. 34. The coronary venous system in the frontal view. *1:* coronary sinus; *2:* great cardiac vein; *3:* anterior interventricular vein; *4:* posterior interventricular vein; *5:* left marginal vein; *6:* small cardiac vein (right marginal); *7:* left atrial vein (oblique vein of Marshall); *8:* ostium of the sinus (Thebesian valve)

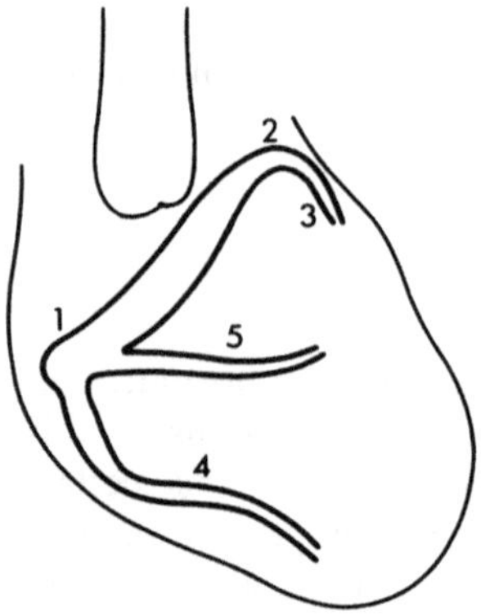

Fig. 35. The coronary venous system in the right anterior oblique view. *1:* coronary sinus; *2:* great cardiac vein; *3:* anterior interventricular vein; *4:* posterior interventricular vein; *5:* left marginal vein

The posterior vein of the LV is less often identifiable. During right coronary arteriography, images of venous return by the posterior interventricular vein and the small cardiac vein are generally not very sharp because much of the contrast medium is drained off directly into the heart chambers by the deep network of Thebesian veins. Only the terminal part of the coronary sinus is distinctly opacified. The posterior interventricular vein is sometimes double.

References

1. Karliner JS, Bouchard RJ, Gault JH (1971) Dimensional changes of the human left ventricle prior to aortic valve opening. A cineangiographic study in patients with and without left heart disease. Circulation 44: 312
2. Leighton RF, Wilt SM, Lewis RP (1974) Detection of hypokinesis by a quantitative analysis of left ventricular cineangiograms. Circulation 50: 121
3. Sniderman AD, Marpole D, Fallen EL (1973) Regional contraction patterns in the normal and ischemic left ventricle in man. Am J Cardiol 31: 484
4. Chaitman BR, Bristow D, Rahimtoola SH (1973) Left ventricular wall motion assessed by using fixed external reference systems. Circulation 68: 1043
5. Besse P, Pruvot C, Choussat A, Bricaud H (1975) La fonction ventriculaire gauche du coronarien: relations entre les troubles de la cinétique ventriculaire et les altérations de la contractilité myocardique. Arch Mal Coeur 68: 125
6. Brower RW, Meester GT (1976) Computer based methods for quantifying regional left ventricular wall motion from cineventriculograms. In: IEEE Computer Society (ed) Comput Cardiol
7. Herman MV, Gorlin R (1969) Implications of left ventricular asynergy. Am J Cardiol 23: 538
8. Scampardonis G, Yang SS, Maranhao V, Goldberg H, Gooch AS (1973) Left ventricular abnormalities in prolapsed mitral leaflet syndrome. Circulation 48: 287
9. Rickards A, Seabra-Gomez R, Thurston P (1977) The assessment of regional abnormalities of the left ventricle by angiography. Eur J Cardiol 5: 167
10. Chaitman BR, De Mots H, Bristow JD, Rosch J, Rahimtoola SH (1975) Objective and subjective analysis of left ventricular angiograms. Circulation 52: 420
11. Pasternac A, Gorlin R, Sonnenblick EH, Haft JI, Kemp HG (1972) Abnormalities of ventricular motion induced by atrial pacing in coronary artery disease. Circulation 45: 1195
12. Nakhjavan FK, Natarajan G, Goldberg H (1975) Comparison of ejection fraction and zonal mean velocity of myocardial fiber shortening. Circulation 52: 264
13. Bertrand M (1978) L'artériographie coronaire. Nomenclature des artères, codification des lésions. Société Française de Cardiologie, Paris

14. Carroll RJ, Verani MS, Falsetti HL (1974) The effect of collateral circulation on segmental left ventricular contraction. Circulation 50: 709
15. Chapman CB, Baker O, Mitchel JH, Collier RG (1966) Experiences with a cinefluorographic method for measuring ventricular volume. Am J Cardiol 18: 25
16. Besse P, Legoff G, Charland R, Le Franc G, Brichaud H (1974) Evaluation angiographique quantitative des volumes et de la cinétique ventriculaires gauches: étude critique. Arch Mal Coeur 67: 1075
17. Greene DG, Carlisle R, Grant C, Bunnell IL (1967) Estimation of left ventricular volume by one-plane cineangiography. Circulation 35: 61
18. Snow JA, Baker LD, Leshin SJ, Messer JV (1969) Validation of the single plane cineangiographic determination of canine left ventricular volume. II: left ventricular dilatation. Fed Proc 28: 517
19. Dodge HT (1971) Determination of left ventricular volume and mass. Radiol Clin North Am 9: 459
20. Crochet D, Petitier H, De Laguerenne J, Bizais Y, De Kersaint-Gilly A, Delumeau J (1980) La mesure des volumes ventriculaires gauches: proposition d'une méthode de calcul de facteur d'agrandissement simple et précise. J Radiol 61: 141
21. Amiel M, Perrin A, Dupont JC, Dahanne R (1975) Etude angiographique des myocardiopathies primitives (quarante et une observations). Ann Radiol 18: 783
22. Arvidsson H (1961) Angiocardiographic determination of left ventricular volume. Acta Radiol 56: 321
23. Brun P, Cannet G, Guichebaron D, Herreman F (1973) Méthode générale de détermination de la contractilité myocardique à l'aide des données de l'exploration fonctionelle. Arch Mal Coeur 66: 95
24. Falsetti HL, Mates RE, Greene DG, Bunnell IL (1971) V max as an index of contractile state in man. Circulation 43: 467
25. Hermann HJ, Bartle SH (1968) Left ventricular volumes by angiocardiography: comparison of methods and simplification of techniques. Cardiovasc Res 2: 404
26. Kennedy JW, Baxley WA, Figley MM, Dodge HT, Blackmon JR (1966) Quantitative angiocardiography. I: The normal left ventricle in man. Circulation 34: 272
27. Petitier H, Crochet D, Lemort JP, Bizais Y (1977) Données quantitatives de la ventriculographie gauche dans les myocardiopathies obstructives. Ann Radiol 20: 389
28. Wynne J, Greene L, Mann T, Levin D, Grossman W (1978) Estimation of left ventricular volumes in man from biplane cineangiograms filmed in oblique positions. Am J Cardiol 41: 726
29. Rackley CE, Dodge HT, Coble YD, Hay RE (1964) A method for determining left ventricular mass in man. Circulation 29: 666
30. Kreulen TH, Gorlin R, Herman MV (1973) Ventriculographic patterns and hemodynamics in primary myocardial disease. Circulation 47: 299
31. Mirsky I, Cohn PF, Levine JA, Gorlin R, Herman MV, Kreulen TH, Sonnenblick EH (1974) Assessment of left ventricular stiffness in primary myocardial disease and coronary artery disease. Circulation 50: 128
32. Ritman EL (1975) Left ventricular function and myocardial contractility. Analysis by roentgen videoangiographic techniques. Mod Med Physiol. Mayo Clin Proc 50: 147
33. Karliner JS, Gault JH, Eckberg D, Mullins CB, Ross J Jr (1971) Mean velocity of fiber shortening: a simplified measure of left ventricular myocardial contractility. Circulation 44: 323
34. McAlpine WA (1975) Heart and coronary arteries. Springer, Berlin Heidelberg New York
35. MacAlpin RN, Abbasi AS, Grollman JH, Eber L (1973) Human coronary artery size during life. A cinearteriographic study. Radiology 108: 567
36. Vieweg WVR, Alpert JS, Hagan AD (1976) Caliber and distribution of normal coronary arterial anatomy. Cathet Cardiovasc Diagn 2: 269
37. O'Reilly RJ (1975) Coronary angiographic nomenclature. Current status and a plea for standardization. Radiology 115: 229

IV Angiographic Explorations: Congenital Anomalies of the Coronary Arteries

With the development of coronary arteriography and myocardial revascularization surgery, and with advances in the surgical repair of congenital cardiopathies, there has been renewed interest in congenital anomalies of the coronary arteries.

1 Anomalies of the Origin, Course and Distribution of Coronary Arteries Arising from the Aorta

The first important study concerning this subject was Ogden's in 1968 [1, 2], and various publications have been devoted to these anomalies [3–13]. A complete review of the literature has been provided by Bertrand [4]. Most coronary anomalies are asymptomatic, although some cases of infarction and even of sudden death have been described [14]. The pathological physiology of these anomalies is discussed: spasm in a single coronary artery; classic atheromatous stenoses, which are all the more serious if they are located in a single artery; and compression of a coronary artery (particularly the left anterior descending artery) coursing abnormally between the aorta and the pulmonary artery. In this last case, arterial compression may be due to increase in cardiac output during exertion, or more simply to dilatation of the aorta in an elderly subject.

A knowledge of congenital coronary anomalies is very useful to the practice of coronary arteriography. When an artery cannot be selectively catheterized, it should not immediately be assumed that there is an ostial obliteration of syphilitic origin or from Takayasu's disease. First, a general aortography should be performed by suprasigmoid injection of contrast medium to detect a possible anomaly in the origin or course of a coronary artery. Knowledge of such anomalies is also useful to the surgeon, particularly in performing a ventriculotomy.

The frequency of anomalies of the origin, course or distribution of coronary arteries arising from the aorta has been estimated at 0.6% by Kimbiris and Amiel on the basis of 7000 examinations [8, 15]. Three main types of anomalies were found:

1. Isolated anomalous vascular origin of one of the two coronary arteries from the ascending aorta at some distance from the sinuses of Valsalva (three cases out of 7000), exceptionally from a branch of the aorta such as the brachiocephalic artery trunk
2. Hypoplastic left anterior descending arteries (5% according to Amiel; 8% according to Ogden)
3. Anomalies of the origin, course or distribution of coronary arteries arising in the sinuses of Valsalva: these are the most common malformations and have been the subject of numerous studies.

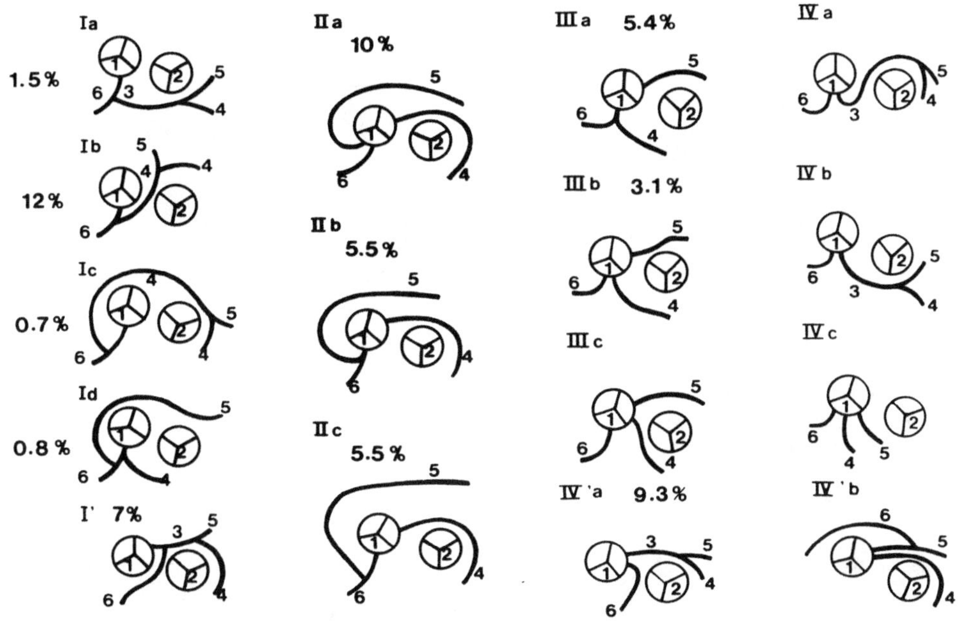

Fig. 1. Diagrammatic representation of variations in the course and origin of the major coronary arteries, according to Bertrand (4). Percentages = incidence of the main types in a group of 129 differing congenital coronary anomalies. *1:* aorta; *2:* pulmonary artery; *3:* left common trunk; *4:* left anterior descending artery; *5:* left circumflex artery; *6:* right coronary artery; *I:* single coronary artery; *II:* aberrant origin of the left circumflex artery; *III:* aberrant origin of the left anterior descending artery; *IV:* multiple orifices in the same coronary sinus (by courtesy of: Ann Cardiol Angeiol 25: 39–58)

It is not possible to give a detailed review here of the variations, which are presented schematically in Fig. 1. These diagrams, taken from a study by Bertrand [4], indicate clearly the respective frequencies of the various anomalies and their polymorphism. From a clinical viewpoint, it should be noted that the most dangerous anatomical conditions for the patient are those in which an important coronary trunk passes between the aorta and the pulmonary artery. This situation gives rise to the most serious disorders: myocardial ischaemia, severe irregularities in ventricular rhythm and sudden death [3]. Figures 2–7 illustrate these anomalies of the origin and course of the coronary arteries.

2 Abnormal Origin of a Coronary Artery from the Pulmonary Artery

The abnormal origin of a coronary artery from the pulmonary artery can be responsible for a very serious form of clinical syndrome that was described remarkably well by Bland, White and Garland in 1963 [16]. The anomaly is very rare (0.5% of congenital cardiopathies), and the seriousness of the clinical signs depends on the presence or absence of intercoronary anastomoses. When the anastomoses are well developed, the malformation may be tolerated without difficulty and be detected only in adult age or fortuitously during an autopsy. Nonetheless, such tolerance is

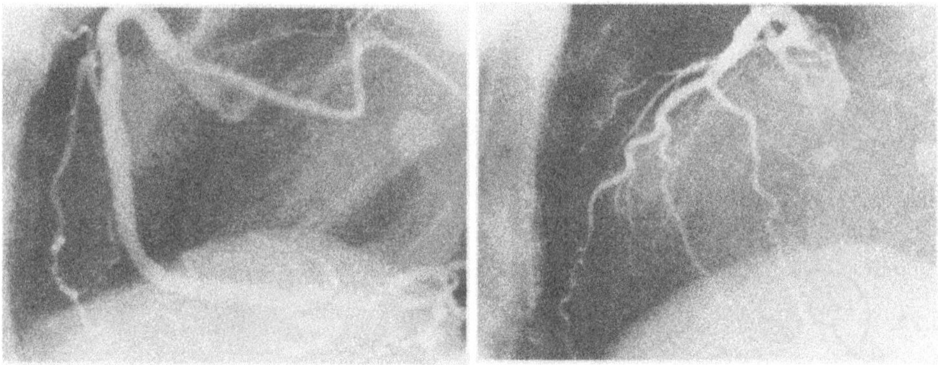

Fig. 2. Type IIb anomaly of origin. The circumflex arises from a common ostium with the right coronary artery (RCA). It reaches the left atrioventricular sulcus by coursing behind the aorta. *(Left):* left anterior oblique view of the RCA, *(right):* transverse view of the left coronary artery

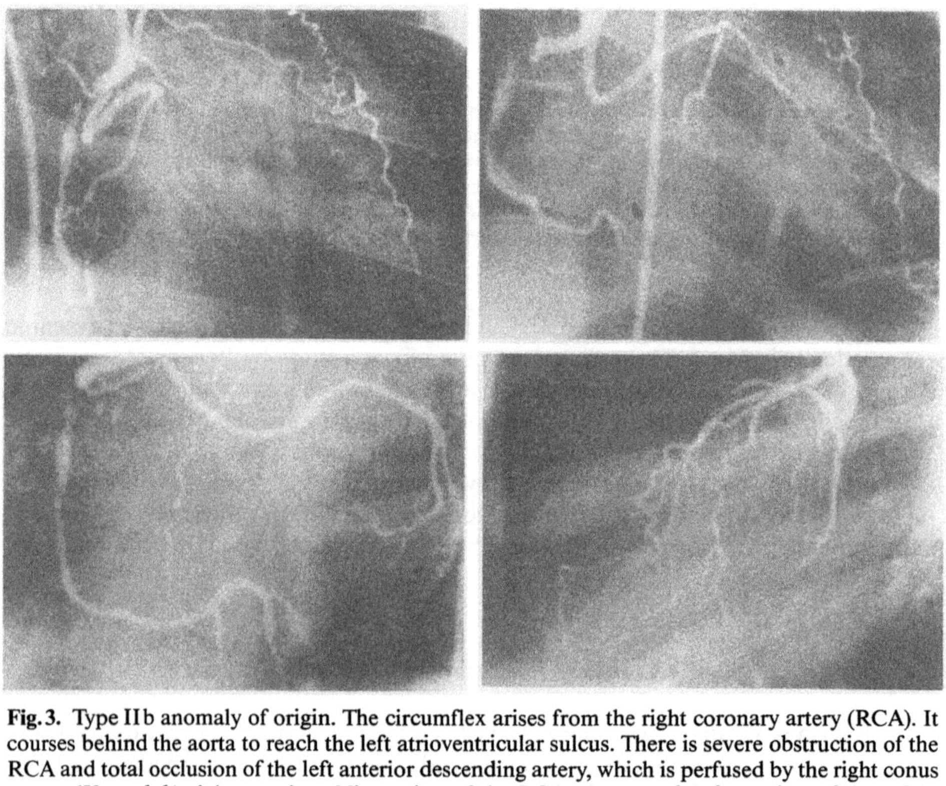

Fig. 3. Type IIb anomaly of origin. The circumflex arises from the right coronary artery (RCA). It courses behind the aorta to reach the left atrioventricular sulcus. There is severe obstruction of the RCA and total occlusion of the left anterior descending artery, which is perfused by the right conus artery. *(Upper left):* right anterior oblique view of the RCA; *(upper right):* front view of the RCA; *(lower left):* left anterior oblique view of the RCA; *(lower right):* transverse view of the left coronary artery

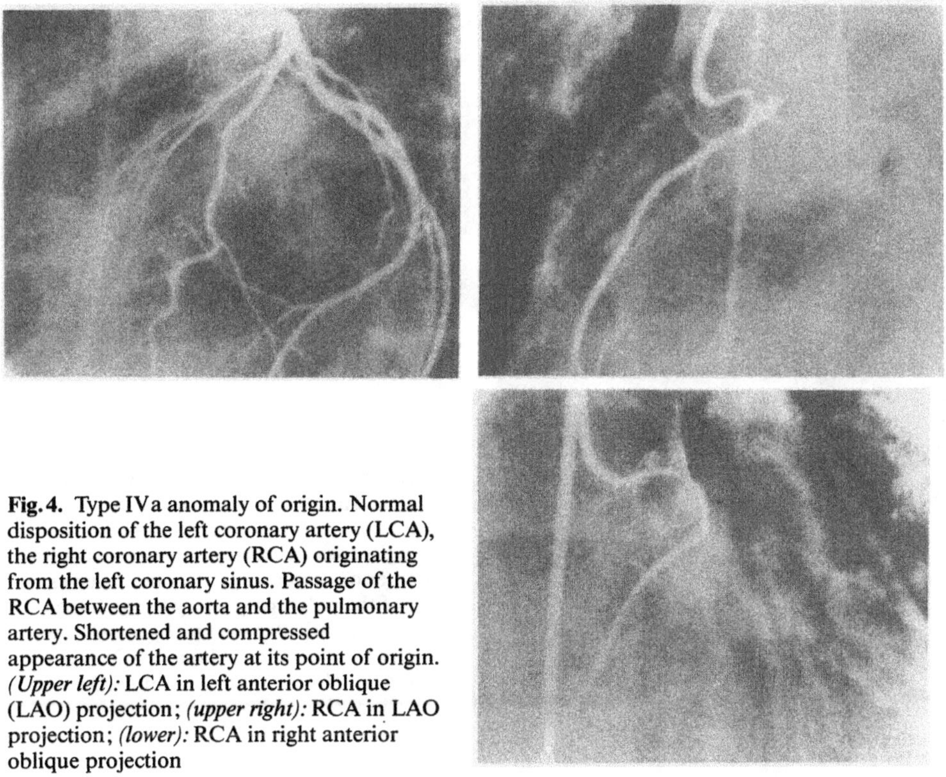

Fig. 4. Type IVa anomaly of origin. Normal disposition of the left coronary artery (LCA), the right coronary artery (RCA) originating from the left coronary sinus. Passage of the RCA between the aorta and the pulmonary artery. Shortened and compressed appearance of the artery at its point of origin. *(Upper left):* LCA in left anterior oblique (LAO) projection; *(upper right):* RCA in LAO projection; *(lower):* RCA in right anterior oblique projection

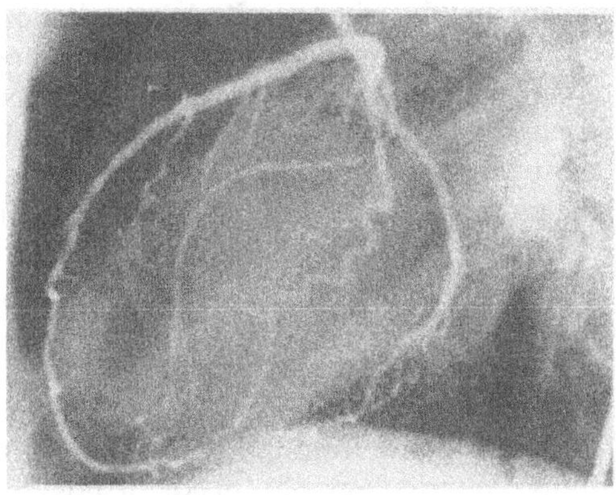

Fig. 5. Single coronary artery of the left type. There is only one coronary ostium, in left position. The left coronary artery is preponderant and its configuration is normal. The right coronary artery arises from the single ostium and reaches the right atrioventricular sulcus by coursing behind the aorta

exceptional. Ordinarily, the collateral supply between the two arteries is insufficient, and a severe myocardial ischaemia syndrome becomes apparent one or two months after birth, when pulmonary arterial resistances drop. The infant's angina pectoris is revealed by cries of pain, pallor, vomiting and hypotension after meals. In the most severe cases, a respiratory distress syndrome may set in, with continual or paroxysmal dyspnoea and cardiac insufficiency. Sudden death can occur more

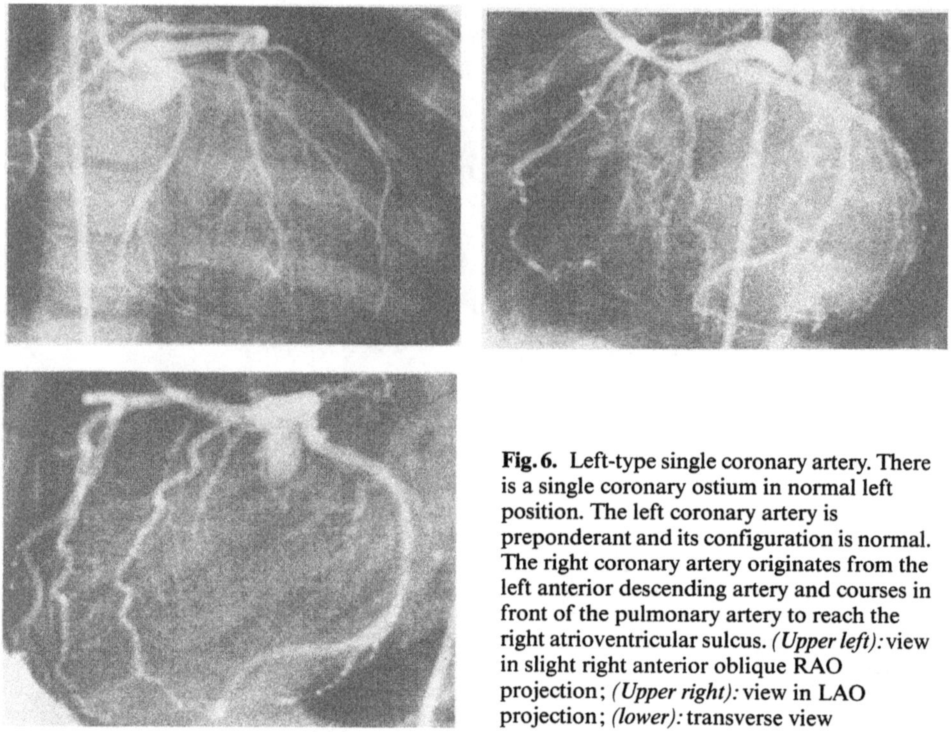

Fig. 6. Left-type single coronary artery. There is a single coronary ostium in normal left position. The left coronary artery is preponderant and its configuration is normal. The right coronary artery originates from the left anterior descending artery and courses in front of the pulmonary artery to reach the right atrioventricular sulcus. *(Upper left):* view in slight right anterior oblique RAO projection; *(Upper right):* view in LAO projection; *(lower):* transverse view

or less immediately. Often the disease takes the form of cardiac insufficiency or of an apparently primary mitral regurgitation, suggesting at that age a diagnosis of fibro-elastosis or myocardiopathy. The mitral regurgitation is due to ischaemic necrosis of a papillary muscle. Catheterization and coronary arteriography show increased left atrial and left ventricular end-diastolic pressure, extensive akinesis, in most cases of the left ventricular anterolateral wall, and an oxygen enrichment in the pulmonary artery trunk, though this sign is quite variable.

In nearly all cases it is the left coronary artery (LCA) which arises abnormally from the pulmonary artery (Figs. 8 and 9), a similar anomaly involving the right coronary artery (RCA) being 20 times less common. The malformation is revealed by suprasigmoid aortography, and occasionally by selective coronary arteriography. In the typical case there is successive opacification of the aorta, of the RCA and of the LCA retrograde from the RCA. The LCA drains partly into the pulmonary artery trunk. Ventriculography makes it possible to determine the degree of alteration of left ventricular contraction and the existence and importance of mitral regurgitation.

3 Anomalies in the Diameter of Coronary Arteries

Reductions in calibre are diffuse or localized. A diffuse luminal narrowing of the coronary network is always difficult to demonstrate. Van Praagh has reported an anatomically verified case in Hurler's disease [17]. In the literature there are a few

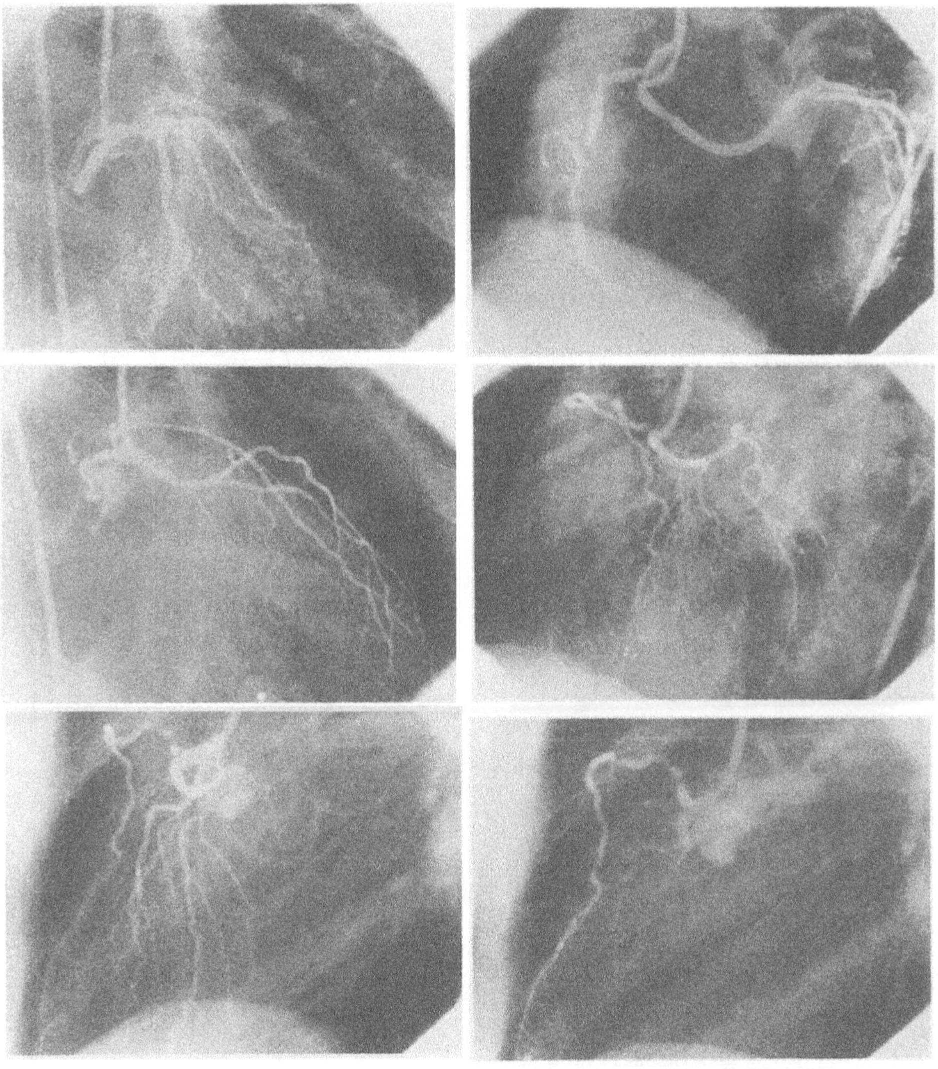

Fig. 7. Both coronary arteries originate from the same sinus. The coronary arteries arise from two adjacent orifices in the right coronary sinus. The first trunk provides the right coronary artery (RCA), in its usual configuration, and the left circumflex (Cx), which courses behind the aorta. The second trunk provides the distal left anterior descending artery (LAD), which heads to the right before crossing the anterior side of the pulmonary infundibulum, and the proximal LAD, which gives off the main septal branch and the main diagonal branches. The course of the proximal LAD passes between the aorta and the pulmonary artery or can be intramyocardial (14). *(upper):* right (RAO) and left anterior oblique (LAO) views of the RCA and Cx; *(middle):* RAO and LAO views of the proximal LAD and distal LAD; *(lower left):* transverse view of both LADs; *(lower right):* transverse view of the distal LAD

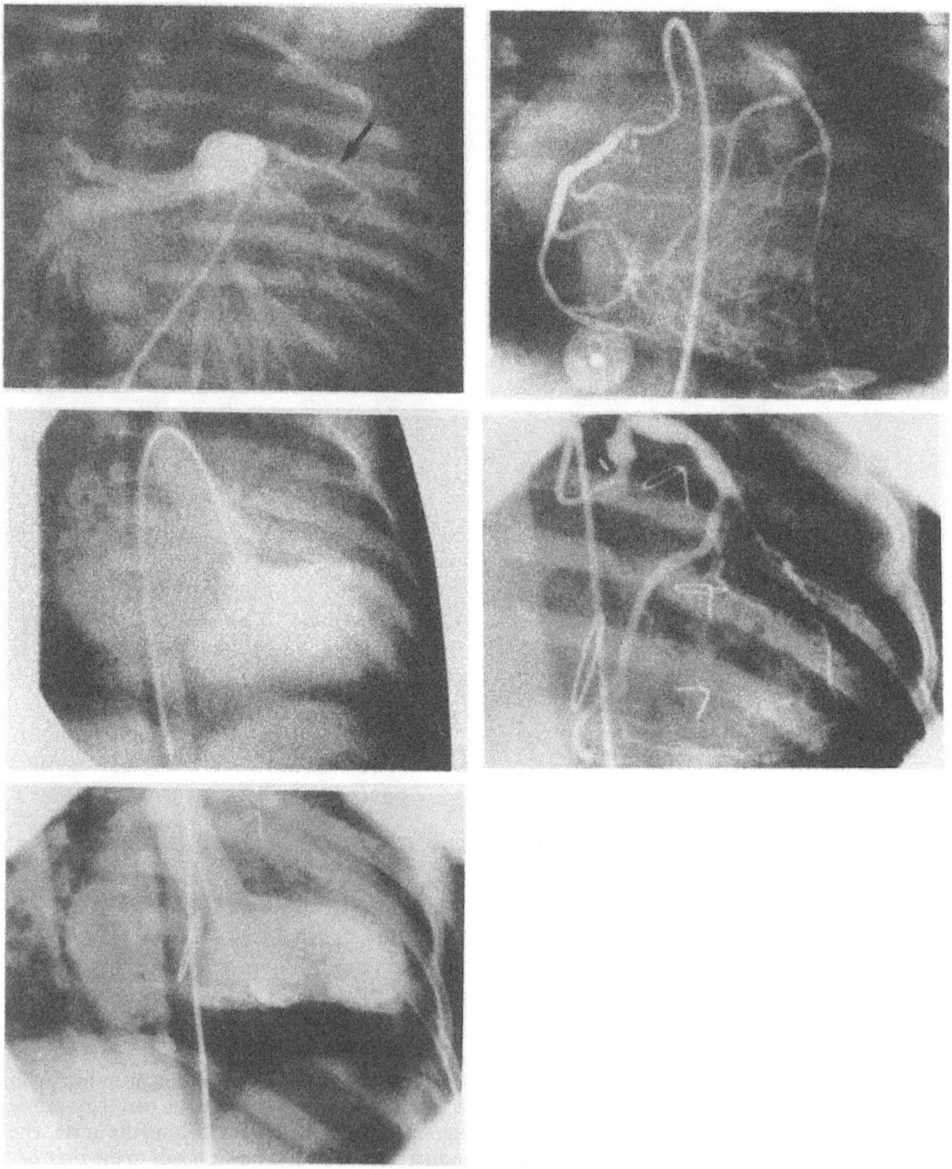

Fig. 8. Aberrant origin of the left coronary artery (LCA). *(Upper left):* right anterior oblique view of the LCA arising from the pulmonary trunk; *(upper right):* selective opacification of the right coronary artery shows that it is anastomosed with the LCA, which partially drains into the pulmonary artery; *(middle left):* severe anterior akinesis of the left ventricular (LV) wall and mitral regurgitation; *(middle right):* the same patient after surgery: good perfusion of the LCA by means of an aortocoronary graft; *(lower):* bioprosthetic replacement of the mitral valve: absence of improvement in LV contraction

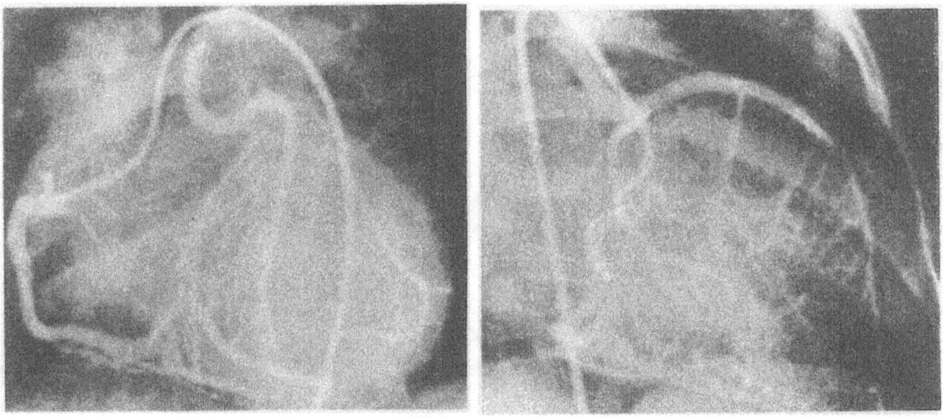

Fig. 9. Selective right coronary arteriography in another case of abnormal origin of the left coronary artery from the pulmonary trunk. *(Right):* right anterior oblique view; *(left):* left anterior oblique view

cases of coronary proximal stenosis that were considered to be congenital. Such a diagnosis can be contemplated in the presence of an isolated proximal stenosis in a young subject, provided that the rest of the coronary system is healthy and that the stenosis does not disappear after intracoronary injection of nitroglycerin.

Increases in calibre are of two types:

1. extensive or diffuse segmentary arterial dilatation corresponding to the dolicho-mega-arteries, and
2. localized arterial ectasia corresponding to true aneurysms.

The dolichomegavessels are generally atheromatous, although according to Van Praagh [17] a congenital origin may be assumed in the particular case of congenital supravalvular aortic stenosis. The congenital origin of aneurysms of the coronary arteries is difficult to maintain and should only be accepted after other possible causes have been excluded and in accordance with the subject's age. The first case in vivo was reported by Sherkat in 1967 in a 9-month-old infant [18]. The diseases to be excluded are atheroma, inflammatory disease and, especially, Kawasaki disease. The subject must not be older than 25. Coronary arteriography permits diagnosis of the aneurysm and specifies its characteristics: RCA localization more often than left; size often large (up to 10 cm in diameter); single or more often multiple in number; and frequent thrombosis downstream from the aneurysm (Fig. 10). Clinical detection is, in fact, generally secondary to an initial infarction rather than to angina. Systolodiastolic murmur is not unusual (50% of cases). When a pathological examination is performed, it can eliminate the possibility of atheromatous or inflammatory lesions and demonstrate a thickening of the intima, a fragmentation of the internal elastic membrane and modification of the media, with disappearance of the elastic and muscle fibres, which are replaced by hyalin tissue.

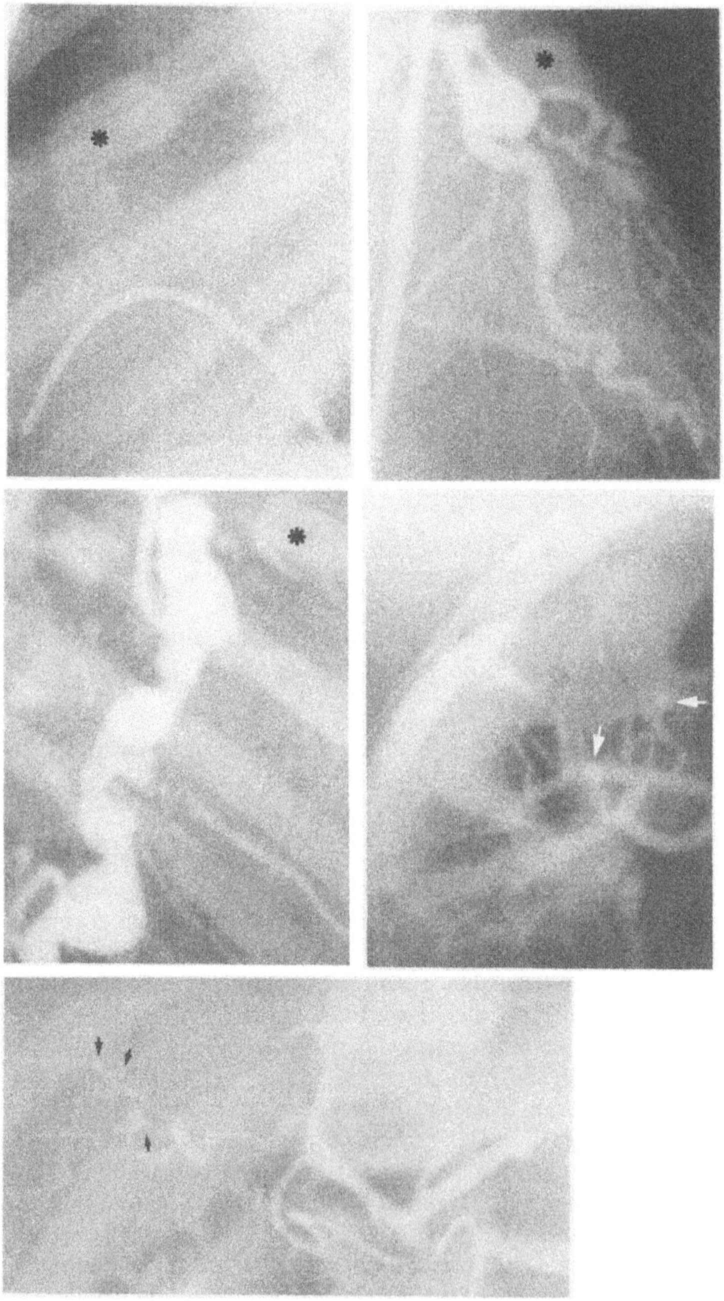

Fig. 10. Multiple arterial aneurysms in a 15-year-old boy who suffered an anterior myocardial infarction. *(Upper left):* transverse view of the calcified left anterior descending artery aneurysm (*), which caused total occlusion of the artery; *(upper right):* front view of the aneurysmal left circumflex; *(middle left):* right anterior oblique view of the aneurysmal right coronary artery; *(middle right):* small aneurysms in the secondary branches of the right renal artery; *(lower):* microaneurysms in the branches of the right hepatic artery

4 Coronary Fistulae

The term "primary coronary fistula" should be reserved for an abnormal communication between a coronary artery and a cardiac cavity, the coronary sinus, the vena cava system or the pulmonary artery system, with anterograde flow maintained in the coronary artery. This definition excludes coronary arteries arising from the pulmonary artery, and so-called Edwards' secondary fistulae observed essentially in certain cases of pulmonary atresia when the interventricular septum is intact, the flow being retrograde in the coronary artery [19].

Three main types of primary coronary fistula have been described. The first comprises coronary-to-cavity fistulae (Figs. 11 and 12), providing communication between one or more coronary arteries and a heart chamber or the vena cava or coronary vein system [4, 20]. The artery concerned is always quite dilated, sometimes enormously. The second type is the coronary to proximal pulmonary artery fistulae, which are related to vascular dysplasias [21]. This type is often a true angiomatous formation located on the anterior wall of the pulmonary artery trunk and sometimes extending along its branches (Fig. 13). This sort of fistula may be associated with other angiomatous localizations (Fig. 14). The third type is rarer. These are the coronary to peripheral pulmonary artery fistulae first reported by Spindola Franco [22].

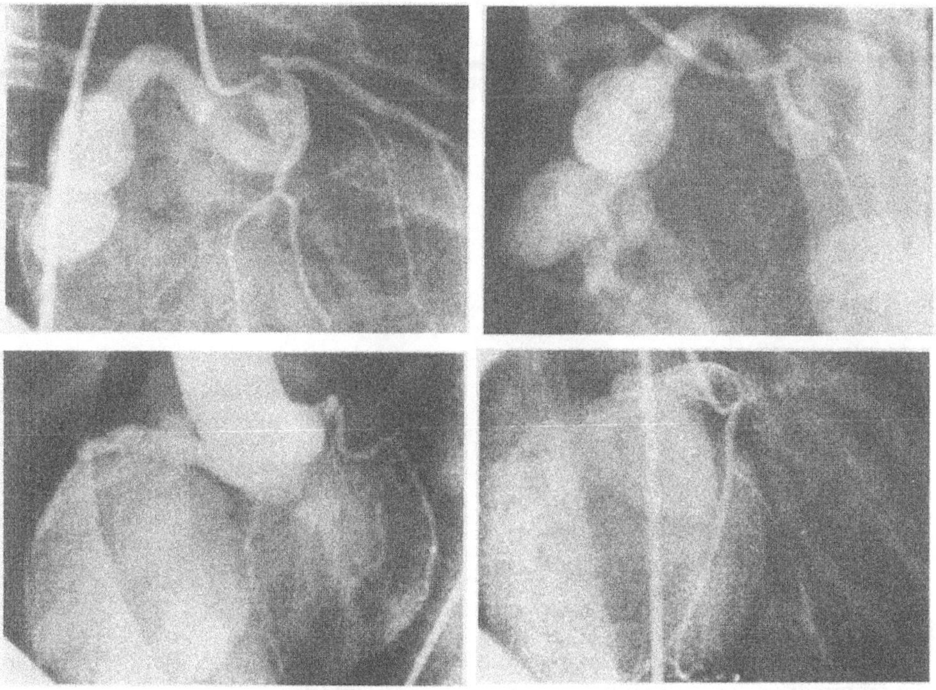

Fig. 11. Coronary-cardiac fistula. *(Upper):* right (RAO) and left anterior oblique (LAO) views of the communication between a right atrial artery arising from the left coronary artery and the right atrium; *(lower left):* LAO view of the communication between a right atrial artery arising from the right coronary artery and the right atrium, as revealed by aortography; *(lower right):* RAO view of the same anomaly as revealed by selective right coronary arteriography

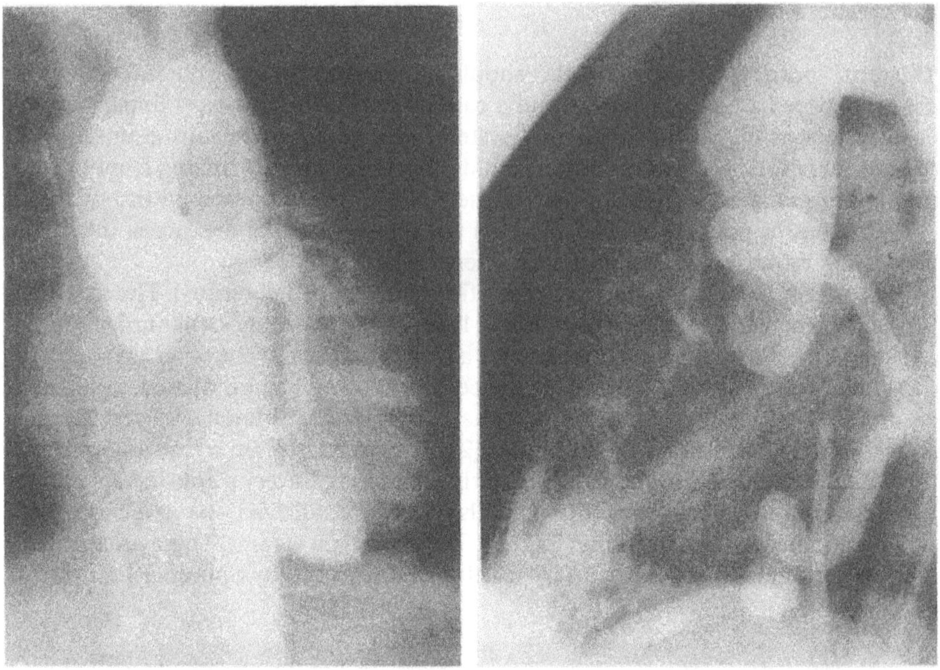

Fig. 12. Coronary-cardiac fistula. The communication between the left circumflex and the right ventricle as revealed by aortography. *(Left):* front projection; *(right):* transverse projection

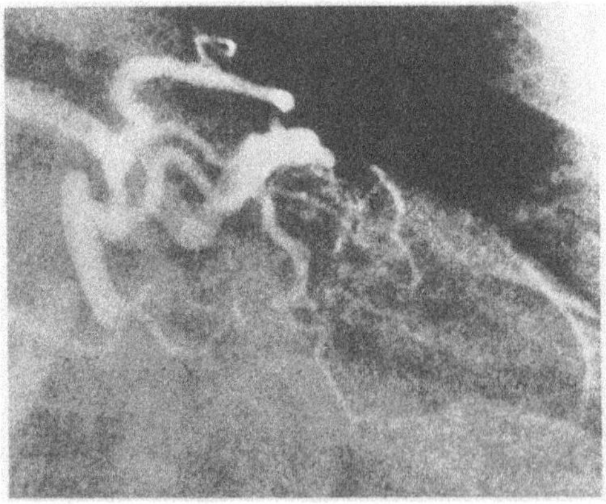

Fig. 13. Proximal coronary-pulmonary fistula: right anterior oblique projection of selective opacification of the right conus artery communicating by numerous branches with the pulmonary trunk and the infundibulum of the right ventricle and providing a right-to-left shunt of no particular significance

This malformation is similar to the shunts between a systemic artery (e.g. an internal mammary artery) and a peripheral pulmonary artery.

Many studies have been devoted to coronary fistulae since 1962. In total, more than 500 cases have been published, with most authors reporting only a few cases. The percentages of involvement relative to the arteries and the heart or vascular cavities with which they communicate are as follows:

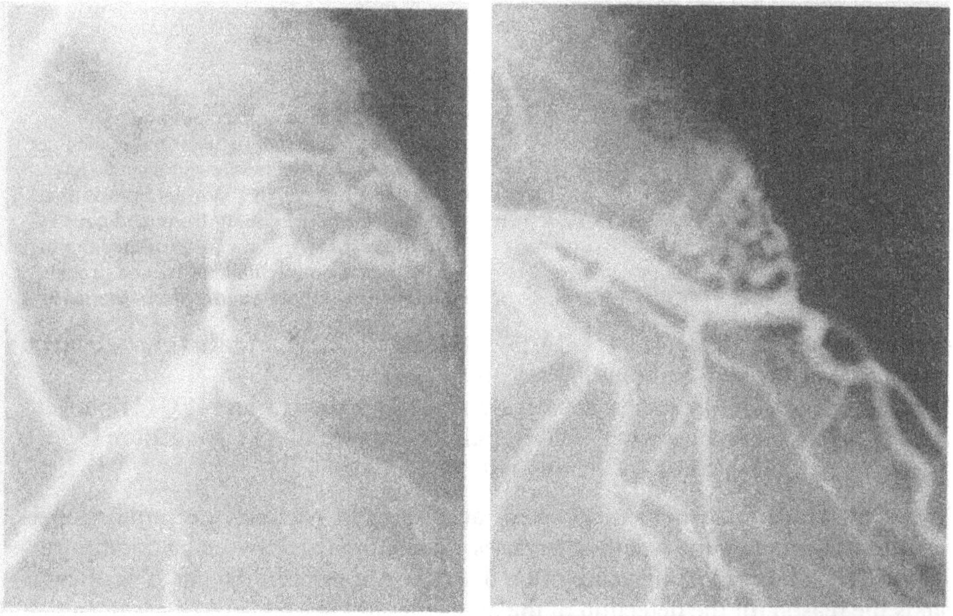

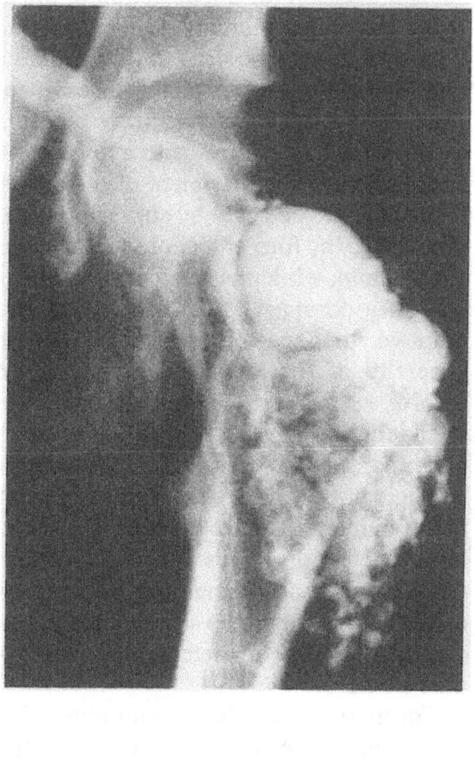

Fig. 14. Proximal coronary-pulmonary fistula *(upper)* associated with an artery-vein fistula on a branch of the left external iliac artery *(lower)*. *(Upper left):* right anterior oblique (RAO) view of right selective coronary arteriography; *(upper right):* RAO view of left selective coronary arteriography. The angiomatous formation in the infundibulum of the right ventricle is perfused by the right and left conus arteries

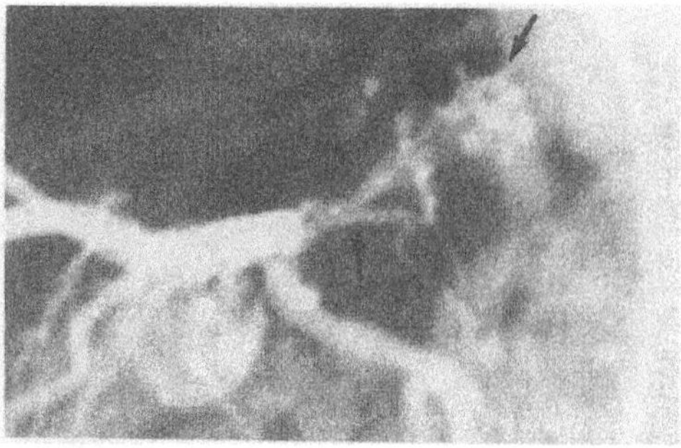

Fig. 15. Distal coronary-pulmonary or coronary-bronchial fistula (same patient as in Fig. 6). Transverse view of a single left coronary artery. An abnormal branch arises from the main coronary trunk and courses to the rear towards the hilus of the lung. It perfuses the bronchial arteries and probably the peripheral pulmonary artery branches

- artery involved: RCA (42%), LCA (37%), both coronary arteries (11.5%), single coronary artery (6%), supernumerary artery (3.5%)
- cavity receiving the artery: vena cava system (1.3%), right atrium (17%), right ventricle (44%), pulmonary artery (17%), pulmonary vein (0.3%), left atrium (3.7%), left ventricle (5%), coronary venous system (10.5%).

In the literature these percentages vary according to whether the population is mainly child or adult and whether the cases are anatomical or based on coronary arteriography. The clinical signs are often discrete. A murmur exists in 70% of cases but is the reason for the detection of the malformation in only 30% of cases. In half of the cases the anomaly is detected during a general examination. Clinical and electrocardiographic signs of myocardial ischaemia are relatively infrequent, occurring late in the course of the disease and nearly always in adults. Most authors attribute myocardial ischaemia to a coronary steal syndrome. In fact, in most cases the artery communicates with a low-pressure cavity which diverts the greater part of arterial flow to the detriment of the collateral branches of the artery in question.

Fistulae are detected by suprasigmoid aortography or by selective coronary arteriography. The former technique is ordinarily satisfactory for the infant and the very young child, while the latter is recommended for older children and adults. In the case of a coronary-to-cardiac fistula, the artery is considerably dilated until the point where it anastomoses with the heart chamber or venous system. The fistula is generally of the lateroterminal type. Most of the coronary-to-cardiac fistulae involve a left-to-right shunt, the left-to-left type being rare. Downstream from the fistula the coronary artery is often poorly opacified because the shunt absorbs most of the contrast material and, as a result, distal coronary flow is weak.

Angiographically, coronary to proximal pulmonary artery fistulae have an entirely different appearance. There are often numerous small arteries which are more or less dilated and sinuous and which collect on the anterior wall of the pulmonary artery to form a sort of angioma. Some branches are very fine and are barely visible, if at all. The angiographic shunt in the pulmonary artery is usually clearly identifiable, whereas its oximetric detection is often not possible. These fistulae provide low-volume shunts.

Coronary to peripheral pulmonary fistulae (Fig. 15) may only be diagnosed angiographically. At the end of the arterial phase of selective coronary arteriography, an abnormal coronary branch is discovered heading off towards a peripheral pulmonary region, where it anastomoses with the pulmonary artery capillary network. The association of a peripheral fistula with a proximal fistula is possible.

References

1. Ogden JA (1968) Congenital variations of the coronary arteries. Thesis, School of Medicine, Yale University
2. Ogden JA (1970) Congenital anomalies of the coronary arteries. Am J Cardiol 25: 474
3. Liberthson RR, Dinsmore RE, Bharati S, Rubenstein JJ (1974) Aberrant coronary artery origin from the aorta: diagnosis and clinical significance. Circulation 50: 774
4. Bertrand ME, Carre A, Ginestet A, Lefebvre JM, Warembourg H (1976) Les anomalies congénitales des artères coronaires. Ann Cardiol Angeiol 25: 39
5. Chaitman BR, Lesperance J, Saltiel J, Bourassa MG (1976) Clinical, angiographic and hemodynamic findings in patients with anomalous origin of the coronary arteries. Circulation 53: 122
6. Engel HJ, Torres C, Page HL Jr (1976) Major variations in anatomical origin of the left coronary arteries: angiographic observations in 4250 patients without associated congenital heart disease. Cathet Cardiovasc Diagn 2: 397
7. Baltaxe HA, Wixson D (1977) The incidence of congenital anomalies of the coronary arteries in the adult population. Radiology 122: 47
8. Kimbiris D, Iskandrian AS, Segal BKL, Bemis CE (1978) Anomalous aortic origin of coronary arteries. Circulation 58: 606
9. Levin DC, Fellows KE, Abrams HL (1978) Hemodynamically significant primary anomalies of the coronary arteries. Angiographic aspects. Circulation 58: 25
10. Liberthson RR, Dinsmore RE, Fallon JT (1979) Aberrant coronary artery origin from the aorta. Report of 18 patients, review of literature and delineation of natural history and management. Circulation 59: 748
11. Liberthson RR, Sazar K, Berkobin JP, Weintraub RM, Levine FH (1979) Congenital coronary arteriovenous fistula. Report of 13 patients, review of the literature, and delineation of management. Circulation 59: 849
12. Lipton MJ, Barry WH, Obrez I, Silverman JF, Wexler L (1979) Isolated single coronary artery: diagnosis, angiographic classification and clinical significance. Radiology 130: 39
13. Bream PR, Souza AS Jr, Elliott LP, Soto B, Curry GC (1979) Right superior septal perforator artery: its angiographic description and clinical significance. AJR 133: 67
14. Cheitlin MD, De Castro CM, Mc Allister HA (1974) Sudden death as a complication of anomalous left coronary origin from the anterior sinus of Valsalva. A not so minor anomaly. Circulation 50: 780
15. Amiel M, Cassagne J, Dalloz C, Age C, Clermont A (1975) Les anomalies congénitales d'origine et de distribution des artères coronaires naissant de l'aorte. Ann Radiol 18: 203
16. Bland EF, White PD, Garland J (1933) Congenital anomalies of the coronary arteries: report of an unusual case associated with cardiac hypertrophy. Am Heart J 8: 787
17. Van Praagh R (1973) Coronary artery anomalies. Anatomic considerations. Annual Meeting of the European Pediatric Cardiology Association, Rhodes
18. Sherkat A, Kavanagh-Gray D, Edworthy J (1967) Localized aneurysms of the coronary arteries. Radiology 89: 24
19. Ogden JA (1971) Secondary arterio-cameral fistula. J Pediatr 78: 78
20. Upshaw CB (1962) Congenital coronary arteriovenous fistula: report of case with an analysis of 73 reported cases. Am Heart J 63: 399
21. Gobel FL, Anderson CF, Baltaxe HA, Amplatz K, Wang Y (1970) Shunts between the coronary and pulmonary arteries with normal origin of the coronary arteries. Am J Cardiol 25: 655
22. Spindola Franco H, Weisel A, Delman AJ (1978) Pulmonary steal syndrome: an unusual case of coronary bronchial pulmonary artery communication. Radiology 126: 25

V Angiographic Explorations: Coronary Atheroma

Ventriculography and coronary arteriography are basic investigative techniques for use in patients with coronary atheroma. They indicate the site of stenoses, assess their severity and determine their operability, as well as sometimes providing positive diagnosis of the disease.

1 Left Ventricle

Myocardial ischaemia and the fibrous sequelae of infarction cause anomalies in left ventricular (LV) contraction and sometimes permanent deformations of ventricular morphology.

1.1 Morphological Anomalies: Bulging and Lacuna-Like Aspects

Left ventricular aneurysms [1–3], or in rare cases pseudoaneurysms [4, 5], appear in the image as a bulge in the ventricular outline which continues to be visible in end-diastole in at least one projection (Fig. 1). This is an important criterion to keep in mind in distinguishing aneurysms from extensive akineses, which may present the same systolic images. Very small aneurysms are sometimes limited to a single one of the six segments of LV outline, though most often two or three segments are involved (Fig. 2). The largest aneurysms leave only a basal ring of healthy myocardium. Paradoxical systolic expansion of the thin-walled aneurysmal sac is the general case, as well as hyperkinesis of adjacent healthy muscle. Infrequently, a thick wall thrombosis makes this sac more rigid and akinetic in systole. Most aneurysms are antero-apical (80%), with or without septal extension. The diagnosis of inferior aneurysms is generally more difficult (Fig. 3). They are very often associated with a mitral regurgitation due to necrosis of the posterior papillary muscle. The aneurysm is a common complication (10%–15%) of infarction. Aneurysms associated with

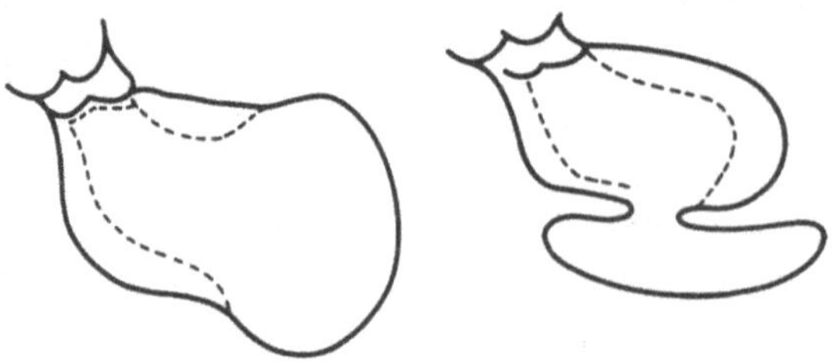

Fig. 1. Schematic representation of true *(left)* and false *(right)* left ventricular aneurysms. The persisting diastolic rupture on the endocardial contour is an important sign

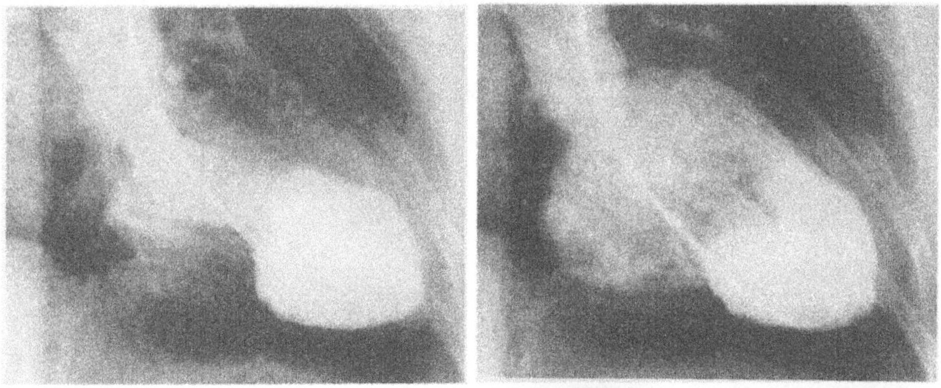

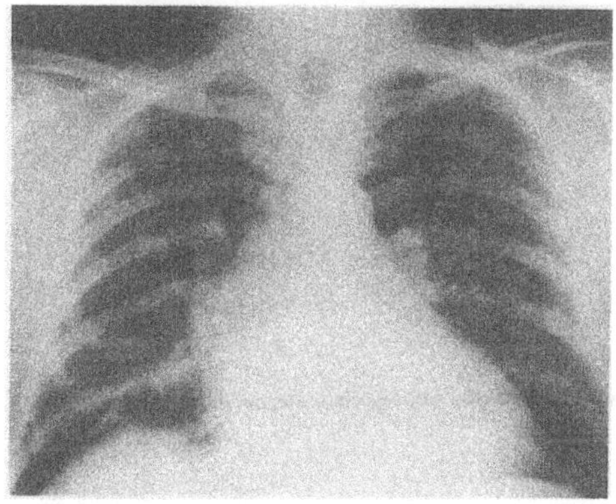

Fig. 2. Antero-apical left ventricular aneurysm. *(Upper):* diastolic and systolic left ventriculographic views; *(lower):* plain film of the chest

cardiac insufficiency, rhythm disturbances or systemic embolisms may require surgical excision, in which case quantitative analysis of the LV, preferably by the biplanar cine-angiographic method, is of considerable value. It is advisable to assess the function of healthy myocardium with respect to the quality of its contraction, its ejection fraction (EF) and its estimated volume after excision of the aneurysm, and to determine the condition of the mitral valve. Measurement of volumes by a method applying Simpson's rule is certainly the most reliable approach [6] for differentiating between the area of healthy myocardium and that of the aneurysm. Surgery can only be recommended if the remaining ventricle is capable of maintaining a normal or moderately lowered systolic ejection volume; otherwise the patient would be condemned to a serious postoperative cardiac insufficiency owing to low output and/or pulmonary venous hypertension. It is not always possible to tell the difference between a true aneurysm and extensive fibrous plaque, even though the determination may be of great importance to the choice of therapy. In these difficult cases, the decision to operate or not depends even more on the size and quality of the remaining ventricle. The pre-operative evaluation of any aneurysm should obviously include coronary arteriography to assess the value of an associated revascularization.

False LV aneurysms are rare (Figs. 4 and 5). They are due to a free wall rupture retained by an adhesive pericardial pouch. Unlike true aneurysms, they are most of-

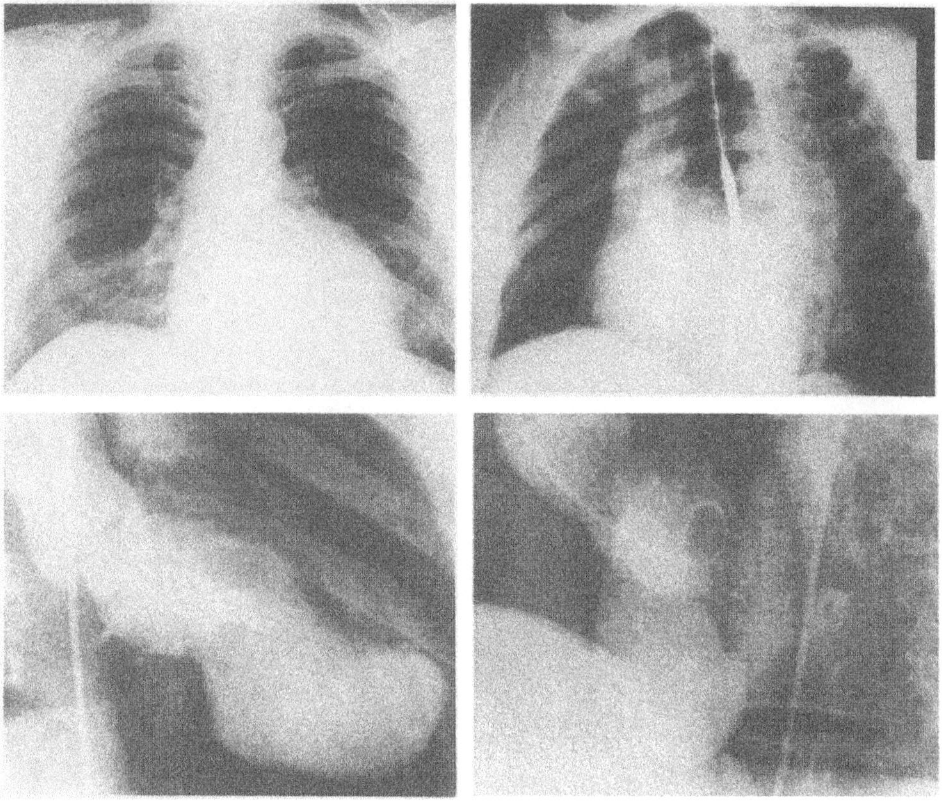

Fig. 3. Inferior left ventricular aneurysm. *(Upper):* frontal and left anterior oblique (LAO) projections of the chest. *(lower):* right anterior oblique and LAO left ventriculographic views showing a surprisingly voluminous aneurysm not easily predictable from plain films

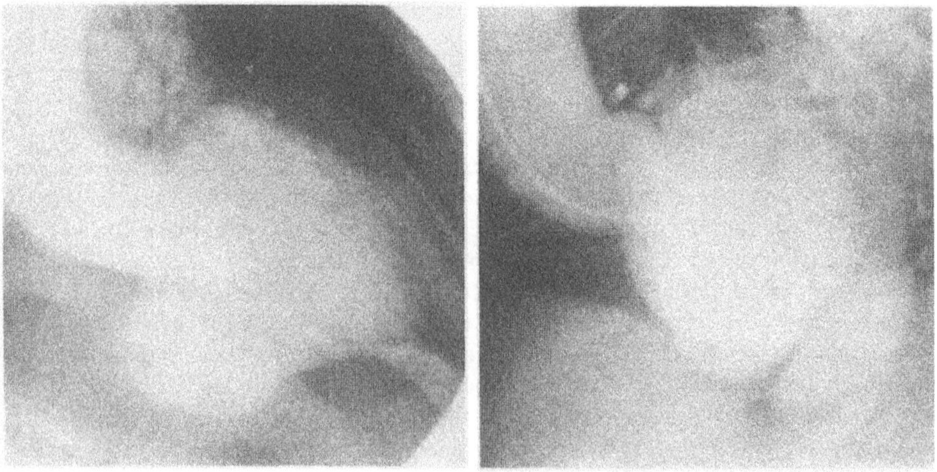

Fig. 4. False inferolateral left ventricular aneurysm. *(Left):* right anterior oblique and *(right):* left anterior oblique (LAO) left ventriculographic projections. The LAO view clearly shows a characteristic collar-like image

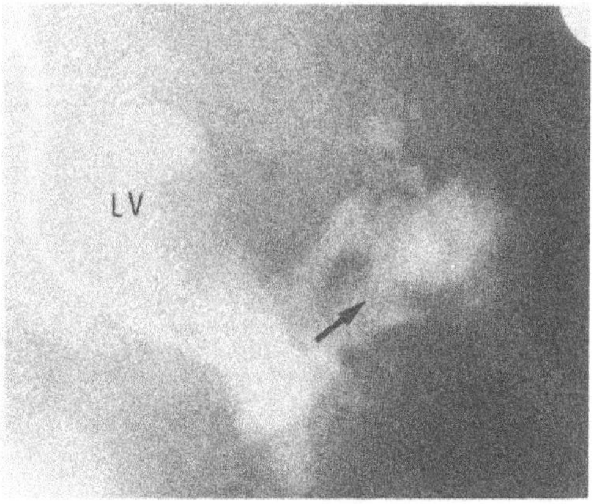

Fig. 5. Right anterior oblique left ventriculographic projection in an adult patient with rupture of the anterior wall occurring 15 days after acute myocardial infarction. Contrast medium is shown spurting out of the left ventricle through the ruptured wall into the pericardial space

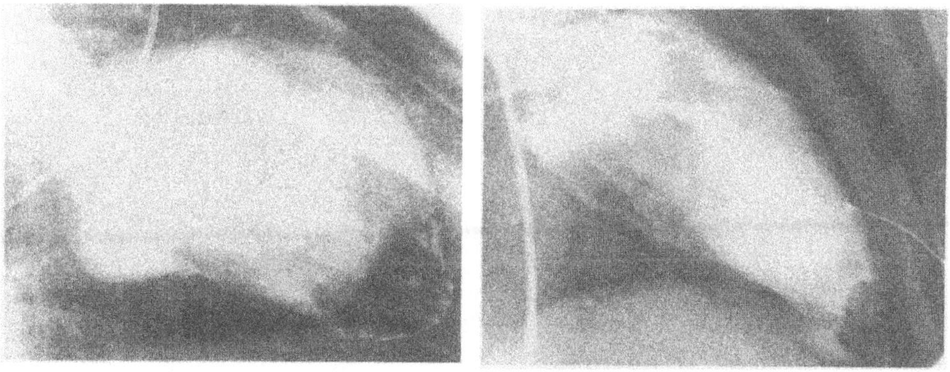

Fig. 6. Two examples of apical, lacuna-like, well-circumscribed mural thrombus

ten inferior or posterolateral and are likely to rupture. Their diagnosis is based on ventriculography and coronary arteriography, which reveal a paraventricular sac having a wall without coronary arteries [7]. Non-invasive methods (ultrasonography, scanning, isotopes) make it increasingly likely that they will be detected early. Intrapericardial rupture is possible in the absence of infarction and of coronary atheroma [1, 4].

Intraventricular thromboses are visualized as radiolucent spaces located centrally or marginally according to radiographic projection. They are now diagnosed mainly by ultrasonography or computed tomography. Their occurrence used to be very frequent as a complication of transmural infarction, but has been reduced considerably by early anticoagulant treatment. They are often discovered fortuitously. The most common are apical (Fig. 6) and appear as a rounded or irregular radiolucent space with sharp outlines, which is more or less floating or moving in the systolo-diastolic flux. The large clots which adhere firmly to the wall may efface the apex in the image. Ventricular aneurysms are commonly filled by stratified organized thromboses which are indirectly identified by angiography due to the fact that the wall of the aneurysmal sac is abnormally thick and sometimes irregular.

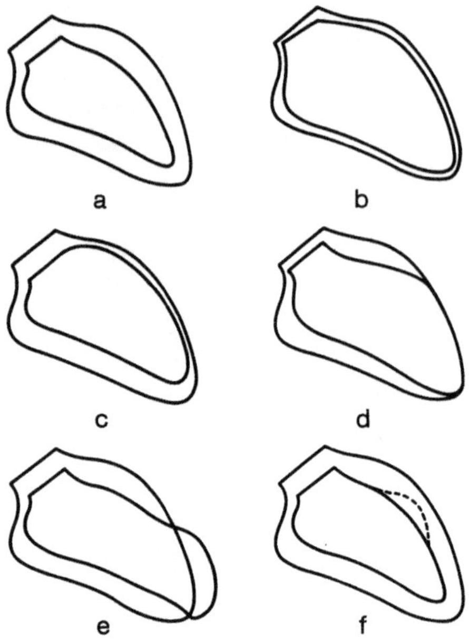

Fig. 7 a–f. Schematic representation of normal and abnormal wall motion. **a** normal; **b** hypokinesis (diffuse); **c** asyneresis (localized); **d** akinesis; **e** dyskinesis (systolic expansion); **f** asynchrony (*dotted line* for illustration of the possible segmentary early relaxation phenomenon). (After Herman [9])

1.2 Anomalies of Contraction and Relaxation

The methods used to analyse and quantify LV contraction have been described earlier (see Part II, Chap. III, Sect. 1.3). In 1969, Herman and Gorlin [8] proposed the first system of classification and precise terminology for contraction anomalies, which until then had been grouped under the general term "asynergies". They suggested the following definitions (Fig. 7):

- asyneresis: localized reduction in contraction
- hypokinesis: general reduction in contraction
- dyskinesis: localized paradoxical systolic expansion
- akinesis: local absence of contraction
- asynchrony: temporal interruption of contraction harmony.

In ordinary practice the term "asyneresis" has generally been abandoned in favour of localized or diffuse hypokinesis. The term "dyskinesis" is questionable for some authors because in its strict etymological sense it should designate all forms of contraction anomalies; however, it is generally used in the sense intended by Herman and Gorlin. These authors from the very beginning of their study [8, 9] stress the important characteristics of these disorders: their high frequency in coronary artery disease (65% of patients explored), their close relationship with myocardial ischaemia and coronary artery lesions, their inconstancy in baseline and resting state, their possible reversibility and their role in causing cardiac insufficiency. Pathological studies show that the severity of contraction alterations is in proportion to the extent of the fibrosis [10]. Akinesis and dyskinesis are ordinarily associated with a condition of extensive myocardial fibrosis, although this is not an absolute rule, for healthy myocardial fibres can continue to exist in the midst of a fibrous plaque [1, 11]. The study of the LV in biplanar projection is quite rewarding [12]. In effect, the customary 30° right anterior oblique (RAO) projection analyses only the anterior and inferior walls, whereas in biplanar projection all the walls can be explored. It is true that the anterior and inferior walls, which are affected equally, have lesions three times as often as the lateral wall or the apex alone [13]. The frequency of septal anomalies is not well known, though it would seem that they are always associated with an anterior or apical affection [12]. Asynergy is not permanent at rest in all patients. Different stress tests [14] are used to detect it: atrial pacing and dynamic or static handgrip exercises (best adapted to catheterization), volume or pressure (angiotensin) overload conditions. These stress tests allow a better assessment of the threat posed by arterial stenoses to the myocardium and thus of their peculiar degree of severity. Some coronary patients have a LV contraction which seems normal when appraised over the entire systolic period, despite the presence of significant coronary stenoses. Studies of the early phase of ejection (first third or first half) show that contraction may be altered at the beginning of systole and above normal and compensatory in the middle or at the end of systole [15–19]. These fractional studies of the ejection phase are also of great value in detecting those subjects whose myocardium is greatly endangered. The protective effect of collateral circulation on wall kinetics, or lack of such effect, will be considered later, as well as the reversibility of contraction disorders as a result of various tests or after surgery.

It is not uncommon to observe an abnormally early relaxation of a wall segment in coronary patients. The frequency of this segmental early relaxation phenomenon (SERP) was estimated as 11% in a group of 535 patients [20]. The SERP concerns especially the anterior wall, though this may simply be due to the fact that the anterior wall is explored the most, and has been noted mainly in left anterior descending artery (LAD) stenoses. However, the phenomenon is not absolutely specific to this lesion. It seems to correspond well to an early phase of contraction change (unsustained contraction) which apparently precedes segmental hypokinesis, in increasing degrees of severity, during exercise and then at rest.

1.3 Alterations in Function

Left ventricular function and contraction are obviously closely related. The former depends on the quality of the latter and on all the stimulating or depressing factors which act upon it. The methods of measuring these angiographic parameters of LV function and their normal values are presented in Part II, Chap. III, Sect. 1.4. The main parameters in ordinary usage are the LV volumes [end-diastolic volume (EDV); endsystolic volume (ESV); systolic volume (SV)], the EF and the mean VCF. The lower limit of the normal value of the EF varies between 0.55 and 0.60 according to author. For purely coronary patients, with no volume or pressure overloading and without associated arrhythmia, the EDV remains normal in the absence of infarction, regardless of the degree of coronary affliction [21]. The EF is also normal in purely anginal patients with single- or double-vessel involvement, but becomes abnormal in patients with triple-vessel involvement [21]. The dilatation of the ventricle is thus related to the presence of infarction, or more exactly of myocardial fibrosis, which is not necessarily transmural but sometimes rudimentarily intramural or subendocardial. The increase in EDV and the decrease in EF are proportional to the extent of the akinetic or hypokinetic areas [22, 23]. The EF is a more sensitive indication of LV function than is the EDV; its diminution reflects an increase in ESV, that is, the incomplete quality of the contraction. Once again the first disorders occur at the beginning of systolic ejection and are compensated for in the middle or second half of systole [16–18]. A certain degree of myocardial hypertrophy, with increased wall thickness, also accounts for these phenomena of compensation for initial or latent ventricular insufficiency [23].

1.4 Physiological and Pharmacological Tests

The performance of left ventriculography during an exercise test is of limited utility. There are various inconveniences: the length of the examination, because it is necessary to wait for a return to baseline values after the first ventriculography; injection of a double amount of contrast medium; patient discomfort; and the customary necessity of leaving the patient in a reclining posture, which does not duplicate well the usual exercise conditions. The exercise can be dynamic (bicycle ergometric) or static and isometric (sustained handgrip). This latter method is not entirely satisfactory, for it acts mainly by means of an increase in systemic arterial resistances. In effect, the non-invasive ultrasonic and radio-nuclide methods of study have supplanted the injection of contrast medium in this area. The ultrasonic and cinegraphic study of markers implanted in the myocardium during surgery is also an interesting technique [24]. Sharma has studied 21 subjects (4 normal and 17 coronary) by left ventriculography [25]. In the normal subject, exercise caused an appreciable increase in EF, with a decrease in ESV and, to a lesser degree, in EDV. In the coronary patient, without angina, EDV, ESV and EF did not vary significantly during effort. In the group of patients with angina, exercise produced a significant increase in EDV and ESV and a significant decrease in EF [25]. The correlation with wall kinetics was evident: in 12 patients with angina, an extension of the areas of localized asynergy was observed six times at rest and six times during exercise. These findings have been confirmed by radio-nuclide studies [17].

The other classic tests for assessing LV function are atrial pacing, the perfusion of isoproterenol and the angiotensin test to increase afterload. To our knowledge, these tests have not been studied methodically by left ventriculography.

Postextrasystolic potentiation has frequently been used to estimate myocardial contractile reserve and the reversibility of segmental contraction anomalies [26, 27]. The long diastole which follows a ventricular extrasystole causes an increase in ventricular filling, that is, in the preload, and an increase in contractility due to the Frank-Starling effect. As a result, there is normally a decrease in ESV, an increase in EF and mean VCF and an improvement in segmental wall contraction. In the coronary patient the improvement in localized asynergies depends on the severity of the coronary lesions and on the quantity of myocardium still intact [26, 28]. The test's predictive value following aorta-to-coronary bypass surgery has been recognized [26]. Although their mechanisms of action are different, postextrasystolic potentiation and nitroglycerin can improve segmental contraction in very similar ways [28, 29].

The test using nitroglycerin administered sublingually or intravenously is relatively easy to carry out during catheterization in order to repeat left ventriculography. In fact, nitroglycerin has the advantage of reducing ventricular preload and of thus neutralizing wholly or partially the results of the first injection of contrast medium. The potential effects of nitroglycerin are reduction of overload and intramyocardial pressure, coronary artery dilatation and a drop in coronary resistances. It can bring about a lowering of myocardial oxygen consumption and an improvement in coronary flow. This test is useful in assessing myocardial reserve and the possible reversibility of ventricular asynergy, one of the major objectives of revascularization surgery. The studies agree in showing that nitroglycerin decreases EDV and ESV, can increase EF and VCF and improves or eliminates a localized hypokinesis [28–30]. Control ventriculographies after aorta-to-coronary bypass surgery have confirmed the rather good predictive value of this test [30].

2 Right Ventricle

In coronary artery pathology, the right ventricle (RV) plays a minimal role and is not involved except when it is the site of an infarction. The diagnosis of RV infarction has been successively anatomic, haemodynamic and scintigraphic, and has practically never involved right ventriculography and coronary arteriography. However, there has been renewed interest in the matter, for RV infarction can be a source of therapeutic problems if ignored, compromising, in particular, the survival of patients with interventricular septal rupture. Rackley has recently made an interesting appraisal of the subject [31]. Approximately 25% of posterodiaphragmatic infarctions involve the RV. The diagnosis is based mainly on elevated RV pressure at baseline state or after filling and on an abnormal uptake of technetium pyrophosphate by the RV free wall. The few studies carried out with coronary arteriography and right ventriculography indicate that RV infarction is generally the result of an association of very severe stenoses ($\geqslant 75\%$) of the right coronary artery (RCA) and the LAD, that the RV is dilated and that its free wall is hypokinetic.

3 Coronary Arteries

Coronary artery stenoses can be described or graded according to different characteristics: number, site, degree of severity, shape, outline, length etc. The site and severity of the narrowing are the most important factors.

3.1 Different Types of Stenosis; Post-stenotic Dilatation

The extent of the stenosis is variable. The shortest have a diaphragm-like appearance (Fig. 8), and the longest measure a few centimetres (Fig. 9). A stenosis which is not very dense though very extended may be misinterpreted and its consequences perhaps underestimated. The stenosis appears concentric (Fig. 8) or eccentric (Figs. 10 and 11). A stenosis appearing concentric in only one projection is more diffi-

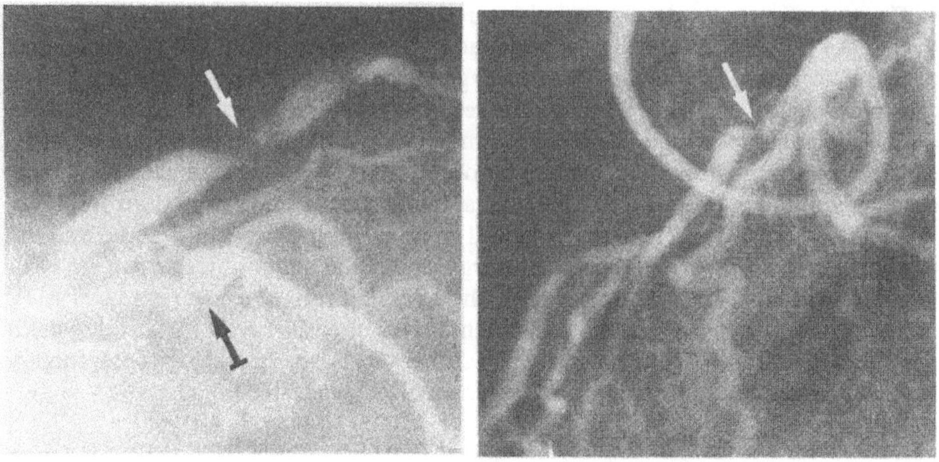

Fig. 8. Concentric and eccentric stenoses. *(Left):* frontal and craniocaudal view of the left coronary artery (LCA) showing a diaphragm-like stenosis of the circumflex *(black arrow)* and an eccentric obstruction of the left anterior descending artery (LAD) *(white arrow); (right):* transverse view of the LCA; concentric severe occlusive lesion of the proximal LAD *(white arrow)*

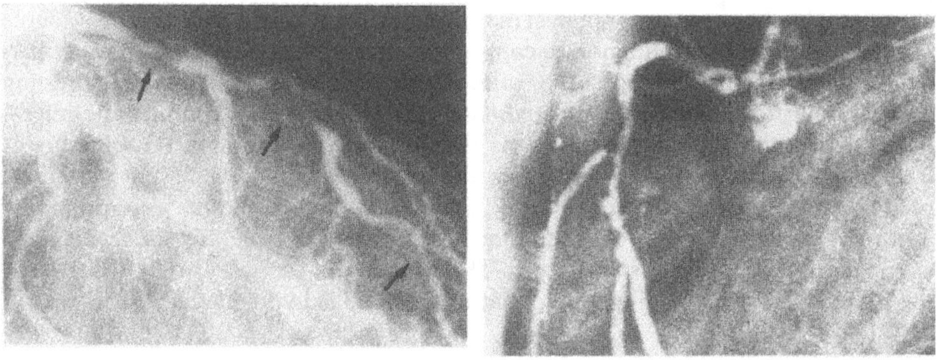

Fig. 9. Examples of long stenoses. *(Left):* right anterior oblique view of the left coronary artery: successive long stenoses *(arrow)* of the left anterior descending artery; *(right):* left anterior oblique view of the right coronary artery (RCA): irregular and long stenosis involving the upper half of the vertical segment of the RCA

cult to appraise (Fig. 12). The outlines of the stenosis are more or less regular. An irregular outline is suggestive of an ulcerated atheromatous plaque (Fig. 13), a particularly progressive lesion, according to Rösch [32]. A severe atheromatous stenosis is often followed by localized dilatation of the artery (Fig. 14). For this reason, an operator noticing a dilated, fusiform and isolated artery segment should suspect post-stenotic dilatation and search carefully for a masked stenosis with the help of additional projections. Sometimes a succession of stenoses in close proximity gives a moniliform appearance to part of an artery segment (Fig. 15). The atheromatous

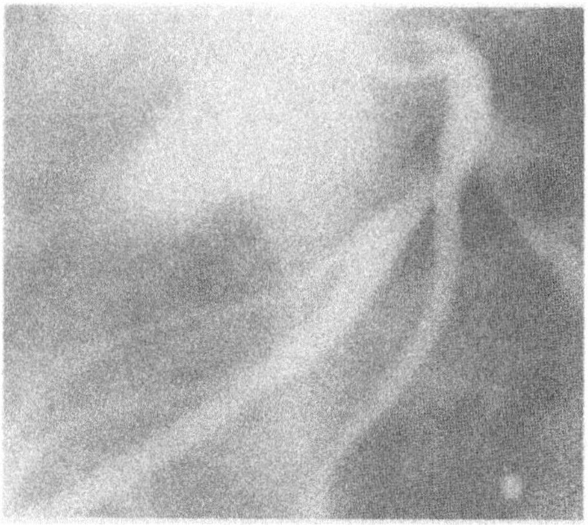

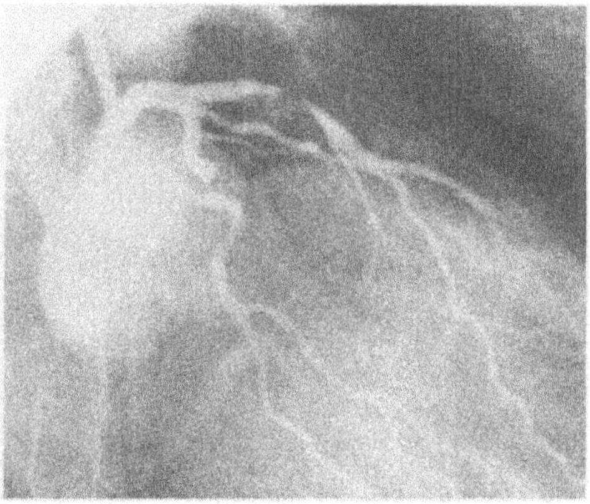

Fig. 10 *(left).* Left anterior oblique and caudocranial view of the left coronary artery: the diaphragm-like eccentric high-degree stenosis located at the origin of the left anterior descending artery is perceptible exclusively in this double-oblique projection. The post-stenotic dilatation had first attracted the operator's attention

Fig. 11 *(right).* Right anterior oblique view of the coronary artery. Slit-like eccentric severe obstructive lesions of the proximal left anterior descending artery and of the circumflex

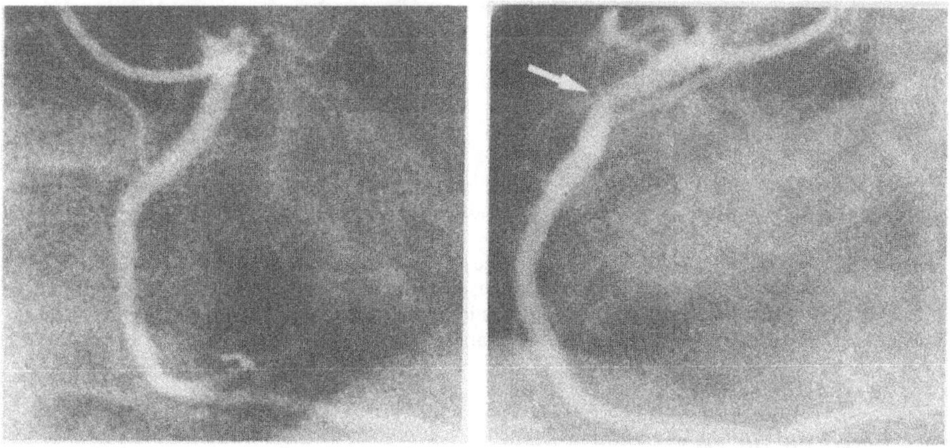

Fig. 12. Obstructive lesion of the proximal right coronary artery, *(left)* not detectable in right anterior oblique view, *(right)* only appearing in left anterior oblique view: this case illustrates one difficulty of determining the exact degree of luminal narrowing

plaques show up as wall irregularities or as images with marginal notches (Fig. 16 left). Many plaques are not stenotic but only stiffen the vessel, as has been confirmed by comparison of the findings of radiological anatomy and surgery [33]. Sometimes there is a segmental rigidity in an artery (Fig. 16 right) joined abruptly with neighbouring, normally mobile segments. This has been described as the "lead pipe effect".

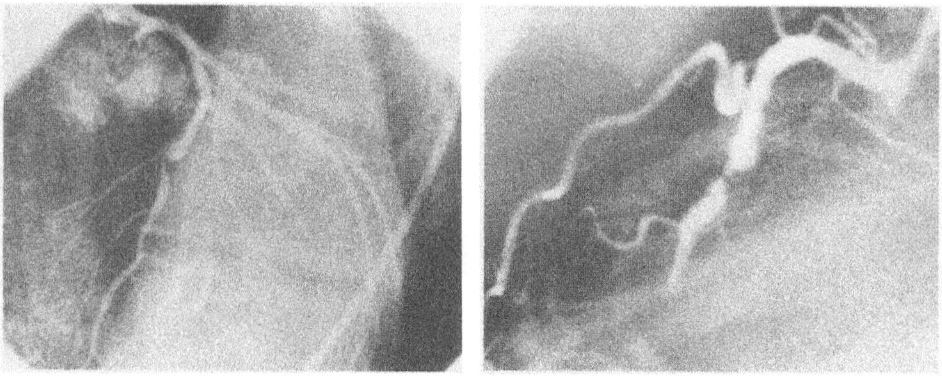

Fig. 13. Atheromatous ulcerations. *(Left):* left anterior oblique (LAO) and caudocranial view of the left coronary artery evidencing this type of lesion on the left anterior descending artery; *(right):* LAO view of a severe atheromatous involvement of the right coronary artery with extreme narrowing and ulcerated plaque preceding total occlusion

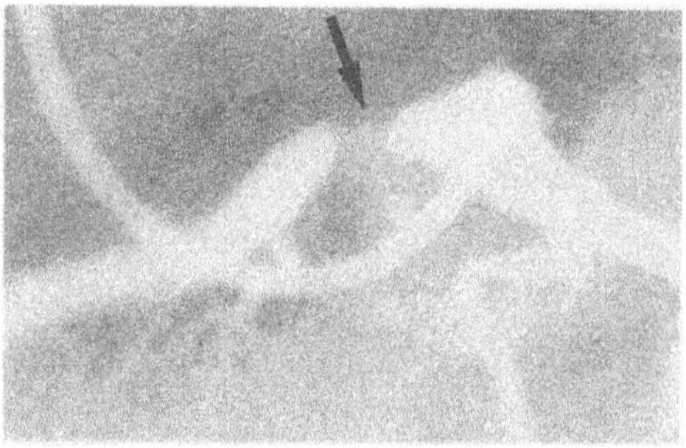

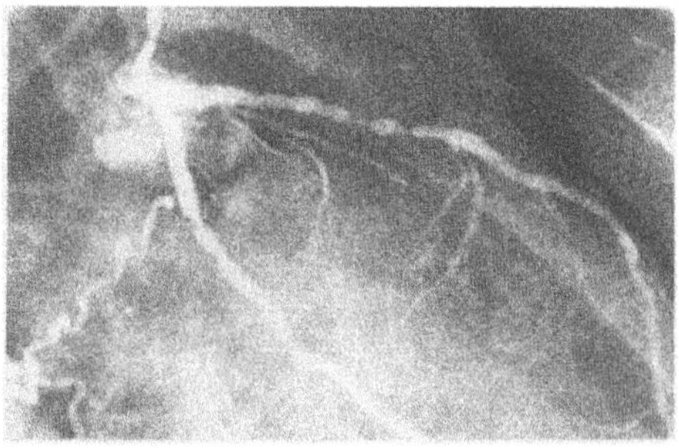

Fig. 14 *(left).* Transverse view of a concentric severe stenosis of the proximal left anterior descending artery with harmonious post-stenotic dilatation of the vessel

Fig. 15 *(right).* Right anterior oblique view of the left coronary artery. Moniliform aspect of the left anterior descending artery and, to a lesser degree, of the circumflex (Cx), due to successive multiple stenoses. A left atrial branch arising from the Cx joins the atrioventricular node artery of the totally occluded right coronary artery (left Kugel-type anastomosis)

3.2 Severity of Stenosis

Opinion is not unanimous as to the best means of assessing severity. Most operators calculate the diameter of the narrowed segment by comparison with the diameter of the adjoining healthy segment, either subjectively and qualitatively, that is approximately, or quantitatively by using a calliper gauge or a compass. The stenosis is then graded by the percentage of narrowing of the calibre or diameter of the vessel. Usually, the greatest degree of narrowing observed is that recorded. Thus a stenosis valued at 75% in RAO and at 50% in left anterior oblique (LAO) projections will be regarded as 75%. Some authors [34, 35] appraise stenoses more exactly according to the reduction in cross-sectional area of the vessel. A stenosis diminishing arterial di-

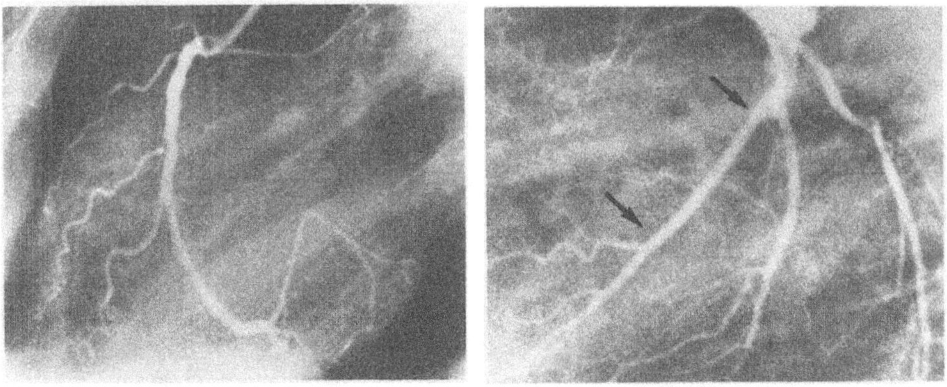

Fig. 16. Moderate atheromatous involvement of coronary arteries. *(Left):* left anterior oblique view of the right coronary artery: usual irregular aspect of the arterial wall without significant stenoses. *(Right):* Transverse view of the circumflex. The *black arrows* delineate, in a major marginal branch, a straight segment appearing wholly rigid on cine film. Its calibre is curiously normal. This is an unusual aspect of atheroma

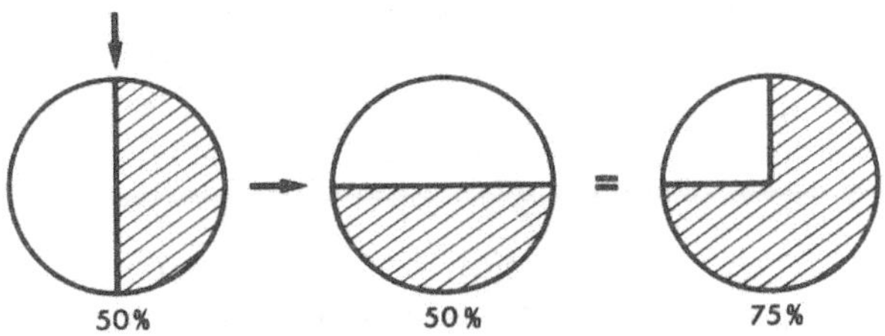

Fig. 17. The appearance of 50% diameter reduction on two opposite angiographic views indicates a true 75% cross-sectional area reduction

ameter by 50% in each of two orthogonal projections is recorded as 75% because it actually narrows the cross-sectional area of the vessel by 75% (Fig. 17). This grading method seems more adequate since, according to Poiseuille's equation, the pressure gradient ΔP necessary to ensure a constant flow F in a vessel of length L is inversely proportional to the length of the radius to the fourth power:

$$P = \frac{8\mu \times L \times F}{\pi r^4} \quad (\mu = \text{the coefficient of viscosity})$$

Hence it is not surprising that small variations in the calibre of a stenosis have a considerable influence on resistance and flow. When the cross-sectional area of a vessel is reduced by 75%, the resistance is multiplied by a factor of 4. The same factor of 4 applies between 75% and 95%, and a factor of 7 between 95% and 99%. These theoretical values have been corroborated by experimental studies [36–38] concerning the relationship between the degree of stenosis and the trans-stenotic pressure gradient (Fig. 18). The greater the severity of the stenosis, the more essential it is to assess it accurately.

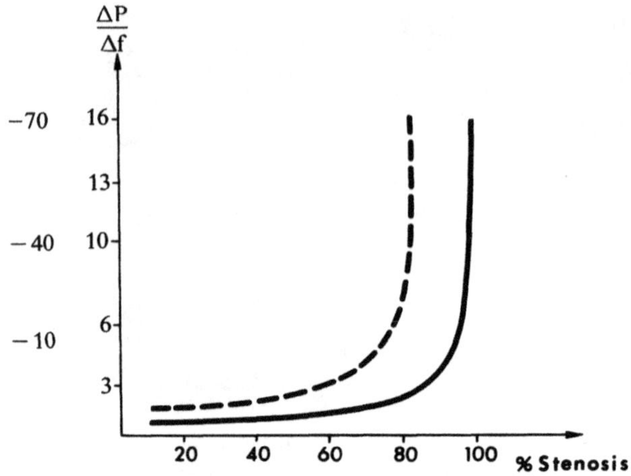

Fig. 18. Effect of the degree of luminal narrowing on resting (——) and hyperaemic reactive (----) coronary flow. Percentage reduction of arterial diameter is shown on the *horizontal axis*. The variation of the arterial resistance (mmHg/ml per minute) is expressed on the *vertical axis: left scale* for hyperaemic flow, *right scale* for resting flow

The difficulties in objective assessment of a narrowing are very real considering the small size of the coronary arteries and the causes of radiological blur [39]. By simulating measurements of small vessels (0.5–3 mm in diameter) in ideal technical conditions, Björk concluded that the error in calculation could be as great as 30% for the tiniest arteries [40]. In most coronary arteriography laboratories, grading is semi-quantitative, with stenoses classified by stages. The following scale has been proposed by the American Heart Association Ad Hoc Committee:

- Normal: absence of narrowing
- 25% stenosis: reduction in luminal diameter not exceeding 25%
- 50% stenosis: reduction in luminal diameter of 26%–50%
- 75% stenosis: reduction in luminal diameter of 51%–75%
- 90% stenosis: reduction in luminal diameter of 76%–90%
- 99% stenosis: lumen as fine as a hair (subtotal occlusion)
- 100% stenosis: occlusion.

This type of grading is the most common, though with slight variations. Thus many authors group together all stenoses below 50%. According to almost unanimous opinion, the stenoses regarded as operable, and thus said to be significant, are those which reduce the lumen by 75%–100%.

3.3 Number and Site of Stenoses

Generally speaking, atheromatous lesions are located mainly in the large artery trunks, and the coronary network is no exception to this rule. The stenoses involve essentially the three main trunks: RCA, LAD and circumflex (Cx). Isolated stenoses are relatively rare, and it is common to observe several stenoses of varying severity in the same vessel and its main branches. In a group of 1550 patients suspected of having coronary artery disease and explored consecutively, Gensini noted the following frequency and distribution of lesions [41]:

- Presence of arterial stenoses: 83.7%
- Significant stenoses (reduction in arterial diameter of more than 75%): 73.6%

- Single-vessel involvement: 30% (LAD 16%, RCA 9%, Cx 5%)
- Double-vessel involvement: 30%
- Triple-vessel involvement: 40%.

In the three main vessels distal stenoses are infrequent (of the order of 5%), whereas proximal stenoses in the large branches (diagonal, marginal and septal) are frequent. Regardless of the artery in question, atheroma preferentially involves the proximal third. In the RCA the stenoses occurring between the main marginal branch and the crux are also very frequent. The preferred sites of stenoses are the bifurcations and branchings (Figs. 19 and 20): LAD-Cx, LAD-diagonal, Cx-marginal, RCA-PDA, PDA-retroventricular. Our observations indicate an average of 2.5 lesions per heart [42], taking into consideration only the main trunks. This is in complete agreement with earlier pathological findings [43, 44]. By counting only ste-

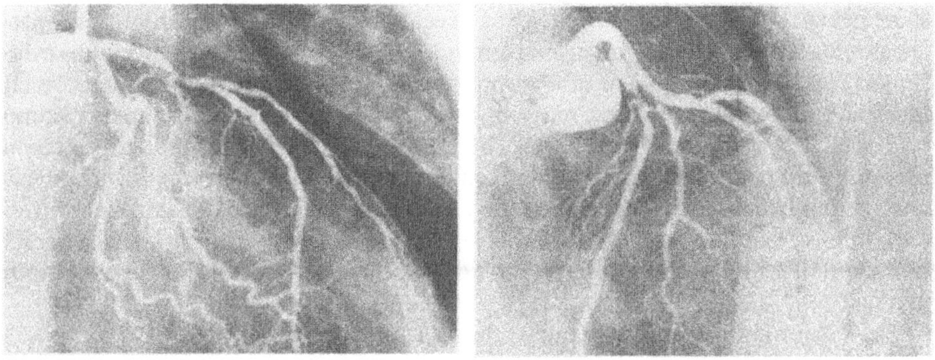

Fig. 19. Preferential localization of stenoses on arterial bifurcations or trifurcations. High-degree stenosis of the proximal left anterior descending artery, affecting the origin of the first septal artery, associated with a severe narrowing of the origin of the first and main diagonal branch. *(Left):* right anterior oblique view; *(right):* left anterior oblique and caudocranial view

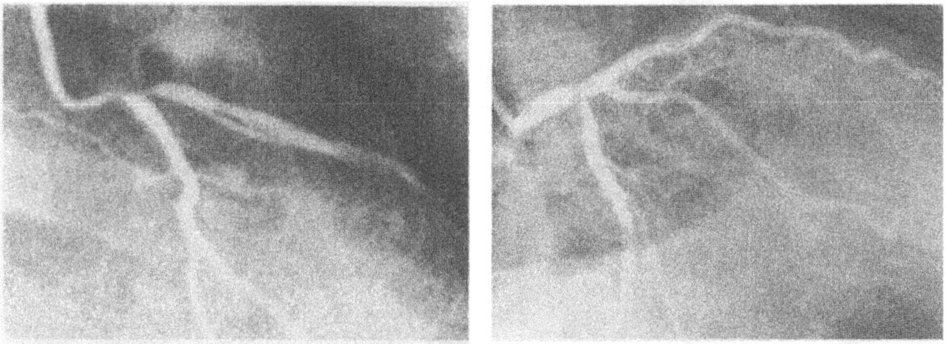

Fig. 20. Stenoses of the bifurcation into left anterior descending artery (LAD) and circumflex (Cx). *(Left):* Standard right anterior oblique (RAO) view of the left coronary artery (LCA): extreme luminal reduction of the left common trunk also involving the origin of LAD and Cx. *(Right):* RAO and craniocaudal view of the LCA. This double-oblique view results in an interesting separation of LAD and Cx at their origin, facilitating the analysis of the bifurcation: severe lesion involving the bifurcation, producing a three-leaf clover appearance

noses greater than 75% relative to the three main trunks, Gensini found 1.85 lesions per heart [41]. The occlusions affect one vessel in 40% of cases, two in 12% and three in 1% [43, 44]. In Gensini's series the frequency of occlusions was 1.5 per patient, with 40% affecting the RCA, 33% the LAD and 27% the Cx [41]. Thus it is apparent that most patients already have double- or triple-vessel involvement when the first clinical signs appear.

3.4 Intercoronary Anastomoses and Coronary Collateral Circulation

The existence of radiologically invisible anastomoses (diameter of around 40 μm) between different branches of the coronary network, and their capacity to develop in pathological conditions, is no longer in doubt owing to the work of Fulton [45] and, especially, Shaper [46]. It is generally admitted that not all individuals have the same genetically determined capacity to develop intercoronary anastomoses. These anastomoses only become functional and increase in size in the presence of a severe stenosis (greater than 75%) or of a coronary artery occlusion. They are then present in 75%–85% of such subjects, reaching their maximum size and diameter (sometimes 500 μm) after a few weeks [46]. The presence and degree of the trans-stenotic pressure gradient has an influence on their appearance, size and possible disappearance, as has been clearly demonstrated by Bourassa [47] in repeated coronary arteriographies of patients with bypasses. They are capable of ensuring the retrograde perfusion of an occluded artery by providing a flow not greater than 18 ml/min in man [47].

Three types of intercoronary anastomosis are found:

1. Homocoronary or intersegmental anastomoses, which directly bypass an obstruction by means of short and very slender vessels (Fig. 21). These are often radiolog-

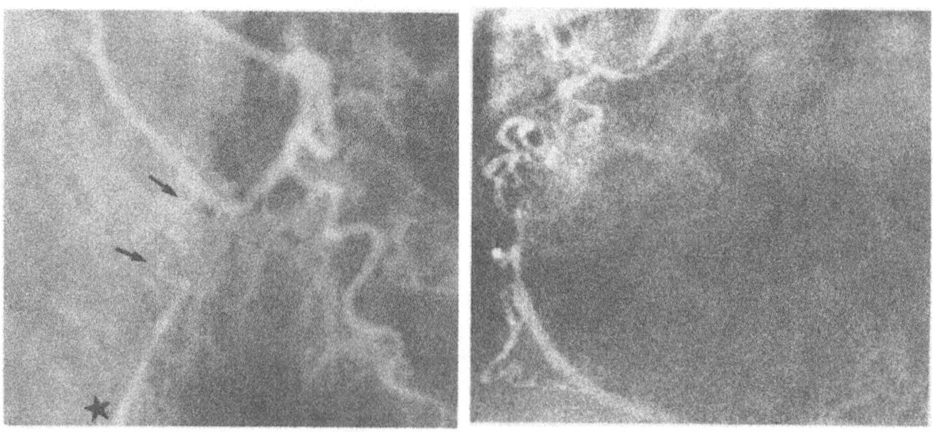

Fig. 21. Intersegmental homocoronary anastomoses. *(Left):* Right anterior oblique view of the right coronary artery (RCA). A total occlusion of the artery beyond a voluminous right atrial branch is bypassed by very fine collaterals *(arrows)* which opacify the distal RCA *(star)*. *(Right):* Left anterior oblique view of the RCA. Double total occlusion at the level of the ostium and on the upper half of the vertical segment. Double bypass by intersegmental collateral channels

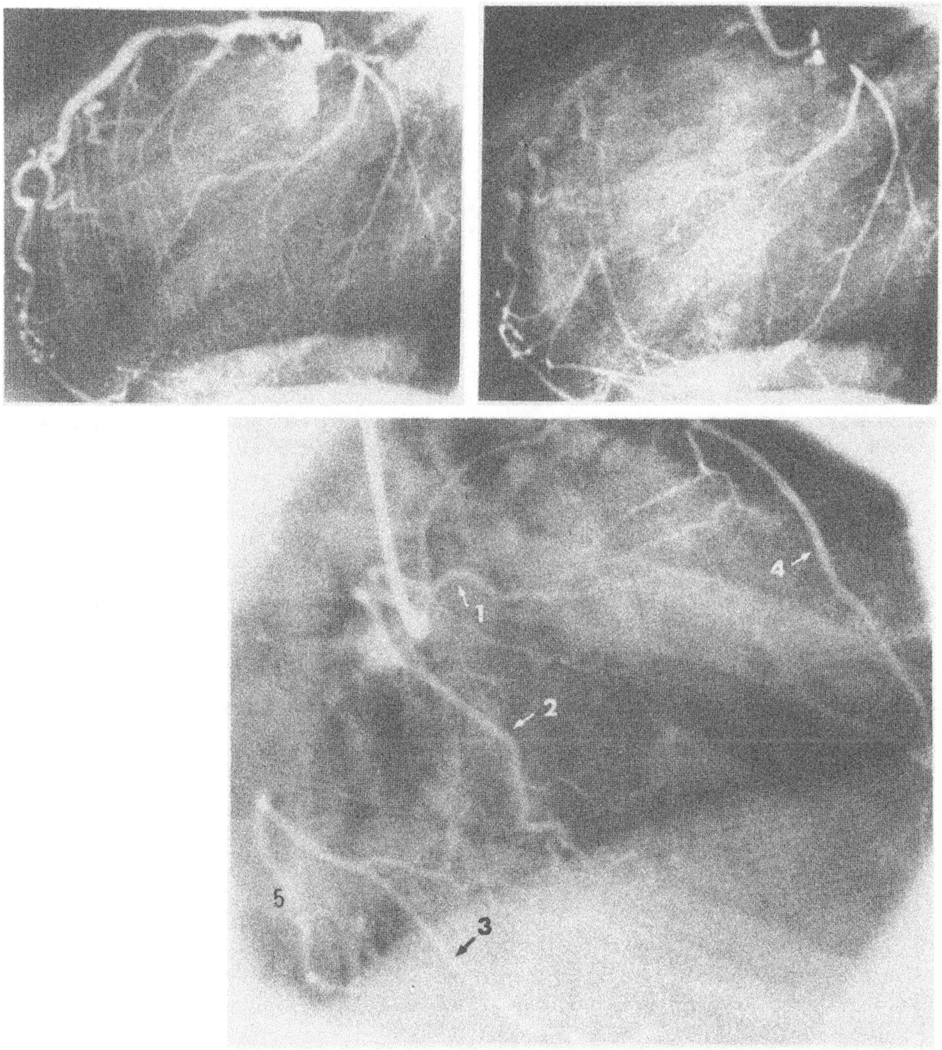

Fig. 22. Homolateral and heterolateral intercoronary anastomoses. *(Upper):* Early and late frames of a left coronary artery angiograph (transverse projection). A left atrial branch bypasses the total occlusion of the circumflex: homolateral anastomosis. The distal part of the dominant right coronary artery (RCA) is opacified by the distal left anterior descending artery (LAD) and the septal branches: heterolateral anastomosis. *(Lower):* Right anterior oblique view of an occluded RCA. The right conus artery *(1)* supplies the LAD *(4)*: heterolateral anastomosis. The right marginal branches *(2* and *3)* are connected and carry blood to the distal RCA *(5)*: homolateral anastomosis

ically invisible or have a localized hair-like appearance, being made up of very tiny epicardial arteries or of vasa vasorum of the occluded artery.

2. Homolateral intercoronary anastomoses, which connect the different branches of the same main artery, either the RCA of the left coronary artery (LCA) (Fig. 22).
3. Heterolateral intercoronary anastomoses, which provide communication between branches of the RCA and those of the LCA (Figs. 23–25).

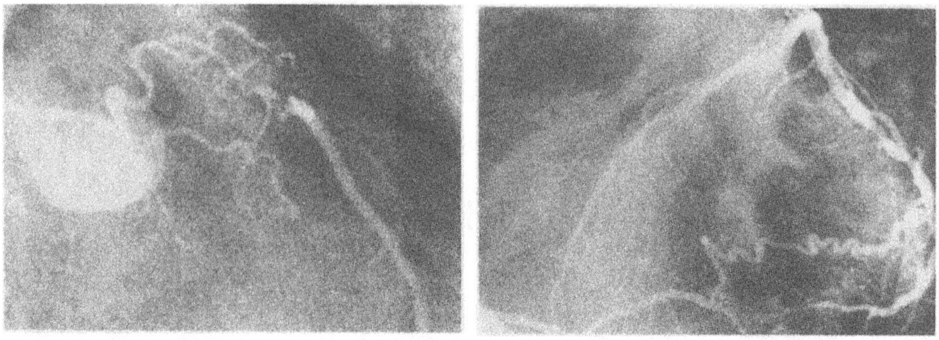

Fig. 23. Heterolateral anastomoses. *(Left):* selective opacification of a right conus artery connected with a completely occluded left anterior descending artery (right anterior oblique view; *(right):* left coronary artery supplying an occluded right coronary artery by way of a full-bore anastomosis between left atrial branches of the two arteries (left anterior oblique view)

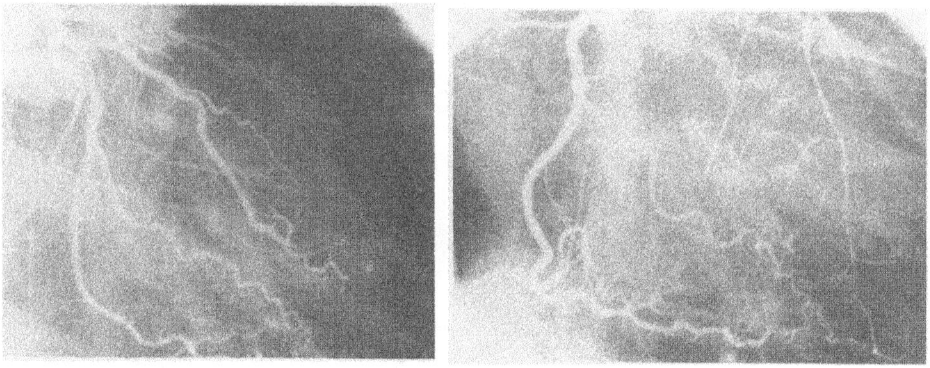

Fig. 24. Heterolateral anastomoses. *(Left):* Right anterior oblique view of left coronary artery showing an occluded left anterior descending artery (LAD). *(Right):* Same projection of the right coronary artery opacification: the LAD is opacified by contrast agent flowing successively through the PDA and inferior and anterior septal branches

An anastomosis may be located at any point in the coronary network. However, the preferential anastomotic pathways are well known [48, 49]. For heterolateral anastomoses, from the LCA to the RCA or vice versa, their order of decreasing frequency is:

- The septal arteries between the LAD and the PDA
- Anastomosis between the LAD and a right marginal branch
- Anastomosis between the Cx and RCA by their terminal branches
- The right conus artery towards the LAD
- The junction between the distal LAD and PDA arteries
- Anastomoses between the LAD or Cx and the RCA by the right and left atrial arteries, the atrioventricular node artery and the Kugel arteries.

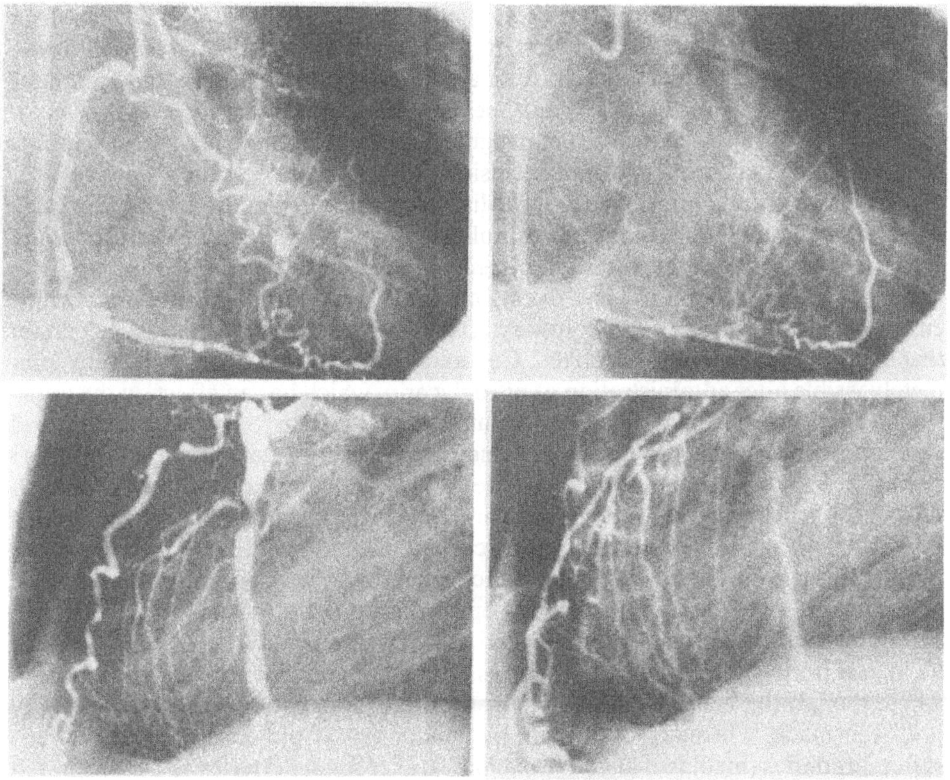

Fig. 25. Heterolateral anastomoses. Early and late frames of right coronary artery (RCA) opacification in *(upper):* right anterior oblique and *(lower):* transverse projections. In spite of double severe stenosis the RCA supplies the occluded left anterior descending artery (LAD) by way of three collateral connections: distal PDA with distal LAD – highly stenosed right marginal branch with distal LAD – inferior septal branches with anterior ones

For left homolateral anastomoses the order is:

- The septal and diagonal arteries between the proximal and distal segments of the LAD
- The marginal and diagonal arteries between the Cx and the LAD, or vice versa
- The left atrial arteries between the proximal and distal segments of the Cx.

The main right homolateral pathways are:

- The right atrial arteries, the right Kugel artery and the right marginal branches between the proximal and distal segments of the RCA
- The right marginal branches between the RCA (before the crux) and the PDA.

Anastomoses of the right Kugel artery are more common angiographically than those of the left Kugel artery [50]. All authors are in agreement that anastomoses are more frequent in patients with a history of infarction. The role of anastomoses in the maintenance of myocardial function, in the degree of severity of coronary disease, in patient survival and in the risk of sudden death has been the subject of many discussions and clinical and experimental studies [49, 52–56]. It has not been clearly demonstrated that LV function during rest is better when there is well-developed collateral circulation, though such a condition ensures a greater vasodilator reserve in the area concerned [57] and seems to limit effectively the extent of myocardial fibrosis [58]. Such factors are in agreement with certain clinico-angiographic observations: total coronary artery occlusions without collateral supply are very often the cause of quite extensive myocardial necrosis and even perhaps of an early aneurysm; and total occlusions not complicated by infarction in the corresponding area are always associated with the presence of compensatory circulation.

From a practical point of view, during coronary arteriography the operator must ensure adequate filling of the coronary artery with contrast medium to be certain that anastomoses are not overlooked. Collateral circulation is better and more completely visible after administration of nitroglycerin, which has an effect on the transstenotic pressure gradient, distal vasodilatation and intramyocardial pressure, and can suppress a spasm. Intercoronary anastomoses very often provide retrograde perfusion in stenosed or occluded arteries and produce images of back-and-forth flow at the junction point of retrograde and anterograde currents or of competitive flow when opacified blood meets with a current of non-opacified blood. The result may be images of radiolucent spaces which should not be confused with segmental arterial gaps. According to James [59], epicardial anastomoses are more effective than intramyocardial anastomoses (septal ones, for example). This would appear to be logical because the systolic resistances of intramyocardial arteries are more elevated, though the hemodynamic demonstration of this hypothesis has apparently not been made. Coronary arteriography cannot reveal the anastomoses between systemic arteries (mediastinal and bronchial) and coronary arteries as demonstrated in anatomical specimens [45].

3.5 Dolichomega-Arteries and Atheromatous Aneurysms [60–65]

The dolichomega-artery image is found more frequently for the RCA than for the LCA. The artery is abnormally and diffusely dilated, elongated, rigid and more or less sinuous, and the flow of contrast medium becomes laminar (Fig. 26), readily lining the wall with an opaque border which washes out slowly. Sometimes the opacifying agent stagnates in an arterial segment. It has not been demonstrated that this apparently slow-moving perfusion of the artery can cause myocardial ischaemia.

Atheromatous aneurysms of the coronary arteries are observed in around 5% of patients explored. They are generally of small size but sometimes reach impressive dimensions (Figs. 27 and 28). They can be multiple in one or two or even three vessels. There are also transitional forms between true aneurysms and very irregular arteries having anfractuous walls.

3.6 Recanalization

Until recently, recanalization images seemed to be rather exceptional. In 200 repeated coronary arteriographies in our experience, there has been only one definite case of repermeabilization of a vessel which was previously totally occluded [66]. Such a

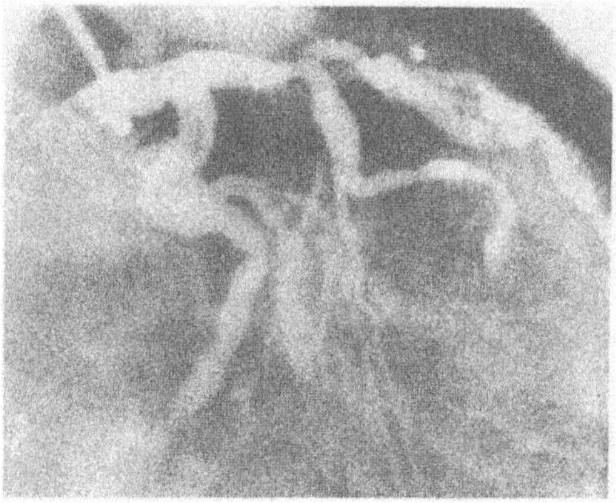

Fig. 26. Right anterior oblique view of a left dolichomega-aneurysmal coronary artery

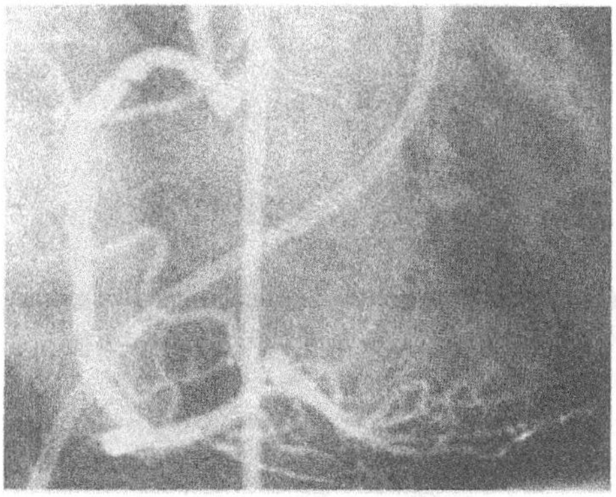

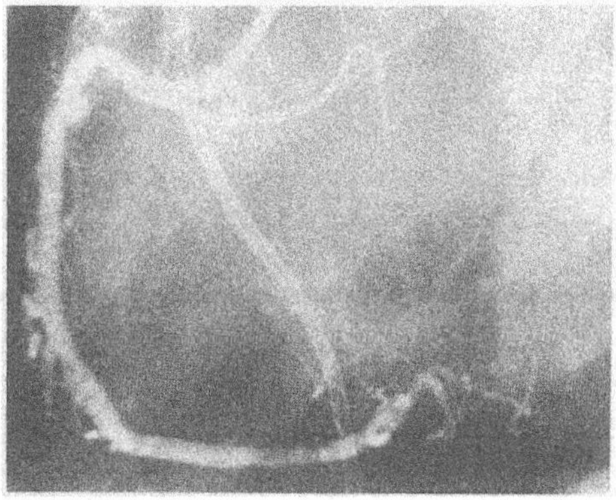

Fig. 27. Small atheromatous aneurysm of the right coronary artery, *(left):* not clearly visible in right anterior oblique projection *(right):* unmasked in left anterior oblique projection

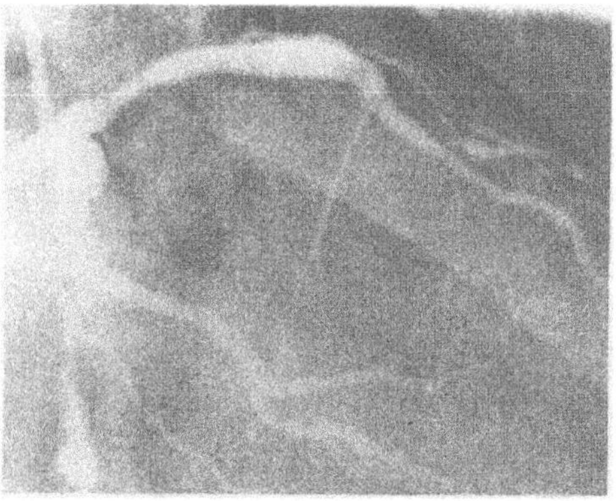

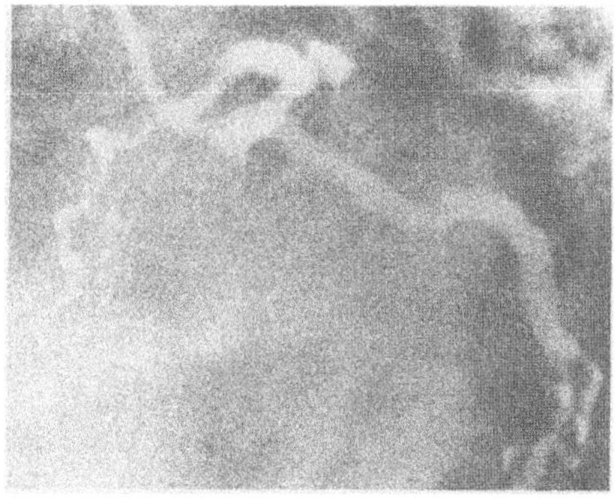

Fig. 28. Irregular atheromatous dilatations and stenoses of the left coronary network. The left anterior oblique view *(right):* shows an aneurysm which was hidden by the opacified left anterior descending artery in right anterior oblique *(left)* projection

case is naturally conducive to the a posteriori diagnosis of thrombosis or embolism [67, 68]. In fact, the recanalization of a thrombosis apparently occurs more frequently than the first coronary arteriography data would lead us to suppose [69]: during autopsy examinations the condition has been observed in 30 out of 75 cases. But the study by De Wood in which coronary arteriography was performed within 24 h after infarction is particularly revealing, as it demonstrates that 87% of patients examined in the first 4 h presented a total arterial occlusion, as compared with only 65% between the 12th and 24th h [70]. Early recanalization has thus been demonstrated, though the exact mechanism has not been made clear – whether spasm or thrombosis or a combination of both factors. The implications of these observations are obviously of considerable importance to vasodilatation and thrombolytic therapy of acute myocardial infarction.

4 Coronary Artery Spasm

Coronary artery spasm is defined angiographically either by local and transient reduction in the calibre of a healthy or slightly affected coronary artery by at least 50% or by significant worsening or total occlusion of a pre-existing stenosis. Evidence of the spasm is sometimes obtained a posteriori once it has disappeared under the influence of a vasodilator. Coronary artery spasm may be iatrogenic, spontaneous or induced. It may be single or multiple and involve one or more vessels. In the presence of a diffuse and reversible reduction in the calibre of the entire coronary network, it would seem more appropriate to speak of vasoconstriction than of vasospasm. The occurrence of iatrogenic spasm, upon contact with the catheter tip, was observed by numerous authors in the early practice of selective coronary arteriography. The hypothesis that spontaneous arterial spasm is a cause of anginal attack was confirmed angiographically by Gensini in 1962 [71]. Later, various authors [72–74] almost simultaneously reported angiographic evidence of the very important role of spasm in the pathogenesis of variant angina as described by Prinzmetal. The relation between spasm and the different varieties of myocardial ischaemia was specified by Maseri [75, 76] and Bertrand [77, 78], the latter having provided a thorough study of the effects of pharmacologically induced spasm [82].

The site of iatrogenic spasm is almost always in the first centimeters of the RCA. The spasm is triggered by the catheter tip, which has generally penetrated too far into the artery. The characteristic image is of a regular, smooth-sided, well-centred progressive proximal narrowing which never completely closes the vessel lumen. The spasm is not accompanied by angina or ECG changes and is ordinarily relieved by sublingual nitroglycerin within 1–3 min (Fig. 29). In rare cases the nitroglycerin must be injected directly into the coronary artery. The frequency of iatrogenic spasm is inversely proportional to the experience and dexterity of the operators. It can currently be estimated, for the RCA, as 1.5%–3% of the cases explored by a competent team. For such a team iatrogenic spasm of the LCA is practically nonexistent.

Spontaneous spasm [79, 80], like spasm induced by a drug [78], generally ergonovine maleate or methylergometrine, is quite different from iatrogenic spasm. It is nearly always the cause of ECG changes (ST segment elevation or depression)

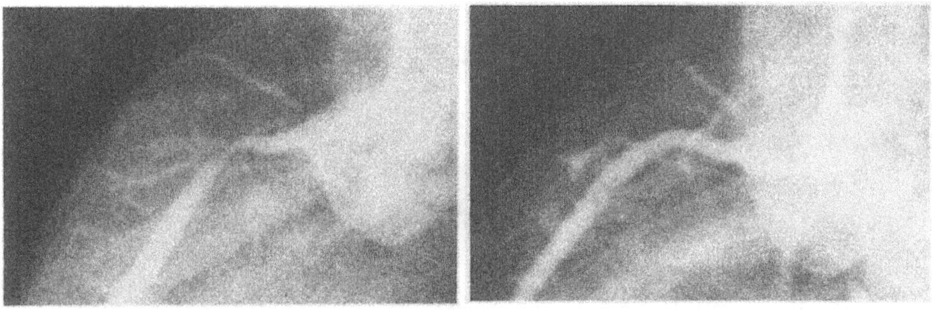

Fig. 29. Left anterior oblique view of an iatrogenic spasm of the right coronary artery *(left):* before and *(right):* after oral administration of nitroglycerin

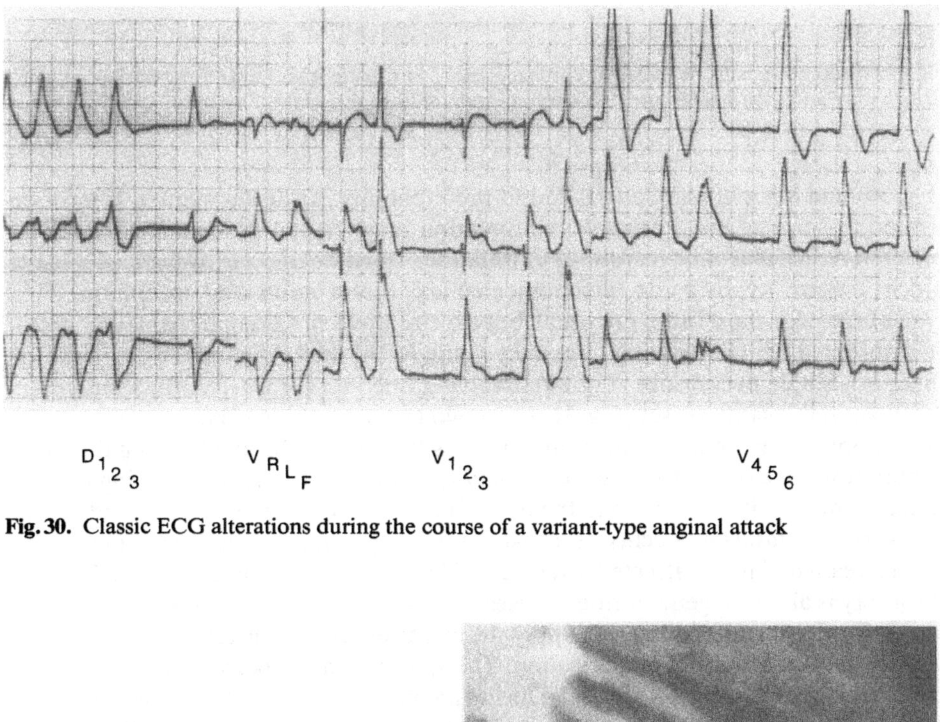

Fig. 30. Classic ECG alterations during the course of a variant-type anginal attack

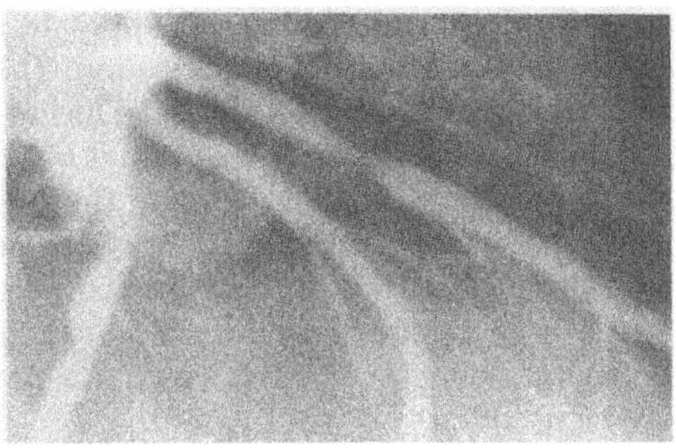

Fig. 31. Right anterior oblique view of a spontaneous spasm of the left anterior descending artery in a patient suffering from variant angina. There is a fixed stenosis of the circumflex

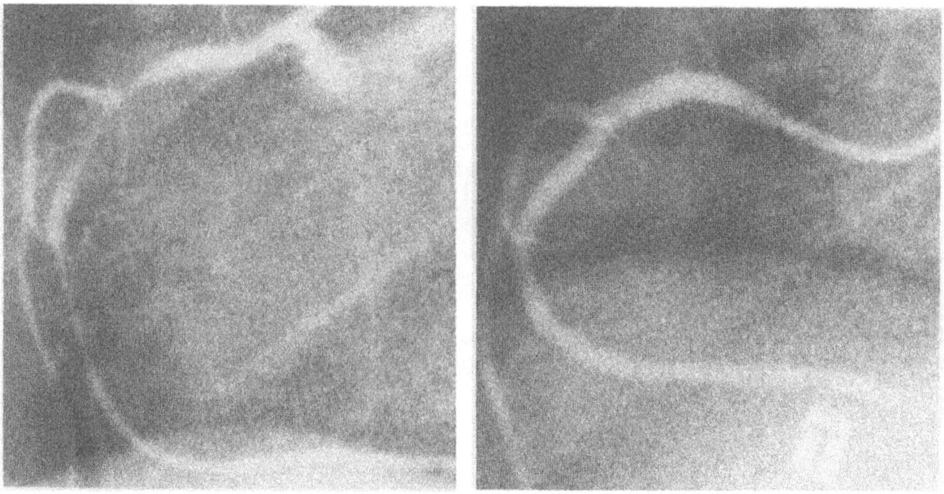

Fig. 32. Multiple spasms of the right coronary artery in a patient suffering from variant angina, *(left):* before and *(right):* after intracoronary injection of nitroglycerin

(Fig. 30) and anginal pain, and is found preferentially in variant angina. It must be treated as soon as possible as its continuation may lead to serious rhythm disturbances (ventricular tachycardia or fibrillation; third-degree atrioventricular heart block), severe hypotension, electromechanical dissociation and infarction. This type of spasm is most often proximal, but a distal site is not exceptional (10%–20%). It is observed with decreasing frequency in the RCA, the LAD and the Cx. Usually, there is a single occurrence (Fig. 31) involving one vessel (85%). Infrequently, it is multiple in the same vessel (Fig. 32) or in two (10%) or three (5%) main vessels. In exceptional cases, spasms with changing sites have been observed during the same exploration. The severity of the spasm may vary with time, and a worsening may be noted from one film sequence to the next. The spontaneous or drug-induced spasm tends to be completely occlusive, causing total angiographic disappearance of the downstream bed in the affected artery (Fig. 33). This obliteration of the distal part of the artery is almost a general rule in cases of variant angina pectoris with normal arteries, for there is no collateral supply. In impaired arteries it tends to be severely stenotic with slight distal opacification. The spasm is more likely to occur in the vicinity of atheromatous lesions [81]. During an anginal attack, whether spontaneous or induced, coronary arterial spasm is observed in almost all patients afflicted with variant angina and in 20%–30% of those with classic angina with ST segment depression. As soon as the spasm has been detected, it should be treated without delay. Administration of oral or intracoronary nitroglycerin (0.3 mg) almost always brings about its disappearance. If this treatment fails, recourse must be had to nifedipine, a calcium antagonist which is a potent coronary dilator. Amiodarone may also be used.

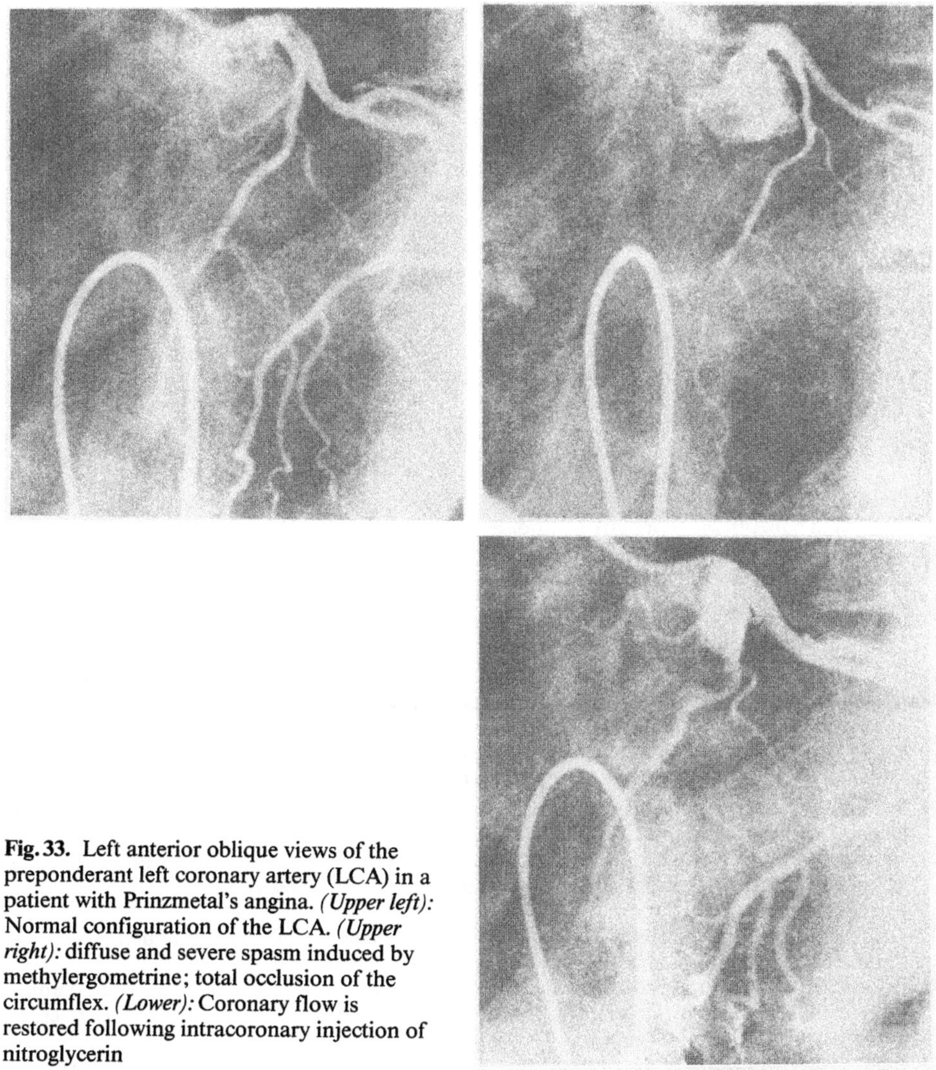

Fig. 33. Left anterior oblique views of the preponderant left coronary artery (LCA) in a patient with Prinzmetal's angina. *(Upper left):* Normal configuration of the LCA. *(Upper right):* diffuse and severe spasm induced by methylergometrine; total occlusion of the circumflex. *(Lower):* Coronary flow is restored following intracoronary injection of nitroglycerin

References

1. Amiel M, Rubet A, Loire R, Diday M, Michaud P, Mikaeloff P, Chassignolle J (1973) Confrontations entre l'angiographie et les données anatomiques per-opératoires ou histologiques dans les anévrysmes du ventricule gauche. Arch Mal Coeur 66: 1135
2. Cheng TO (1971) Incidence of ventricular aneurysm in coronary artery disease. An angiographic appraisal. Am J Med 50: 340
3. Lenegre J, Guize L, Lucsko M (1973) Les anévrysmes ventriculaires. Arch Mal Coeur 66: 7
4. Swanson DA, Chean Ming Liu, Alexander CS, Kieffer SA (1973) Posterior left ventricular pseudoaneurysm. Angiographic pathologic correlation. Radiology 106: 275
5. Higgins CB, Lipton MJ, Johnson AD, Peterson KL, Vieweg WVR (1978) False aneurysms of the left ventricle: identification of distinctive clinical, radiographic, and angiographic features. Radiology 127: 21

6. Cribier A, Cazor JL, Letac B, Soyer R (1980) Quantitative angiographic evaluation in left ventricular aneurysm. Eur J Cardiol 11: 367
7. Dachman AH, Spindola-Franco H, Solomon N (1981) Left ventricular pseudoaneurysm. Its recognition and significance. JAMA 246: 1951
8. Herman MV, Gorlin R (1969) Implications of left ventricular asynergy. Am J Cardiol 23: 538
9. Herman MV, Heinle RA, Klein MD, Gorlin R (1967) Localized disorders in myocardial contraction, asynergy and its role in congestive heart failure. N Engl J Med 277: 222
10. Ideker RE, Behar VS, Wagner GS, Starr JW, Starmer CF, Lee KL, Hackel DB (1978) Evaluation of asynergy as an indicator of myocardial fibrosis. Circulation 57: 715
11. Gorlin R, Klein MD, Sullivan JM (1967) Prospective correlative study of ventricular aneurysm; mechanistic concept and clinical recognition. Am J Med 42: 512
12. Cohn PF, Gorlin R, Adams DF, Chahine RA, Vokonas POS, Herman MV (1974) Comparison of biplane and single plane left ventriculograms in patients with coronary artery disease. Am J Cardiol 33: 1
13. Baxley WA, Reeves TJ (1971) Abnormal regional myocardial performance in coronary artery disease. Prog Cardiovasc Dis 13: 405
14. Slutsky R, Watkins J, Peterson K, Karliner J (1981) The response of left ventricular function and size to atrial pacing, volume loading and afterload stress in patients with coronary artery disease. Circulation 63: 864
15. Leighton RF, Pollack MEM, Welch TG (1975) Abnormal left ventricular wall motion at mid-ejection in patients with coronary heart disease. Circulation 52: 238
16. Johnson LL, Ellis K, Schmidt D (1975) Volume ejected in early systole. A sensitive index of left ventricular performance in coronary artery disease. Circulation 52: 378
17. Slutsky R, Battler A, Karliner JS, Froelicher V, Ashburn W (1980) First-third ejection fraction at rest compared with exercise radionuclide angiography in assessing patients with coronary artery disease. Radiology 136: 197
18. Slutsky R, Karliner JS, Battler A, Peterson K, Ross J Jr (1980) Comparison of early systolic and holosystolic ejection phase indexes by contrast ventriculography in patients with coronary artery disease. Circulation 61: 1083
19. Sniderman AD, Marpole D, Fallen EL (1973) Regional contraction patterns in the normal and ischemic left ventricle in man. Am J Cardiol 31: 484
20. Trieb G (1980) Segmental early relaxation phenomenon (SERP) versus exercise-induced hypokinesia: a correlation study. Clin Radiol 3: 211
21. Moraski SE, Russel RO, Mc Smith K, Rackley CE (1975) Left ventricular function in patients with and without myocardial infarction and one, two or three vessel coronary artery disease. Am J Cardiol 35: 1
22. Feild BJ, Russel RO, Dowling JT, Rackley CE (1972) Regional left ventricular performance in the year following myocardial infarction. Circulation 46: 679
23. Besse P, Pruvot C, Choussat A, Bricaud H (1975) La fonction ventriculaire gauche du coronarien: relations entre les troubles de la cinétique ventriculaire et les altérations de la contractilité myocardique. Arch Mal Coeur 68: 125
24. Caldwell JH, Stewart DK, Dodge HT, Frimer M, Kennedy JW (1978) Left ventricular volume during maximal supine exercise. Circulation 58: 732
25. Sharma B, Goodnin JF, Raphael MJ, Steiner RE, Rainbow RG, Taylor SH (1976) Left ventricular angiography on exercise. A new method of assessing left ventricular function in ischaemic heart disease. Br Heart J 38: 59
26. Popio KA, Gorlin R, Bechtel D, Levine JA (1977) Postextrasystolic potentiation as a predictor of potential myocardial viability. Preoperative analyses compared with studies after coronary bypass surgery. Am J Cardiol 39: 944
27. Cohn PF (1980) Evaluation of inotropic contractile reserve in ischemic heart disease using postextrasystolic potentiation. Circulation 61: 1071
28. Banka VS, Bodenheimer MM, Helfant RH (1975) Determinants of reversible asynergy. The native coronary circulation. Circulation 52: 810
29. Klausner SC, Ratshin RA, Tyberg JV, Lappin HA, Chatterjee K, Parmley WW (1976) Similarity of changes in segmental contraction patterns induced by postextrasystolic potentiation and nitroglycerin. Circulation 54: 615
30. Helfant RH, Pine R, Meister SG, Feldman MS, Trout RG, Banka VS (1974) Nitroglycerin to unmask reversible asynergy. Correlation with post-coronary bypass ventriculography. Circulation 50: 108

31. Rackley CE, Russel RO Jr, Mantle JA, Rogers WJ, Papapietro SE, Schwartz KM (1981) Right ventricular infarction and function. Am Heart J 101: 215
32. Rosch J, Antonovic R, Trenouth RS, Rahimtoola SH, Sim DN, Dotter CT (1976) The natural history of coronary artery stenosis. Radiology 119: 513
33. Mikaeloff P, Amiel M, Delaye J, Saint Pierre A, Dupont JC, Rubet A, Cuisenier J, Boissel JP, De Castro O (1972) Incidence des lésions coronariennes et des données de la cinéventriculographie sur les résultats de la chirurgie de pontage veineux aorto-coronarien. Ann Chir Thorac Cardiovasc 11: 737
34. Amiel M (1977) Quelques difficultés dans l'interprétation de la coronarographie. Ann Cardiol Angeïol 26: 455
35. Brandt PWT, Partridje JB, Wattie WJ (1977) Coronary arteriography; method of presentation of the arteriogram report and a scoring system. Clin Radiol 28: 361
36. Gould KL, Lipscomb K (1974) Effects of coronary stenoses on coronary flow reserve and resistance. Am J Cardiol 34: 48
37. Lipscomb K, Gould KL (1975) Mechanism of the effect of coronary artery stenosis on coronary flow in the dog. Am Heart J 89: 60
38. Gould KL (1978) Pressure-flow characteristics of coronary stenoses in unsedated dogs at rest and during coronary vasodilation. Circ Res 43: 242
39. Brown BG, Bolson E, Frimer M, Dodge HT (1977) Quantitative coronary arteriography. Estimation of dimensions, hemodynamic resistance, and atheroma mass of coronary artery lesions using arteriogram and digital computation. Circulation 55: 329
40. Bjork L, O'Keefe A (1976) Estimation of coronary artery stenosis. Acta Radiol [Diagn] 17: 777
41. Gensini GG (1975) Coronary arteriography. Futura, New York
42. Amiel M, Delaye J, Rubet A, Janin A, Normand J, Pinet F (1972) Inventaire par l'artériographie coronaire sélective de l'athérome dans l'angor coronarien. Ann Radiol 15: 419
43. Lenegre J, Himbert J (1958) Les lésions anatomiques de l'angine de poitrine commune. Arch Mal Coeur 51: 481
44. Lenegre J, Himbert J, Beaumont JL, Froment R, Normand J, Perrin A (1961) Athérosclérose et insuffisance coronarienne. In: XXXIIIe Congrès français de Médecine. Masson, Paris
45. Fulton WFM (1965) The coronary arteries. Thomas, Springfield
46. Shaper W (1971) The collateral circulation of the heart. North Holland, Amsterdam
47. Bourassa MG, Solignac A, Goulet C, Lesperance J (1974) Regression and appearance of coronary collaterals in humans during life. Circulation 50 [Suppl II]: 127
48. Gensini GG, Dacosta BCB (1969) The coronary collateral circulation in living man. Am J Cardiol 24: 393
49. Levin DC, Sos TA, Lee JG, Baltaxe HA (1973) Coronary collateral circulation and distal coronary runoff: the key factors in preserving myocardial contractility in patients with coronary artery disease. AJR 119: 474
50. Soto B, Jochem W, Karp RB, Barcia A (1973) Angiographic anatomy of the Kugel's artery. AJR 119: 503
51. Cohn PF, Maddox DE, Holman BL, See JR (1980) Effect of coronary collateral vessels on regional myocardial blood flow in patients with coronary artery disease. Relation of collateral circulation to vasodilatory reserve and left ventricular function. Am J Cardiol 46: 359
52. Gorlin R (1976) Coronary artery disease. Saunders, Philadelphia
53. Helfant RH, Kemp HG, Gorlin R (1970) The interrelations between extent of coronary artery disease, presence of collaterals, ventriculographic abnormalities and hemodynamics. Am J Cardiol 25: 102
54. Helfant RH, Vokonas PS, Gorlin R (1971) Functional importance of the human coronary collateral circulation. N Engl J Med 284: 1277
55. Levin DC (1974) Pathways and functional significance of the coronary collateral circulation. Circulation 50: 831
56. Tanabe M, Fujiwara S, Ohta N, Shimamoto N, Hirata M (1980) Pathophysiological significance of coronary collaterals for preservation of the myocardium during coronary occlusion and reperfusion in anaesthetised dogs. Cardiovasc Res 14: 288
57. Flameng W, Schwarz F, Hehrlein F (1978) Intra-operative evaluation of the functional significance of coronary collateral vessels in patients with coronary artery disease. Am J Cardiol 42: 187

58. Schwarz F, Schaper J, Becker V, Kubler W, Flameng W (1982) Coronary collateral vessels: their significance for left ventricular histologic structure. Am J Cardiol 49: 291
59. James TN (1970) Angina without coronary disease. Circulation 42: 189
60. Befeler B, Aranda JM, Embi A, Mullin FL, El Sherif N, Lazara R (1977) Coronary artery aneurysms. Study of their etiology, clinical course and effect on left ventricular function and prognosis. Am J Med 62: 597
61. Lipton MJ, Pfeifer FJ, Lopes MG, Hultgren HN (1975) Aneurysms of the coronary arteries in the adult. Clinical and angiographic features. Radiology 117: 11
62. Markis JE, Joffe CD, Cohn PF, Fee DJ, Herman MV, Gorlin R (1976) Clinical significance of coronary arterial ectasia. Am J Cardiol 37: 217
63. Falsetti HL, Carroll RJ (1976) Coronary artery aneurysm; a review of the literature with a report of 11 new cases. Chest 69: 630
64. Sherkat A, Kavanagh Gray D, Edworthy J (1967) Localized aneurysms of the coronary arteries. Radiology 89: 24
65. Vasile N (1975) Anévrysmes congénitaux des coronaires. Ann Radiol 18: 213
66. Amiel M, Mikaeloff Ph, Chassignolle J, Delaye J, Allard D (1976) Angiographic studies after revascularization. In: Lichtlen PR (ed) Coronary angiography and angina pectoris. Thieme, Stuttgart
67. Bourassa MG, Goulet C, Lesperance J (1973) Progression of coronary arterial disease after aortocoronary bypass grafts. Circulation 47–48 [Suppl III]: 127
68. Henderson R, Rowe G (1973) The progression of coronary atherosclerotic disease as assessed by cine-coronary arteriography. Am Heart J 86: 165
69. Levin DC, Baltaxe HA, Lee JG, Sos TA (1975) Potential sources of error in coronary arteriography. II. In interpretation of the study. Am J Roentgenol 124: 386
70. De Wood MA, Spores J, Notske R, Mouser LT, Burroughs R, Golden MS, Lang HT (1980) Prevalence of total coronary occlusion during the early hours of transmural myocardial infarction. N Engl J Med 303: 897
71. Gensini GG, Di Giorgi J, Murad Netto J, Black A (1962) Arteriographic demonstration of coronary artery spasm and its release after the use of a vasodilator in a case of angina pectoris and in the experimental animal. Angiology 13: 550
72. Dhurandhar RW, Watt DL, Silver MD, Trimble AS, Adelman AG (1972) Prinzmetal's variant form of angina with arteriographic evidence of coronary arterial spasm. Am J Cardiol 30: 902
73. Froment R, Normand J, Amiel M (1973) Angine de poitrine de type Prinzmetal. Coronaires perméables mais spasme de l'interventriculaire antérieure en cours de crise. Arch Mal Coeur 66: 755
74. Oliva PB, Potts DE, Pluss RG (1973) Coronary arterial spasm in Prinzmetal angina: documentation by coronary arteriography. N Engl J Med 288: 745
75. Maseri A, Mimmo R, Chierchia S, Marchesi C, Pesola A, L'Abbate A (1975) Coronary artery spasm as a cause of acute myocardial ischemia in man. Chest 68: 625
76. Maseri A, Severi S, De Nes M, L'Abbate A, Chierchia S, Marzilli M, Ballestra AM, Parodi O, Biagini A, Distante A (1978) "Variant" angina: one aspect of a continuous spectrum of vasospastic myocardial ischemia. Pathogenetic mechanisms, estimated incidence and clinical and coronary arteriographic findings in 138 patients. Circulation 42: 1019
77. Bertrand ME, Laisne C, Lefebvre JM, Carre A, Warembourg H Jr, Lekieffre JP (1977) Le spasme des artères coronaires. Arch Mal Coeur 70: 1233
78. Bertrand ME, Lablanche JM, Tilmant PY, Thieuleux FP, Delforge MR (1981) Methergine, provocative testing, experience in 321 cases. In: Bertrand ME (ed) Coronary arterial spasm. Dausse, Paris, p 320
79. Bory M, Benichou M, Sacerdote P, Egre A, Djiane P, Serradimigni A (1981) Les aspects coronarographiques au cours de l'accès ischémique spontané. In: Bertrand ME (ed) Coronary arterial spasm. Dausse, Paris, p 146
80. Maseri A, Persola A, Marzilli M, Severi S, Parodi O, L'Abbate A, Ballestra AM, Maltinti G, De Nes DM, Biagini A (1977) Coronary vasospasm in angina pectoris. Lancet 1: 713
81. Mac Alpin RN (1980) Relation of coronary arterial spasm to sites of organic stenosis. Am J Cardiol 46: 143
82. Bertrand ME, Lablanche JM, Tilmant PY, Thieuleux FA, Delforge MR, Carre AG, Asseman P, Berzin B, Libersa C, Laurent JM (1982) Frequency of provoked coronary arterial spasm in 1089 consecutive patients undergoing coronary arteriography. Circulation 65: 1299

VI Angiographic Explorations: Critical Appraisal of Coronary Arteriography

1 Introduction

The degree of reliability of angiographic documents for analysis depends on several factors

- the film quality of the images (mastery of the techniques of radiological filming and development);
- knowledge of the enlargement factor (choice of a precise method for its measurement);
- certainty that no part of the ventricle or coronary arteries escapes observation (correct centring on the film, and panning, if necessary);
- the possibility of obtaining a complete spatial representation of the left ventricle (LV) (LV filmed in two complementary projections, and simultaneously, if possible – that is, preferably with a biplanar system;
- certainty that all arterial segments are clear, in at least one projection, of any superimposition of an adjacent artery (sufficiently numerous projections and suitable angulations);
- lack of doubt about the atheromatous or vasospastic nature of a stenotic or occlusive lesion (judicious use of nitroglycerin);
- the validity of the methods of measurement chosen;
- and the vigilance, objectivity and competence (level of theoretical knowledge and degree of experience) of the person analysing the ventriculography and coronary arteriography documents.

The problems raised by film technology and development will not be discussed here, as they depend in great part on the knowledge of engineers and technicians. Suffice it to say that the physician must be able to detect shortcomings in their abilities. In the pages which follow, the problems treated will be essentially those directly dependent on physicians or on the inherent limits of the method.

2 Reliability of the Examination

2.1 *Operational Reliability*

A certain number of technical faults likely to produce artefacts or hamper evaluation of arterial segments or the LV should be avoided. Left ventriculography should be performed using a flow of contrast medium in accordance with LV volume and cardiac output. For a normal volume [end-diastolic volume (EDV) = 70 ml/m^2] and

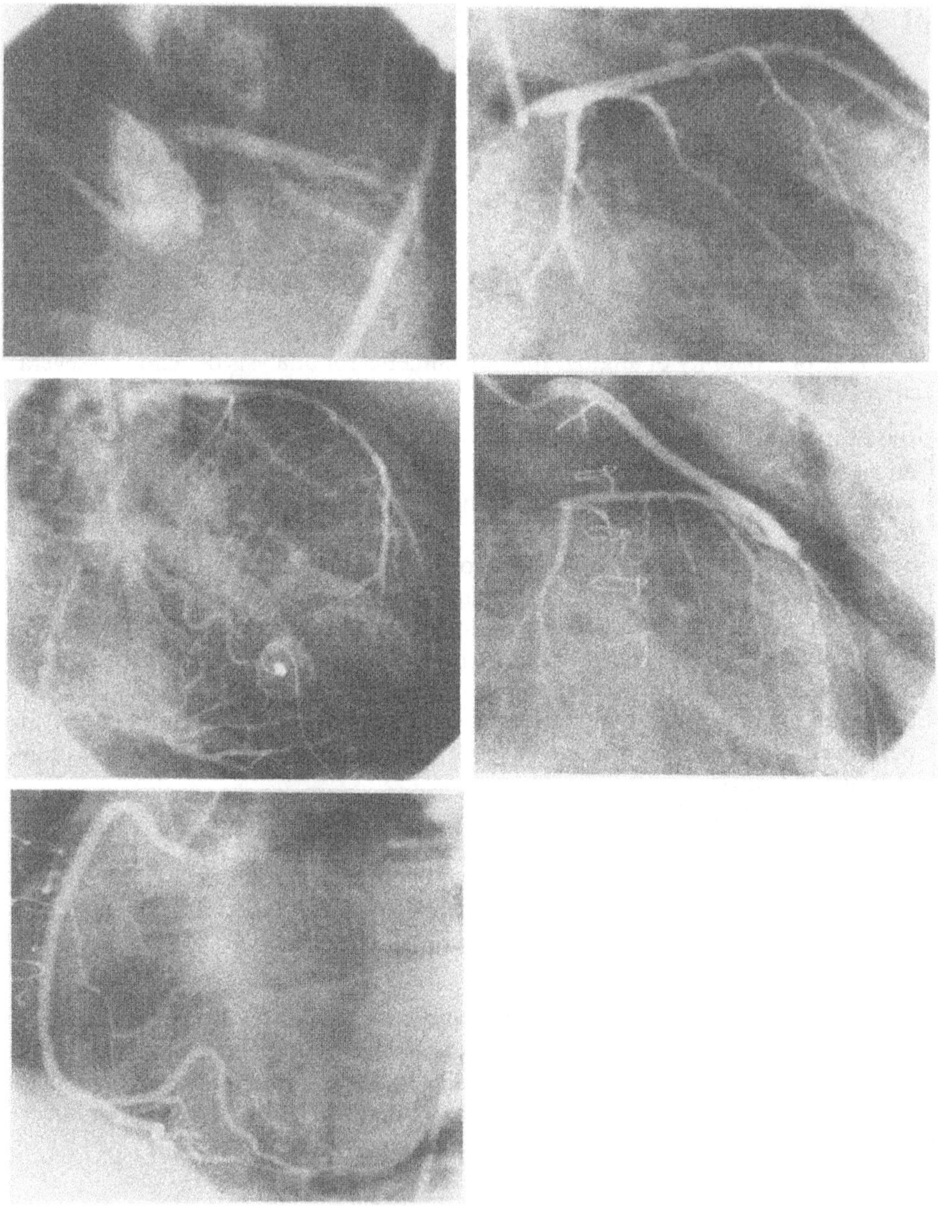

Fig. 1. Subtotal occlusion of the left main coronary trunk. *(Upper left):* Semi-selective injection of the left coronary artery (LCA) by opacification of the left coronary sinus. *(Upper right):* Selective left coronary arteriography: the resemblance to the mouthpiece of a flute and the absence of backward flow of the contrast medium into the aorta are signs indicative of ostial or para-ostial stenosis. *(Middle left):* Selective right coronary arteriography: there is a delayed opacification of the LCA by means of multiple heterolateral intercoronary anastomoses. *(Middle right):* Aortocoronary bypass on the left anterior descending artery: good perfusion of the entire LCA. *(Lower):* Right coronary examination after surgery: the anastomoses with the LCA are no longer functional

a normal cardiac frequency ($\leqslant 75$/min), injection of 45 ml contrast medium during 3 or 4 s generally makes it possible to avoid extrasystoles and to obtain good highlighting of the endocardial outline, without which calculation of LV wall thickness and mass is impossible. In case of cardiac erethism with rapid wash-out of the ventricle, of a small heart (a young woman), or of a very dilated LV (pseudomyocardiopathy), the volume and flow of the contrast medium must be adjusted as necessary.

During coronary arteriography, the operator should adapt the volume and rate of injection of contrast medium to the size and flow of each coronary artery [1]. He should obtain a complete filling of the vessel without lacuna-like images (radiotransparent areas) or a laminar or heterogeneous flow suggestive of false narrowing. The injection should be stopped only when the entire vessel is opacified from its orifice to its most distal branches. The operator should avoid overinjection of contrast medium, which can flow back into the aorta and the sinuses of Valsalva and conceal the proximal part of the artery like a smoke-screen. A slight backflow of the product is nevertheless useful in evaluating the coronary ostium correctly, and a total absence of backflow suggests the possibility of ostial stenosis (Fig. 1). A semi-selective injection in a sinus can thus be helpful. The operator should be careful not to insert the catheter too far beyond the ostium for fear of overlooking a para-ostial lesion. Visualization of the left anterior descending artery (LAD) or circumflex (Cx) alone is indicative of possible side by side origin of the two arteries or of a very short common trunk. Only after these possibilities have been eliminated will the operator search for a truly abnormal origin of these arteries (see Part II, Chap. IV). When the downstream bed of a totally occluded LAD is not visible after opacification of the left coronary artery (LCA) and right coronary artery (RCA), it may be necessary to do selective injection of a right conus artery originating separately from the aorta (Fig. 2; see also Fig. 23 in Part II, Chap. V). Once the exploration is completed, the operator should go over the entire video recording and verify that the most crucial areas have been filmed and displayed correctly and without ambiguity: the left

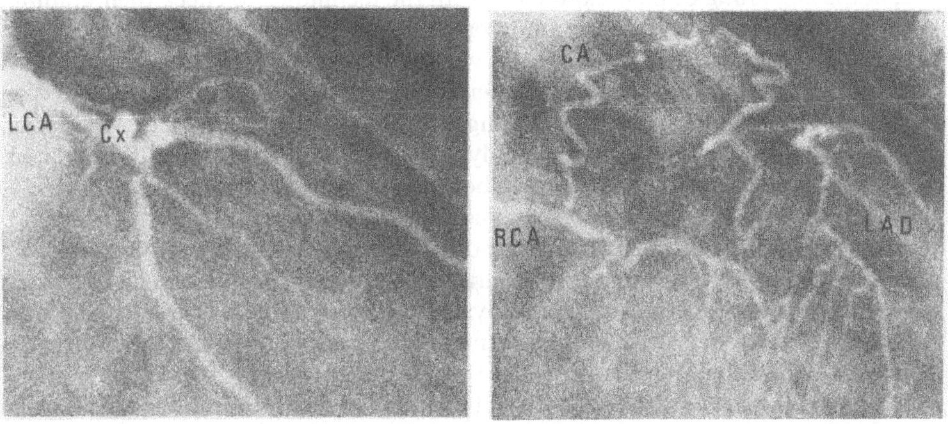

Fig. 2. Total occlusion of the left anterior descending artery *(LAD)* at its point of origin. *(Left):* Left coronary arteriography: the operator may suppose that there is isolated origin of the *LAD*. *(Right):* Right coronary arteriography: the right conus artery supplies the normally located *LAD*

main coronary trunk; the LAD-Cx bifurcation; the origin of the LAD, the Cx and the main diagonal and left marginal branches; the bifurcation of the RCA at the level of the crux; and the origin of the PDA.

2.2 Reliability of the Method and Correlations Between Anatomical and Angiographic Findings

Many authors have compared the findings of coronary arteriography with those of intra-operative or postmortem anatomical analysis [2–5]. As a result, the notion has become widespread that coronary arteriography tends to underestimate atheromatous lesions, particularly stenoses of the proximal LAD, of the RCA in the region of the crux, and all those located at a bifurcation. The smaller the diameter of the vessel, the greater the risk of error. On the other hand, overevaluation of a stenosis, indicating a possibly unnecessary surgical intervention, is rare. The general underestimation may be due to the fact that in spite of multiple projections the smallest diameter of a stenosis is not always detected [6]. The vasodilator effects of the contrast medium and sometimes of the nitroglycerin or of the drugs taken by the patient are also probably involved. In our opinion, the lack of vessel distention by intraluminal blood pressure is, on the contrary, a cause of overestimation of the narrowings in postmortem studies.

2.3 Reliability of Interpretation

Every practitioner of coronary arteriography knows that his own analysis of the same film can vary in two interpretations separated by a period of time and, especially, that his assessment of the stenoses can differ from those of his colleagues. Even the nearly universal adoption of a semi-quantitative method of grading lesions has not avoided these difficulties. It is a good idea for all the operators and analysts in the same laboratory to spend one or more sessions together interpreting films and, at the beginning of their experience with the technique, to check their grading quantitatively with a compass or a micrometric magnifying glass. Various authors have evaluated as exactly as possible this variability in coronary arteriography interpretation for the same analyst and between different analysts [7–10]. The rate of disagreement among four analysts in grading a stenosis of the LAD can be as great as 50% [8]. The rate of error for a single analyst is 18%, and a 75% stenosis is evaluated incorrectly 31 times out of 100. The collaboration of three analysts makes it possible practically to eliminate these errors [9]. The majority opinion is not always right and can be wrong half the time, with false positives being sometimes more numerous than false negatives [10]. A report by Bourassa [11], as part of the National Institutes of Health Coronary Artery Surgery Study, indicates that as far as variations among analysts are concerned there is significantly conflicting opinion on 15% of the lesions analysed, with clinical consequences for 7% of the lesions. The number of errors is proportional to fatigue, to the number of examinations interpreted during the same session and to the number of lesions present in the same coronary network. Knowledge of patient history (myocardial infarction, for example) sometimes leads to overevaluation of a lesion.

3 Significance of Lesions

3.1 The Concept of Significant Stenosis

The concept of significant stenosis should be related to that of myocardial ischaemia. In our opinion, a stenosis is to be considered significant when it reduces the lumen diameter of the vessel by 75% or more, which corresponds to a reduction in cross-sectional area of 90%–95%. This definition of the significant quality of a stenosis would appear to be rather accurate. The experimental studies of Gould and Lipscomb [12–14] have in fact demonstrated that a stenosis causes the appearance of a pressure gradient and of a reduction in coronary flow during rest when it reaches 80% in the case of a short stenosis and merely 60% in the case of a long stenosis. As long as this degree of severity is not reached, the coronary reserve flow (hyperaemic reaction due to vasodilatation downstream from the stenosis) ensures preservation of sufficient local output during rest. However, the coronary reserve flow begins to diminish when the vessel lumen is reduced by 30%–45%, which explains why myocardial ischaemia can occur during exercise in the presence of stenoses of less than 80%. The coronary reserve flow drops very rapidly when the stenosis is greater than 85%, and becomes nil at 95%.

The true quantitative evaluation of stenosis severity would be very useful in determining its exact physiopathological significance. The first attempts at this consisted in measuring the exact diameter of the stenosis and of the healthy artery by reference to the known diameter of the catheter. A greater degree of precision was obtained by measuring the reduction in cross-sectional area of the vessel [1, 15, 16]. Current research is directed towards videodensitometric measurements and computer-assisted spatial reconstruction of the stenosis [17–19]. In the future, thanks to techniques of digitization of the video image and automatic analysis, experiments currently limited to a few research laboratories will become part of routine practice.

3.2 The Concept of a Global Lesional Score

Various authors [20–24] have worked out scoring systems in an effort to provide an overall assessment of the severity of coronary artery disease in patients. Their purpose has been twofold: to appraise future risks better and thus determine the prognosis for survival and operability of a given patient, and to search for possible similarities in the lesions of identical clinical groups. These scoring systems take into account the number of coronary lesions, their severity, their site, the quality of the downstream bed, the collateral circulation, the LV contraction anomalies, and, for some authors, the area of myocardium either subject to necrosis or necrosed.

4 Pitfalls in Interpretation [25]

In 30° right anterior oblique (RAO) projection, a total obstruction of the LAD, with no distal opacification by collateral arteries, may at first glance go undetected because the main diagonal artery is mistaken for the LAD. However, in the absence of right ventricular hypertrophy, the diagonal artery always runs along the anterosupe-

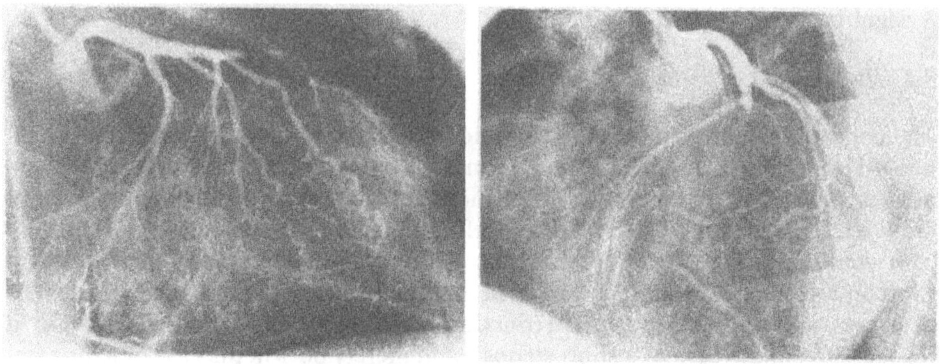

Fig. 3. Complementary nature of the orthogonal projections for exact identification of the arteries. *(Left):* Right anterior oblique view of the left coronary artery (LCA): probable total occlusion of the left anterior descending artery (LAD) and possible opacification of the PDA by anastomoses from the circumflex (Cx). *(Right):* left anterior oblique view of the LCA: confirmation of occlusion of the LAD; the Cx is opacifying a diaphragmatic artery of the left ventricle and not the PDA

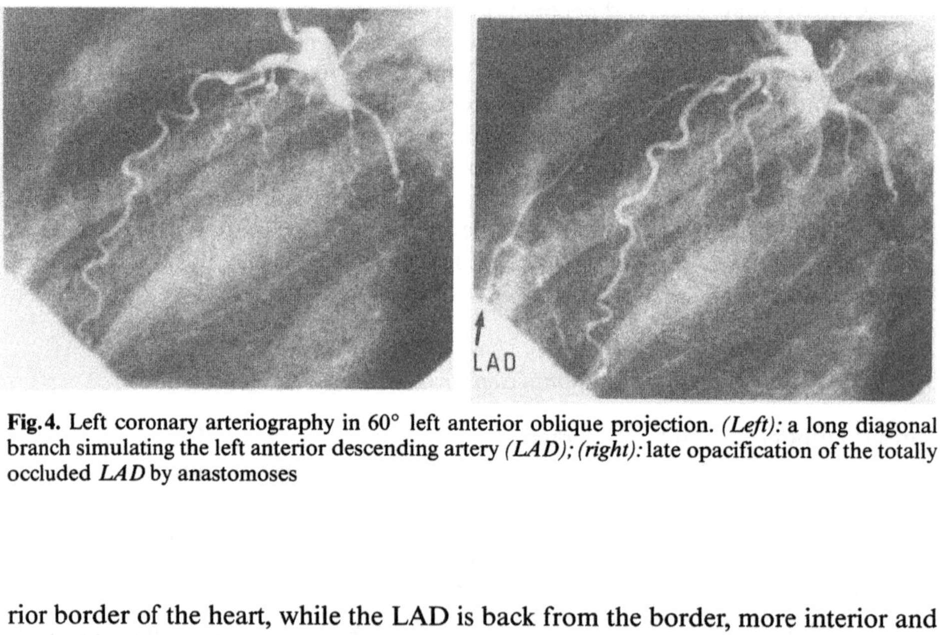

Fig. 4. Left coronary arteriography in 60° left anterior oblique projection. *(Left):* a long diagonal branch simulating the left anterior descending artery *(LAD); (right):* late opacification of the totally occluded *LAD* by anastomoses

rior border of the heart, while the LAD is back from the border, more interior and vertical in the cardiac mass, and terminates in two small branches behind the apex. Moreover, a search for the septal arteries should lead to the realization that the distal LAD is not visualized. Left anterior oblique (LAO) and transverse projections readily indicate the early total occlusion of the LAD (Figs. 3 and 4).

Also in RAO projection a first or second septal artery of very large calibre may be initially mistaken for a diagonal or marginal branch. This error is immediately rectified once the coronary network is observed in transverse projection. The superimposition of diagonal branches, and sometimes of the first left marginal branches, on the proximal LAD should not result in the overlooking of a stenosis concealed by

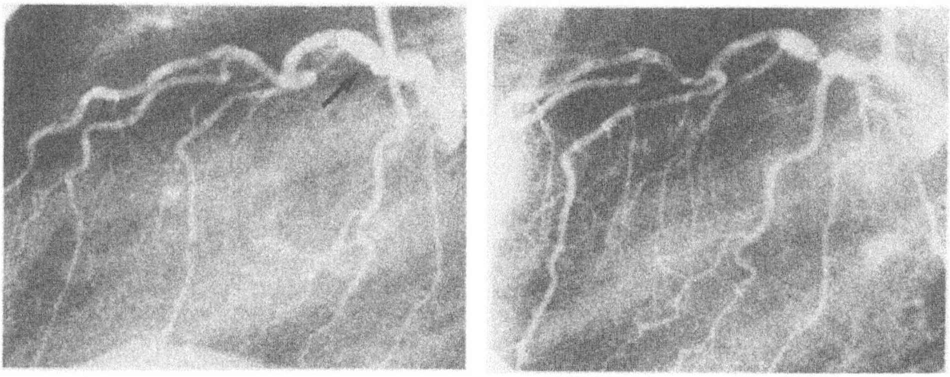

Fig. 5. Transverse view of the left coronary artery. Very severe proximal stenosis of the left anterior descending artery *(left):* poorly visible in transverse projection *(arrow)* but *(right):* clearly visible with the addition of a caudocranial projection

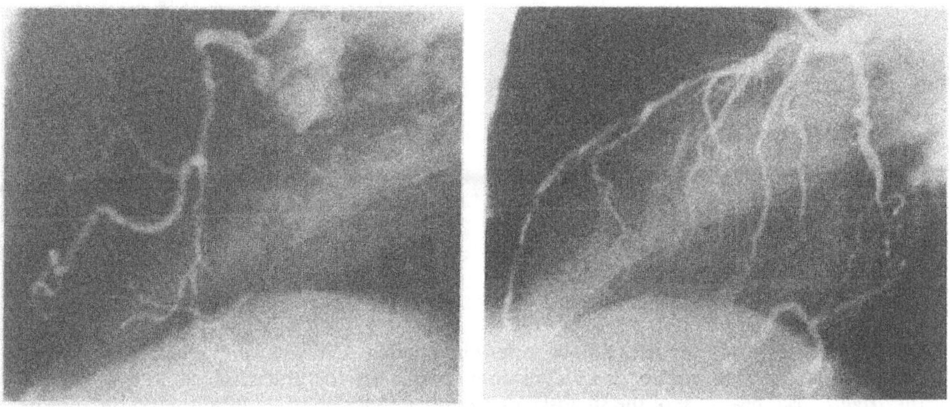

Fig. 6. Total occlusion of a preponderant right coronary artery (RCA). *(Left):* Transverse view of the RCA. Diffuse atheromatous deposits responsible for the pseudohypotrophic appearance of the artery. *(Right):* Transverse view of the left coronary artery. The circumflex is opacifying the distal part of the preponderant RCA

this artery if the operator systematically performs multiple projections and has recourse to double-oblique projections (Fig. 5).

Certain total obstructions of the left marginal branches at their point of origin can only be detected late in the film sequence when there is slight revascularization from the diagonal branches or the RCA. A total early obstruction of the RCA immediately downstream from the point of origin of a main marginal branch may make it appear, in the absence of distal revascularization, that the RCA is hypotrophic (Fig. 6). In RAO projection a proximal stenosis of the PDA may be mistaken for a large diaphragmatic branch of the LV. This error may be avoided if caudocranial 30°–40° LAO projection is performed (Fig. 7). Administration of nitroglycerin should clear up any possible confusion between a spasm and an atheromatous stenosis (Fig. 8).

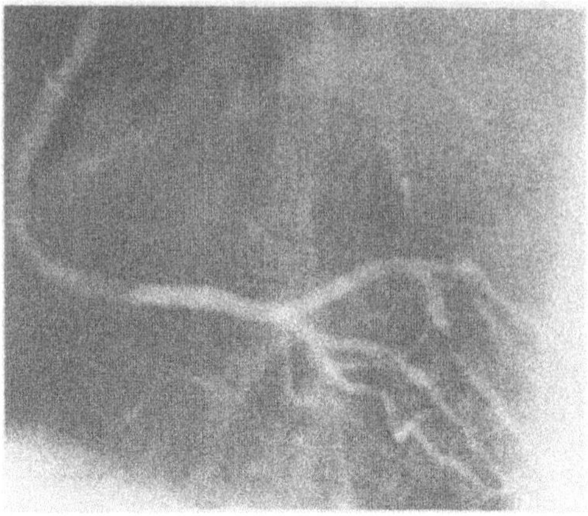

Fig. 7. Thirty- to forty-degree left anterior oblique and 20°–25° caudocranial double-oblique projection providing good separation, identification and analysis of the distal branches of the right coronary artery: PDA and diaphragmatic branches

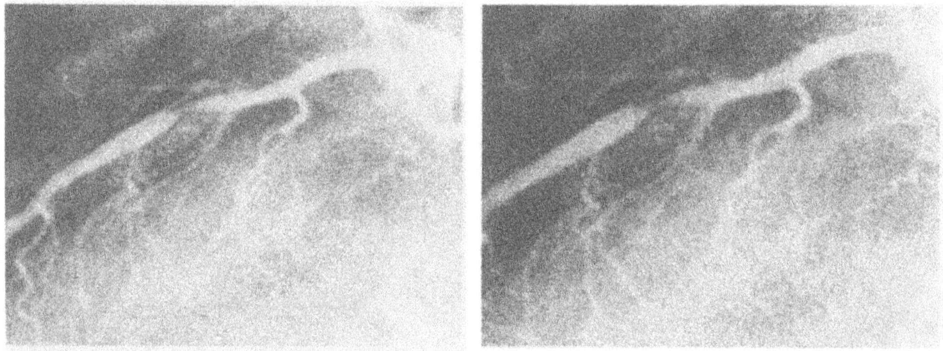

Fig. 8. Transverse view of the left coronary artery in a patient afflicted with variant angina. *(Left):* severe stenosis of the left anterior descending artery persisting after oral administration of nitroglycerin; *(right):* disappearance of the stenosis after intracoronary injection of nitroglycerin, thus demonstrating the spastic nature of the lesion

The other pitfalls in interpretation are mainly related to congenital anomalies or anatomical variants. Before concluding that there is total obstruction of a main vessel at its origin, the operator should search for one of the following conditions, either using aortography involving the Valsalva manoeuvre or selective opacification:

- a side by side origin of the LAD and the Cx
- an elevated origin of the LCA or the RCA
- a LAD or Cx originating from the RCA
- a single coronary artery.

Still other anomalies are possible (see Part II, Chap. IV). The principal anatomical variants more or less likely to cause confusion are a double PDA, a PDA originating from a right marginal branch, a short LAD, the origin of an anterior septal artery from a diagonal branch or from the RCA, a double LAD, and a LAD associated with a large parallel diagonal branch.

5 Methodology of Coronary Arteriographic Analysis

The need to apply strict rules of interpretation to coronary arteriography analysis is obvious to radiologists, cardiologists and surgeons. The prognosis for the patient and the choice of treatment depend on it. The following is a list of the rules that in our opinion are fundamental:

- a perfect knowledge of the patient's case history
- an examination which is reliable radiologically and for surgery (see above)
- identification of the anatomical type of coronary circulation: right- or left-preponderant or balanced
- systematic analysis of each vessel over its entire length, from beginning to end, followed by similar analysis of its main branches
- identification of stenoses, of their proximal or distal site, and of their severity (taking complementary projections into consideration)
- observation of collateral circulation and anastomoses
- assessment of the quality of the arterial runoff and vessel diameter
- recognition of the existence of a myocardial bridge
- evaluation of the anatomical suitability of each vessel for surgery
- determination of the extent of the non-perfused or underperfused vascular areas and correlation of these findings with the quantitative analysis of wall kinetics and LV function.

In all cases, the physician who performs coronary arteriography analysis should weigh matters carefully and proceed without haste. He should not concentrate on the severest lesions or an interesting anomaly to the point of neglecting analysis of some arterial segments. Whenever possible, there should be at least two persons viewing the film; if alone, the operator should re-examine the same film with a delay of 24 h or more. The requirement of reporting his analysis on a chart or, for example, filling in a microcomputer form, is a useful means of maintaining the vigilance of the analyst [20–24].

References

1. Amiel M (1977) Quelques difficultés dans l'interprétation de la coronarographie. Ann Cardiol Angeïl 26: 455
2. Grondin CM, Dyrda I, Pasternac A, Campeau L, Bourassa MG, Lesperance J (1974) Discrepancies between cineangiographic and postmortem findings in patients with coronary artery disease and recent myocardial revascularization. Circulation 49: 703
3. Hutchins GM, Bulkey BH, Ridolfi RL, Griffith LSC, Lohr FT, Piasio MA (1977) Correlation of coronary arteriograms and left ventriculograms with postmortem studies. Circulation 56: 32
4. Isner JM, Kishel J, Kent KM, Ronan JA Jr, Ross AM, Roberts WC (1981) Accuracy of angiographic determination of left main coronary arterial narrowing: angiographic-histologic correlative analysis in 28 patients. Circulation 63: 1056
5. Vlodaver Z, Frech R, van Tassel RA, Edwards JE (1973) Correlation of the antemortem coronary arteriogram and the postmortem specimen. Circulation 47: 162
6. Bourassa MG (1980) In: chap. 11 exploration de la circulation coronarienne par la coronarographie. Cachera JP, Bourassa MG (eds) La maladie coronarienne. Flammarion, Paris, p 233
7. Detre KM, Wright PH, Murphy ML, Takaro T (1975) Observer agreement in evaluating coronary angiograms. Circulation 52: 979

8. Zir LM, Miller SW, Dinsmore RE, Gilbert JP, Harthorne JW (1976) Interobserver variability in coronary angiography. Circulation 53: 627
9. De Rouen TA, Murray JA, Owen W (1977) Variability in the analysis of coronary arteriograms. Circulation 55: 324
10. Galbraith JE, Murphy ML, De Soysa N (1978) Coronary angiogram interpretation. Interobserver variability. JAMA 240: 2053
11. Bourassa MG (1980) In: chap. 11 exploration de la circulation coronarienne par la coronarographie. Cachera JP, Bourassa MG (eds) La maladie coronarienne. Flammarion, Paris, p 235
12. Gould KL, Lipscomb K (1974) Effects of coronary stenoses on coronary flow reserve and resistance. Am J Cardiol 34: 48
13. Lipscomp K, Gould KL (1975) Mechanism of the effect of coronary artery stenosis on coronary flow in the dog. Am Heart J 89: 60
14. Gould KL (1978) Pressure-flow characteristics of coronary stenoses in unsedated dogs at rest and during coronary vasodilation. Circ Res 43: 242
15. Fester A, Mildner FJ (1977) Cross-sectional coronary artery stenosis. Cathet Cardiovasc Diagn 3: 107
16. Conti CR, Pepine CJ, Feldman RL, Curry RC, Christie LG, Nichols WW (1979) Angiographic definition of critical coronary stenosis. Adv Cardiol 26: 100
17. Brown BG, Bolson E, Frimer M, Dodge HT (1977) Quantitative coronary arteriography. Estimation of dimensions, hemodynamic resistance, and atheroma mass of coronary artery lesions using arteriogram and digital computation. Circulation 55: 329
18. Crawford DW, Brooks SH, Barndt R, Blankenhorn DH (1977) Measurement of atherosclerotic luminal irregularity and obstruction by radiographic densitometry. Invest Radiol 12: 307
19. Cherrier F, Booman F, Serruys PW, Cuilliere M, Danchin N, Reiber JHC (1981) L'angiographie coronaire quantitative. Application à l'évaluation des angioplasties transluminales coronaires. Arch Mal Coeur 74: 1377
20. Friesinger GC, O'Neal Humphries J, Ross RC (1973) Prognostic significance of coronary arteriography. In: Kaltenbach M (ed) Coronary heart disease. Thieme, Stuttgart
21. Gensini GG (ed) (1975) Coronary arteriography. Futura, New-York, p 271
22. A reporting system on patients evaluated for coronary artery disease. Report of the Ad Hoc Committee for Grading of Coronary Artery Disease, Council on Cardio-vascular Surgery (1975) American Heart Association. Circulation 51: 5
23. Brandt PWT, Partridge JB, Wattie WJ (1977) Coronary arteriography: method of presentation of the arteriogram report and a scoring system. Clin Radiology 28: 361
24. Alderman EL, Hamilton KK, Silverman J, Harrison DC, Sanders WJ (1982) Anatomically flexible, computer-assisted reporting system for coronary angiography. Am J Cardiol 49: 1208
25. Levin DC, Baltaxe HA, Sos TA (1975) Potential sources of error in coronary arteriography. II. In interpretation of the study. A J R 124: 386

VII Angiographic Explorations: Natural History of Coronary Atheroma and Clinico-Angiographic Correlations

The fact that atheroma impairs the coronary arteries at an early age has been well known since Enos in 1953 reported his autopsy observations in young American men killed in Korea. It is also well known that there is no parallel between the anatomical and clinical severity of the disease, which, in the case of one or more identical arterial stenoses, can be revealed by sudden death, infarction or anginal attack.

1 Beginning and Progression of the Disease

1.1 Coronary Arteries

Lenegre's anatomical studies [1] showed originally that there was no very marked difference between coronary lesions due to infarction and those due to angina. The first coronary arteriography studies, reported by major centres between 1965 and 1974 [2–10], confirmed this notion and demonstrated that the severity and diffusion of the lesions were not necessarily proportional to the length of the patient's clinical history. Since then it has been imperative to assess the mode of onset and progression of coronary lesions by means of repeated coronary arteriographic examinations of the same subject. The first study of this type was carried out by Bemis [11]. Seventy-three patients underwent coronary arteriography at mean intervals of 24 months. The group was heterogeneous both clinically and therapeutically and had been selected on the criterion that all the patients remained symptomatic or became symptomatic again between the two examinations. A worsening of the disease was noted in 52% of cases, consisting either in a progression of the pre-existing lesions (58%) or the appearance of new plaques or atheromatous stenoses in arterial segments previously intact (30%) or impaired (12%). The progression of the lesions was the same for the three main vessels, affecting the proximal segments and the bifurcations in 98% of cases and being more marked in patients under 40 years of age, in those who initially had had a severer disease and in those with an abnormal glucide or lipid metabolism. Development of collateral circulation was related to an increase in the severity of the stenoses. Studies by Bruschke [12] and Kimbiris [13], including respectively 37 and 35 patients, are in agreement with Bemis' but introduce the idea that lesions can regress and that an infarction can occur without apparent worsening of the lesions.

Amiel studied 75 patients (50 were treated surgically, 25 were not, with a mean interval of 25 months between the two coronary arteriography examinations [14]. He evaluated the rate of progression per patient at 2.5% per month and per vessel at 1% per month. In other words, a patient who is not operated upon runs a 10% per year risk that a pre-existing lesion will worsen and a 5% per year risk that a new lesion will appear. The progression of the lesions depends neither on the vessel involved nor on the severity of the stenosis, and it is greater in younger subjects. Rösch's study [15], including 58 coronary patients explored a second time after a mean interval of 28 months, showed that almost all the stenoses which progressed and the total occlusions which appeared were recorded in 66% of the subjects, whereas 34% remained almost entirely unaffected. The progression of the lesions was slightly related to general risk factors, being a little greater for stenoses with collateral circulation and for the right coronary artery (RCA). Tubular stenoses with ulcerating plaques showed a high tendency to progress.

The major criticism to be made about the above works is that they essentially included subjects with severe coronary artery disease, that is potential candidates for surgery, some of whom were in fact operated on. More recently, the Montreal Heart Institute group [16] had the opportunity of repeating coronary arteriography in 48 patients with normal (22 cases) or not significantly impaired (26 cases) arteries. Two coronary arteriography examinations were performed with a mean time interval of 42 months. No atherosclerotic lesions developed in the group of 22 patients with normal arteries, even though two of them had suffered myocardial infarction. Among the 26 patients with less than 50% narrowing, worsening of the stenoses was observed in 27% of cases. For two arteries occlusion became total. In this group two patients also suffered myocardial infarction, one with and the other without angiographic evidence of a worsening of his coronary disease. Thus it would seem that over a period 3 years a middle-aged adult with healthy arteries has the maximum chance of maintaining this anatomical advantage. On the other hand, an adult with mild coronary atheroma has a 25% chance of his disease worsening, a probability which is proportionally higher for the younger adult.

As far as the progression of significant stenoses (greater than or equal to 50%) in non-surgical coronary patients is concerned, the very important recent work of Bruschke [17] provides quite useful additional information. This study includes 256 non-surgical coronary patients (mean age 49.2 years) with a relatively low number of women (7%), as is the case in all series excluding subjects over 60 or 65 years of age. The mean interval between the two coronary arteriographic examinations was greater than a year for 213 patients. Many were logical candidates for surgery, and 92 were undergoing repeated examinations systematically because the waiting period before surgery was too long. A progression in lesions was noted in one arterial segment in at least 56.3% of the total group of patients. The number of patients whose condition worsened was in proportion to the length of the interval between two explorations: 40% for an interval of less than a year and 92% for an interval greater than 5 years. The tendency for stenoses to progress was greatest for the RCA, the left anterior descending artery (LAD) distal from the first septal branch and the first diagonal branch, and the main left marginal branch. The angiographic progression of lesions was not related to age, sex, tobacco use or lipid disorders; however, it must be remembered that this was a short- or middle-term study. Most of the patients who suffered infarction between the two examinations had a worsening of their lesions, although this was not an absolute rule. The two most significant factors determining lesion progression were the degree of initial severity of the stenoses and the length of time between two coronary arteriographic examinations. In

12 (4.7%) of the 256 patients a regression of the lesions was observed. In five of these cases an occlusion was transformed into a narrowing, and recanalization of a thrombus would seem likely to have occurred. In the other seven cases the reduction in the degree of arterial narrowing was indubitable. All the examinations without exception were performed after administration of nitroglycerin; thus the reality of regression of a stenosis is a plausible notion. Moreover, it does not exclude the progression of stenoses in a subject's other branches (three cases).

The contemporary study by Kramer [18] is in perfect agreement with Bruschke's, although the results are expressed in slightly different form. Kramer studied 335 subjects, including 262 with at least one stenosis (greater than or equal to 50%) in at least one major artery. The second coronary arteriographic examination was performed after a mean interval of 36 months. In the 262 subjects with stenoses a progression of lesions was observed in 1.3 arteries per patient, corresponding to an annual impairment rate of 14%; that is, each year 14% of the group was exposed to a worsening of lesions. Most often progression affected one (71%) vessel, and less frequently two (25%) or three (4%). A regression of stenoses was detected in 20 patients (6%). The development of the lesions was more marked in subjects under 50 years of age and did not seem to be influenced by the customary risk factors: family history, blood pressure, diabetes, tobacco use, weight and lipid disorders.

1.2 Left Ventricle

The appearance and progression of left ventricular (LV) lesions is closely related to the severity and spread of coronary lesions [16–20]. However, the correspondence is not strict. A progression of arterial lesions was noted in only 73.3% of patients who presented a transmural infarction between the first and second coronary arteriographic examinations in Bruschke's series [17] and in 62% in Kramer's series [18]. Markis [20] studied 36 patients explored twice with a mean interval of 26 months whose LV function was practically unaltered. He notes that the ejection fraction (EF) was stable in subjects without progression of coronary lesions, whereas it dropped from 0.60 to 0.52 for those with impaired coronary lesions. The general opinion, confirmed by Markis, is that LAD occlusion plays a more negative role than that of the RCA or circumflex (Cx) in the drop in EF and the deterioration in LV function. This is due, as shown by Bertrand [21], to the sole fact that more LV wall segments are generally affected by occlusion of the LAD. All authors are in agreement with the fact that alteration of LV function depends in part on the increase in the degree of stenoses but especially on their multiplication and spread to several vessels. In most cases LV dysfunction is also closely related to occurrence of transmural or subendocardial infarction. However, alteration of wall kinetics would sometimes appear to be independent of the degradation of stenoses or of an identifiable intercurrent infarction. Such observations suggest the possible influence of different factors: transient myocardial ischaemia, underestimated or unrecognized arterial lesions, recanalized occlusion, or progressive development of myocardial fibrosis due to recurrent ischaemia [20]. The role of collateral circulation remains poorly explained: it is always indicative of severe arterial stenoses, and it sometimes seems to ensure the viability of myocardium dependent on a totally occluded artery.

It is difficult not to imagine the functioning of such a safeguard in patients whose wall contraction remains normal despite the existence of very severe stenoses, sometimes in the three major vessels.

2 Arteriographic Findings Related to Clinical Status

The search for clinico-angiographic correlations is a tempting and logical undertaking which has proved rather disappointing. At the time of the first coronary arteriographic study based on a large population (1 000 cases) in 1967, Proudfit concluded that there was no pattern of arterial involvement pathognomonic of a clinical syndrome [22]. Analysis of the arteriographic alterations of the main clinical groups of coronary artery disease has been untertaken to assess as well as possible the risks of progression in these groups. It should, of course, be kept in mind that no transfer of a statistical tendency from a group to a particular individual case is warranted.

2.1 Chronic Angina

In the chronic angina (stable angina) group, involvement of one, two or three vessels is practically of equal frequency: 31%, 37% and 32% respectively in Fuster's study [23]. There is no significant difference between patients with exertional angina and those with resting angina as far as the severity and distribution of stenoses and the existence of anastomotic collateral circulation are concerned. This type of circulation was detected in 75% of patients with stenoses greater than 50% [24]. Stenoses or occlusions of the left main coronary trunk (LMCT) are exceptional [25, 26]. The rate of stenoses of less than 75% has been reported as 20% and of total occlusion of at least one vessel as 42% [23].

Left ventricular contraction anomalies are rare in patients with no history of myocardial infarction. Their perfect detection is only provided by biplanar ventriculography [27]. Most often they are due to spontaneous or induced myocardial ischaemia, characterized by its reversibility under the effect of nitrates or inotropic intervention (see Part II, Chap. V). However, non-reversible segmental asynergy can be secondary to prolonged or repeated severe ischaemia without infarction: it indicates replacement of normal tissue with fibrous tissue [28].

2.2 Unstable Angina

Unstable angina has been described over the years by a variety of terms: impending myocardial infarction snydrome, pre-infarction angina, intermediate coronary syndrome, coronary failure, acute coronary insufficiency, impending coronary occlusion, status anginosus etc. More recently it has been referred to as crescendo angina, accelerated angina, de novo angina, progressive angina etc. In certain countries, including France, there is a tendency to include the subgroup Prinzmetal's angina in this syndrome. This would appear logical to the extent that the term "unstable angina" is used to stress the notion of destabilization in the course of coronary artery disease, with high risk, in the absence of treatment, of sudden death or myocardial infarction. A good discussion of the difficulties in defining the syndrome is provided by Chahine [29]. Today most authors include the following characteristics in the profile of unstable angina:

- sudden or progressive (more intense and/or longer and/or more frequent attacks) worsening of a known anginal condition
- development of resting angina in a patient who previously suffered from exertional angina
- appearance of angina having at the onset the characteristics of severity described above for a subject until then in good health
- occurrence of one or more anginal attacks lasting more than 15 min, despite administration of nitroglycerin
- persistence or worsening of angina during the month following occurrence of infarction

Angiographic studies of unstable angina [30–36] show distribution of lesions in the three vessels similar to that for stable angina. Alison's study [34] can be taken as a point of reference. This author found 34% single-, 38% double- and 26% triple-vessel involvement in a series of 188 patients. However, the anatomical severity of the disease can be regarded as greater than that of stable angina, as indicated by the following observations: 83% of patients had severe stenoses greater than 70%; 10.6% of such patients had stenoses of the LMCT; and 75% of patients were potential candidates for surgery. It is somewhat surprising to note the high rate of normal coronary arteries: 10.6% according to Alison [34]; 19% in a series reported by Scanlon [30]. These figures now seem questionable and may be attributable to an era in which the nature of spastic angina had not yet been well defined. In our current experience, excluding Prinzmetal's angina in order to keep within the strict profile of unstable angina defined above, patients with normal arteries are extremely infrequent. Conti's series corroborates our findings, indicating less than 2% of cases [31]. Conti also notes that collateral circulation is present in 50% of subjects [31].

A French multicentre study [36] grouping together 581 patients, including 99 cases of Prinzmetal's angina, reports only six cases of isolated spasm in normal arteries without associated atheromatous stenosis. Stenoses of the LMCT were observed in 10.8% of patients, and one-, two- and three-vessel involvement respectively in 24%, 39% and 33% of cases. On the whole, it would thus appear that coronary arteriographic features of stable and unstable angina are not fundamentally different.

Left ventriculography demonstrates an EF of less than 50% in a third of cases [33]. Study of myocardial uptake of technetium-99-pyrophosphate suggests that examined patients suffer from subendocardial infarctions of which clinical, biological and ECG examinations give no hint [33].

2.3 *Variant Angina*

The angiographic features of variant angina (Prinzmetal's angina) are well known today [37–40]. The pathological physiology of this particular form of angina [41–43] and the role of spasm in its onset [44] have been specified. The vast majority of patients have arteriosclerotic lesions identical to those found in the other clinical varieties of angina. Four angiographic features are characteristic of this group of patients: subjects with atheromatous stenoses generally have at least one extremely severe proximal stenosis; compensatory collateral circulation is little developed or non-existent; the rate of normal coronary arteriographic examinations is higher; and spontaneous or induced coronary artery spasm in a healthy or diseased artery is quite frequent (see Part II, Chap. V).

2.4 Myocardial Infarction

2.4.1 Angiographic Findings

Coronary arteriographic studies concerning the range of coronary artery lesions responsible for the occurrence of infarction are relatively divergent in their findings and limited in number [45–49]. Only one author has been able to perform coronary arteriography during the 1st day of infarction [47] in a large series of patients. The usual mean interval between infarction and examination is 12–30 days in other series. All these studies are quite commendable because they are difficult to carry out, yet their results must be interpreted with regard to certain methodological shortcomings. An inevitable drawback common to all these studies is that they concern only survivors. Also, as a rule it is not possible to include systematically all the patients consecutively admitted to hospital. The highest rate of inclusion (91%) was obtained by Betriu [49], but this author excluded subjects over 60 years of age, and there fore women because most of those admitted are over that age limit. His series is based on a population whose rate of survival at 1 month was very high (94.6%), which may be explained by the lower proportion of patients with stenosis of the LMCT or three-vessel involvement (Table 1). The following notions may be drawn from these studies as a whole: total arterial occlusion with (and perhaps because of) thrombosis is the most frequently detected anomaly during the first hours of infarction; and there is at least one stenosis of a major vessel greater than 90% in around 75% of patients. Stenoses of less than 50% are detected in around 7% of cases, with normal coronary arteries being involved in around 3% of cases, almost exclusively in young subjects (see following paragraph). Some 25%–30% of patients have involvement of one vessel, 30% of two vessels and 30%–40% of three vessels. The oc-

Table 1. Findings in early coronary arteriography after myocardial infarction

Authors	No. of patients	Percentage inclusion	Time of arteriography	Vessels diseased (%)			Stenosis of left stem (%)
				1	2	3	
Bertrand [45]	106		16 days	23	43	32	0
Betriu [49]	259	91	30 days	34	33	26	1.1
De Wood [47]	322	27	4–24 h	–	–	–	–
Taylor [46]	106	39	12 days	27	20	53	11
Turner [48]	196	70	30 days	25	32	30	10

currence of a second infarction is generally associated with the presence of three- or two-vessel involvement. One month after infarction collateral circulation is present in 44% of patients, being well developed in 23% and providing total revascularization of obstructed arteries in 11% [44]. The great variability in the frequency of stenoses of the LMCT (1%–10%) is no doubt a good indicator of the bias entering deliberately or otherwise into the selection of patients. It is certain that studies presently being undertaken concerning intracoronary thrombolytic treatment of myocardial infarction will provide valuable additional angiographic data (see Part. II, Chap. XI).

The work of De Wood [47] seems to be of capital importance because it demonstrates that only very early angiographic study is capable of assessing the true frequency of occlusive coronary thrombosis, which drops from 87% to 65% between the 4th and the 24th h. This poses the problem as to the possible intervention of early spasm, partial spontaneous thrombolysis and recanalization.

As for subjects who die during the acute phase of infarction, descriptive pathological studies are the only source of valid information. Autopsies performed later than the very first hours of infarction enabled Davies [50] to demonstrate that occlusive thrombosis is the rule in localized transmural infarction (95% of cases), whereas it is infrequent in subendocardial infarction (20%), which is due particularly to diffuse severe stenoses involving two or more vessels. According to Roberts [51], coronary thrombosis is less frequent and may be a secondary and not a primary phenomenon. This divergence of opinion apparently results from the author's examination of a larger group of coronary patients who died suddenly or within the very first hours of infarction and for whom a ventricular arrhythmia or an excessive myocardial exertional demand played a predominant harmful role in the attack.

2.4.2 Mechanical Complications

The rupture of the free wall is almost always fatal, unless there is a preliminary buildup of pericardial adhesions and formation of a false aneurysm (see Part II, Chap. V). Some classic ruptures have nevertheless been operated on with success.

The rupture of the septal wall is complicated by congestive heart failure in which LV failure predominates over that of the right ventricle. When medical treatment fails to control the situation adequately, ventriculography and coronary arteriography using intra-aortic balloon counterpulsation must be performed. This is one of the best indications, and the beneficial effect of the circulatory assistance is usually remarkable [52, 53]. The balloon is introduced through one femoral artery, either by arteriotomy or by the percutaneous approach [54], at the beginning of catheterization, the second femoral artery being used to introduce catheters. Left ventriculography in caudocranial left anterior oblique (LAO) projection visualizes clearly the intraseptal anfractuous course of the rupture. The septum, mainly in low and posterior sites, is sometimes aneurysmal. According to ECG localization of the infarct, a moderate left angulation (30°–40°) is chosen for inferobasal septal defects, a wider one (50°–60°) for antero-apical septal defects. Once again, the biplanar system can be of considerable advantage. Indeed, the contralateral right anterior oblique

(RAO) projection simultaneously assesses LV contraction and detects possible associated mitral and/or tricuspid regurgitation.

Mitral regurgitation occurring during the acute phase of infarction is usually fatal when due to rupture of an entire papillary muscle, most often the posterior one. Some patients are able to survive if operated on immediately and with no preliminary exploration [53]. Mitral regurgitations not immediately fatal [55, 56] are secondary to partial or total rupture of the head only of a papillary muscle. During the recovery phase and later, rupture of the chordae tendineae or dysfunction of a papillary muscle is generally involved. Mitral regurgitation causes acute or subacute LV failure, which is controlled more or less well by medical treatment, particularly vasodilators, and by circulatory assistance. Angiographic exploration is important in assessing the functional capability of the LV and the severity of coronary lesions and in estimating surgical curability. The haemodynamic and angiographic picture of acute mitral regurgitation is very characteristic, almost specific, when the pumping function of the LV is still good [56]. This is mitral regurgitation with a small non-compliant left atrium (LA). The contrast medium flows back very far into the distended pulmonary veins. In RAO projection it is common for the contrast medium to swirl around in the LA with either a clockwise or a counter-clockwise movement, depending on whether the prolapse or the eversion involves the posterolateral or septal leaflet of the mitral valve. When LV function and contraction are greatly altered, mitral regurgitation is either central or diffuse and non-localizable. In these cases the clinical picture is no longer dominated by pulmonary oedema but by peripheral signs of cardiogenic shock. Sometimes mitral regurgitation is a late and relatively unobtrusive complication of a coronary artery disease developing either silently, like a cardiomyopathy, or by repeated infarctions with gradual dilatation of the LV and the LA and severe and diffuse LV hypokinesis.

2.5 Angina and Myocardial Infarction with "Healthy" Coronary Arteries

Angina and myocardial infarction with "healthy" coronary arteries require little commentary as far as their coronary arteriographic diagnosis is concerned: it is obviously imperative to have films of excellent quality taken in multiple projections, if necessary in double-oblique projection, and free from any grounds for disagreement in the interpretation of any segment of the coronary artery network.

2.5.1 Angina with Angiographically Normal Coronary Arteries

The diagnosis of angina with normal coronary arteries can only be maintained in the presence of a painful thoracic syndrome simulating a true angina, accompanied by exertional and sometimes resting ECG anomalies and associated with ischaemic-type myocardial metabolic abnormalities during atrial pacing [57–61]. This type of angina is infrequent, and its cause remains obscure. It is more frequent in women and is transient by nature; its long-term prognosis is generally very promising. Vasospastic angina with healthy arteries is not part of this syndrome: a test to induce spasm must be performed to eliminate this possibility.

2.5.2 Infarction with Angiographically Normal Coronary Arteries

Infarction with angiographically normal coronary arteries is observed in 1%–2% of all patients suffering infarction and in around 15% of those under 36 years of age [62–64]. This infarction of the young adult is normally not preceded by angina. It occasionally occurs during intense effort, notably in athletes. The proportion of women involved is much higher than for infarction due to coronary atheroma. Its long-term prognosis is rather favourable. The cause of the infarction is sometimes detected by coronary arteriography: coronary embolism [65], spasm in addition to an atheromatous lesion [66] or an anomaly of the origin or course of a coronary artery (see Part II, Chap. IV). More often the cause remains hypothetical: a recanalized thrombosis [67] or a prolonged spasm [68]. The use of tobacco and the use of oral contraceptives are two conductive factors frequently cited [69].

3 Predictive Value of Coronary and Ventricular Lesions

The prognosis is most definitely related to the severity, number and site of arterial lesions. If the changes in the whole of a population subjected to coronary arteriography are considered, without taking indications into account, the annual mortality is respectively 2%, 7% and 11% in cases of more than 50% stenosis of one, two and three vessels [70]. The most dangerous stenoses are those of the LMCT, which are responsible for 15%–25% of the annual death rate [7, 71]. According to Humphries [72], the order of increasing severity of coronary involvement is as follows: isolated obstruction of the Cx, RCA, LAD; double obstruction of the RCA-Cx, LAD-Cx, LAD-RCA; obstruction of three vessels; obstruction of the LMCT. Stenoses of the LAD have a markedly poorer prognosis when the narrowing is located proximal to the origin of the first main septal artery. In cases of double-vessel involvement concerning the LAD and the RCA or Cx, death within 5 years is four times as frequent when the LAD is stenosed above the first septal artery [72]. As Kent [73] has justly pointed out, the above-cited studies were carried out at a time when our current powerful medicinal means were unavailable, so that the mortality figures are probably too pessimistic.

It is not possible to determine a valid and precise prognosis for an isolated patient on the basis of coronary arteriographic data. Table 2 presents the results of three authors [7, 74, 75] whose non-surgical patients were followed up over at least 5 years. The rate of survival at 5 years was of the order of 85%, 65% or 50%, depend-

Table 2. Five-year percentage survival rate related to the number of vessels involved (reduction in luminal diameter of 50% or greater)

Authors	No. of vessels involved		
	1	2	3
Bruschke [7]	85	62	46
Burggraf [74]	92	65	55
Webster [75]	85	64	45

ing on whether one, two or three major vessels were stenosed. When there was involvement of the LMCT, the mortality at 5 years was 50%–75% according to the degree of stenosis and the associated lesions in the other vessels. The degree of stenosis severity is an unfavourable influence on the prognosis of patients with two- or three-vessel involvement [74], and their course is particularly subject to recurrence of complications: angina, infarction or heart failure. There is good correlation between the severity of coronary lesions and that of LV contraction alterations, which probably constitutes the most significant prognostic factor. The rate of survival at 5 years is 93% in the case of a normal LV and 58% if it is abnormal [74]; and it is 69% in the case of localized hypokinesis or akinesis, 36% in the case of a LV aneurysm and 29% in the case of diffuse LV contraction alterations [7]. The incidence of LV contractile quality was determined in a group of 231 patients not selected for revascularization surgery [76]. The rate of survival at 3 years was 90% when the EF was greater than 0.34, but dropped to 59% when it was below 0.35. Involvement of one, two or three vessels and the quality of the downstream bed were comparatively less influential factors on mortality [76]. The same prognostic tendencies are apparent when survival is analysed over a 10-year period [77] as indicated in Table 3.

The predictive value of non-significant lesions (stenoses of less than 50%) and of the absence of lesions (arteries strictly normal) is also of interest. A total of 521 subjects satisfying these criteria were followed up over 10 years by Proudfit [78]. The rate of survival at 10 years was 93.6% in the group with normal arteries or stenoses of less than 30%, and 74.6% in the group with 30%–50% stenoses. In comparison, the rate of survival at 10 years of an American population sample with the same mean age is 92.3%. The risk of occurrence of a coronary event – death, infarction, significant angiographic worsening of a lesion – during these 10 years was determined as 2.1% for those with normal arteries, 13.8% for those with stenoses of less than 30% and 33% for stenoses of 30%–50% [78]. Thus for the third group only, the prognosis at 10 years must be relatively cautious. The particular case of patients afflicted with acute myocardial infarction has been studied by Taylor [46], who followed the course of 106 patients who underwent coronary arteriography within 12 days after their admission. Taylor excluded from the study subjects over 66 years of age, those with cardiogenic shock, interventricular communication or rupture of

Table 3. Five- and 10-year survival rates related to the type of obstructive coronary involvement, according to Proudfit [77]

		5 years	10 years
One-vessel disease	RCA	89.5%	70.4%
	LAD	80.8%	53.7%
	Cx	87.1%	62.5%
	LMS	51.2%	22.5%
Two-vessel disease		61.8%	45.4%
Three-vessel disease		46.7%	23.6%

RCA: right coronary artery; *LAD:* left anterior descending artery; *Cx:* circumflex; *LMS:* left main stem a papillary muscle and, of necessity, those who died early. The follow-up was carried out over 30 months. During this period 19 patients (18%) underwent an aortocoronary bypass operation because of unstable or intolerable angina (17 cases) or of stenosis of the LMCT (two cases). Among the 87 patients treated medically, 68 continued to suffer from angina (64%), 12 presented a new infarction (11%) and 13 died (12%), 11 suddenly. The number of subjects in danger of another serious coronary event or of a fatal complication is thus considerable, and it would be of capital importance to be able to determine who they are, so that they may be examined by coronary arteriography and benefit, if possible, from revascularization surgery. The prognostic value of spontaneous symptoms seems insufficient for the choice of these subjects. Friesinger [79] found no significant difference in the severity and spread of lesions between asymptomatic subjects and those with angina in a group of 104 patients explored within the year following their first infarction. In a group of 108 patients suffering from infarction of the inferior wall, Chaitman [80] determined that triple-vessel involvement and proximal stenoses of the LAD were significantly more frequent in subjects with Canadian class II–III angina [81] than in class 0–I subjects, and that five patients with stenosis of the LMCT were all in class II–III. However, a relatively high proportion (21%) of class 0–I patients had triple-vessel involvement and 6% left main equivalent disease in a group of 31 patients with class 0–I postinfarction angina. In practice, the best method of identifying high-risk patients consists in taking several variables into account [73, 80, 82]: age over 55 years, permanent alteration of the ECG ST-T segments, cardiomegaly, presence of one or more risk factors and, most importantly, a positive exercise test. This last variable is definitely the most decisive. Myocardial thallium scintigraphy and radio-nuclide angiography are useful complementary methods. As for strictly angiographic variables, that is coronary and LV involvement, these have relatively little predictive value when considered in isolation. Taylor [46] has nonetheless shown that association of triple-vessel involvement with a proximal stenosis of the LAD and an EF of less than 0.30 is predictive of sudden death; that association of a previous infarction with an EF of less than 0.40 is predictive of a fatal complication; and that three-vessel involvement is predicitive of recurrence of infarction within 30 months.

References

1. Lenegre J, Himbert J, Beaumont JL, Froment R, Normand J, Perrin A (1961) Athérosclérose et insuffisance coronarienne. In: XXXIIIe Congrès français de Médecine. Masson, Paris
2. Cohen LS, Elliot WC, Klein MD, Gorlin R (1966) Coronary heart disease: clinical, cinearteriographic and metabolic correlation. Am J Cardiol 17: 153
3. Proudfit WL, Shirey EK, Sones FM (1966) Selective cinecoronary arteriography: correlation with clinical findings in 1000 patients. Circulation 33: 901
4. Elliot WC, Gorlin R (1966) The coronary circulation, myocardial ischemia and angina pectoris. Mod Concepts Cardiovasc Dis 35: 117
5. Gensini GG, Kelley AE (1972) Incidence and progression of coronary artery disease. An angiographic correlation in 1,263 patients. Arch Intern Med 129: 814
6. Bruschke AVG, Proudfit WL, Sones FM Jr (1973) Clinical course of patients with normal and slightly or moderately abnormal coronary arteriograms. A follow-up study on 500 patients. Circulation 47: 936

7. Bruschke AVG, Proudfit WL, Sones FM Jr (1973) Progress study of 590 consecutive non-surgical cases of coronary disease followed 5–9 years. I. Arteriographic correlations. Circulation 47: 1147
8. Bourassa MG, Goulet C, Lesperance J (1973) Progression of coronary arterial disease after aortocoronary bypass grafts. Circulation 48 [Suppl III]: 127
9. Delaye J, Pincon B, Janin A, Beaune J, Amiel M, Gonin A (1974) Les données de l'artériographie coronarienne contemporaines des premières manifestations angineuses. Arch Mal Coeur 67: 173
10. Humphries JO, Kuller L, Ross RS, Friesinger GC, Page EE (1974) Natural history of ischemic heart disease in relation to arteriographic findings. Circulation 49: 489
11. Bemis CE, Gorlin R, Kemp HG, Herman MV (1973) Progression of coronary artery disease – a clinical arteriographic study. Circulation 47: 455
12. Bruschke AVG, Proudfit WL, Sones FM Jr (1973) Progress study of 590 consecutive non-surgical cases of coronary disease followed 5–9 years. II. Ventriculographic and other correlations. Circulation 47: 1154
13. Kimbiris D, Lavine P, Van der Broek H, Najmi M, Likoff W (1974) Devolutionary pattern of coronary atherosclerosis in patients with angina pectoris. Am J Cardiol 33: 7
14. Amiel M, Thevenin P (1979) Progression des lésions coronariennes étudiée par coronarographies itératives chez des patients opérés ou non. Ann Radiol 22: 525
15. Rosch J, Antonovic R, Trenouth RS, Rahimtoola SH, Sim DN, Dotter CT (1976) The natural history of coronary artery stenosis. A longitudinal angiographic assessment. Radiology 119: 513
16. Marchandise B, Bourassa MG, Chaitman BR, Lesperance J (1978) Angiographic evaluation of the natural history of normal coronary arteries and mild coronary atherosclerosis. Am J Cardiol 41: 216
17. Bruschke AVG, Wijers TS, Kolsters W, Landmann J (1981) The anatomic evolution of coronary artery disease demonstrated by coronary arteriography in 256 nonoperated patients. Circulation 63: 527
18. Kramer JR, Matsuda Y, Mulligan JC, Aronow M, Proudfit WL (1981) Progression of coronary atherosclerosis. Circulation 63: 519
19. Ben-Zvi J, Hildner FJ, Javier R (1974) Progression of coronary artery disease. Cinearteriographic and clinical observations in medically and surgically treated patients. Am J Cardiol 34: 295
20. Markis JE, Joffee CD, Roberts BH, Ransil BJ, Cohn PF, Herman MV, Gorlin R (1980) Evolution of left ventricular dysfunction in coronary artery disease: serial cineangiographic studies without surgery. Circulation 62: 141
21. Bertrand ME, Rousseau MF, La Blanche JM, Carre AG, Lekieffre JP (1979) Cineangiographic assessment of left ventricular function in the acute phase of transmural myocardial infarction. Am J Cardiol 43: 472
22. Proudfit WL, Shirey EK, Sones FM Jr (1967) Distribution of arterial lesions demonstrated by selective cinecoronary arteriography. Circulation 36: 54
23. Fuster V, Frye RL, Connolly DC, Danielson MA, Elveback LR, Kurland LT (1971) Arteriographic patterns early in the onset of the coronary syndromes. Br Heart J 33: 863
24. Gorlin R (1976) Coronary collaterals. In: Gorlin R (ed) Coronary artery disease. Saunders, Philadelphia
25. De Mots H, Bonchek LI, Rosch J, Anderson RP, Starr A, Rahimtoola SH (1975) Left main coronary artery disease. Risk of angiography, importance of coexisting disease of other coronary arteries and effects of revascularization. Am J Cardiol 36: 136
26. Goldberg S, Grossman W, Markis JE, Cohen MV, Baltaxe HA, Levin DC (1978) Total occlusion of the left main coronary artery. A clinical, hemodynamic and angiographic profile. Am J Med 64: 3
27. Cohn PF, Gorlin R, Adams DF, Chahine RA, Vokonas PS, Herman MV (1974) Comparison of biplane and single-plane left ventriculography in patients with coronary artery disease. Am J Cardiol 33: 1
28. Bodenheimer MM, Banka VS, Hermann GA, Trout RG, Pasdar H, Helfant RH (1976) Reversible asynergy: histopathologic and electrocardiographic correlations in patients with coronary artery disease. Circulation 53: 792
29. Chahine RA (1975) Unstable angina: the problem of definition. Br Heart J 37: 1246

30. Scanlon PJ, Nemickas R, Moran JF, Talano JV, Amirparviz F, Pifarre R (1973) Accelerated angina pectoris – clinical, hemodynamic, arteriographic, and therapeutic experience in 85 patients. Circulation 47: 19
31. Conti CR, Brawley RK, Griffith LSC, Pitt B, Humphries JO, Gott VL, Ross RS (1973) Unstable angina pectoris – morbidity and mortality in 57 consecutive patients evaluated angiographically. Am J Cardiol 32: 745
32. Bertolasi C, Tronge JE, Carreno CA, Jalon J, Vega MR (1974) Unstable angina. Prospective and randomized study of its evolution with and without surgery – preliminary report. Am J Cardiol 33: 201
33. Donsky MS, Curry GC, Parkey RW, Meyer SL, Bonte FJ, Platt MR, Willerson JT (1976) Unstable angina pectoris. Clinical, angiographic, and myocardial scintigraphic observations. Br Heart J 38: 257
34. Alison HW, Russell RO Jr, Mantle JA, Kouchoukos NT, Moraski RE, Rackley CE (1978) Coronary anatomy and arteriography in patients with unstable angina pectoris. Am J Cardiol 41: 204
35. Rafflenbeul W, Smith LR, Rogers WJ, Mantle JA, Rackley CE, Russel RO Jr (1979) Quantitative coronary arteriography. Coronary anatomy of patients with unstable angina pectoris reexamined 1 year after optimal medical therapy. Am J Cardiol 43: 699
36. Delaye J (1980) Le risque de la coronarographie dans l'angor instable. Enquête du groupe de travail de la Société Française de Cardiologie. Arch Mal Coeur 73: 211
37. Higgins CB, Wexler L, Silverman JF, Schroeder JS (1976) Clinical and arteriographic features of Prinzmetal's variant angina: documentation of etiology factors. Am J Cardiol 37: 831
38. Weiner L, Kasparian H, Duca PR, Walinsky P, Gottlieb RS, Hanckel F, Brest AN (1976) Spectrum of coronary arterial spasm. Clinical, angiographic and myocardial metabolic experience in 29 cases. Am J Cardiol 38: 945
39. Cherrier F, Neimann JL, Groussin P, Aliot E, Cuilliere M, Beissel J (1978) Prinzmetal angina: a study of 100 cases. In: Kaltenbach M (ed) Coronary heart disease. Thieme, Stuttgart, p 131
40. Johnson AD, Stroud HA, Vieweg WVR, Ross J Jr (1978) Coronary angiographic patterns and results of medical and surgical therapy in 42 consecutive patients with variant angina pectoris. In: Kaltenbach, M (ed) Coronary heart disease. Thieme, Stuttgart, p 181
41. Yasue H, Touyama M, Shimamoto M, Kato H, Tanaka S, Akiyama F (1974) Role of autonomic nervous system in the pathogenesis of Prinzmetal's variant form of angina. Circulation 50: 534
42. Yasue H, Nagao M, Omote S, Takizawa A, Miwa K, Tanaka S (1978) Coronary arterial spasm and Prinzmetal's variant form of angina induced by hyperventilation and Tris-buffer infusion. Circulation 58: 56
43. Maseri A, Severi S, De Nes M, L'Abbate A, Chierchia S, Marzilli M, Ballestra AM, Parodi O, Biagini A, Distante A (1978) "Variant" angina: one aspect of a continuous spectrum of vasospastic myocardial ischemia. Pathogenetic mechanisms, estimated incidence and clinical and coronary arteriographic findings in 138 patients. Circulation 42: 1019
44. Bertrand ME (ed) (1981) Coronary arterial spasm. Dausse, Paris
45. Bertrand ME, Lefebvre JM, Rousseau MF, Carre AG, Lekieffre JP (1979) Coronary arteriography in acute transmural myocardial infarction. Am Heart J 97: 61
46. Taylor GJ, Humphries JON, Mellitis ED, Pitt B, Schulze RA, Griffith LSC, Achuff SC (1980) Predictors of clinical course, coronary anatomy and left ventricular function after recovery from acute myocardial infarction. Circulation 62: 960
47. De Wood MA, Spores J, Notske R, Mouser LT, Burroughs R, Golden MS, Lang HT (1980) Prevalence of total coronary occlusion during the early hours of transmural myocardial infarction. N Engl J Med 303: 897
48. Turner JD, Rogers WJ, Mantle JA, Rackley CE, Russell RO Jr (1980) Coronary angiography soon after myocardial infarction. Chest 77: 58
49. Betriu A, Castaner A, Sanz GA, Pare JC, Roig E, Coll S, Magrina J, Navarro-Lopez F (1982) Angiographic findings 1 month after myocardial infarction: a prospective study of 259 survivors. Circulation 65: 1099
50. Davies MJ, Woolf N, Robertson WB (1976) Pathology of acute myocardial infarction with particular reference to occlusive coronary thrombi. Br Heart J 38: 659
51. Roberts WC, Buja LM (1972) The frequency and significance of coronary arterial thrombi and other observations in fatal acute myocardial infarction. A study of 107 necropsy patients. Am J Med 52: 425

52. Gold HK, Leinbach RC, Sanders CA, Buckley MJ, Mundth ED, Austen WG (1973) Intraaortic balloon pumping for ventricular septal defect or mitral regurgitation complicating acute myocardial infarction. Circulation 47: 1191
53. Slama R, Piwnica A, Masquet C, Beaufils P, Bouvrain Y (1977) Traitement d'urgence des complications mécaniques de l'infarctus myocardique aigu. Perforations septales et insuffisances mitrales. Arch Mal Coeur 70: 557
54. Bregman D, Nichols AB, Weiss MB, Powers ER, Martin EC, Casarella WJ (1980) Percutaneous intraaortic balloon insertion. Am J Cardiol 46: 261
55. Baxley WA, Kennedy JW, Feild B, Dodge HT (1973) Hemodynamics in ruptured chordae tendineae and chronic rheumatic mitral regurgitation. Circulation 48: 1288
56. Petitier H, Wanlin P, Crochet D, Bizais Y, De Laguerenne J, Grossetete R (1981) Fonction ventriculaire gauche des insuffisances mitrales aiguës d'origine ischémique et par rupture de cordage idiopathique. Ann Cardiol Angeiol 30: 325
57. Bemiller CR, Pepine CJ, Rogers AK (1973) Long term observations in patients with angina and normal coronary arteriograms. Circulation 47: 36
58. Kemp HG, Vokonas PS, Cohn PF, Gorlin R (1973) The original syndrome associated with normal coronary arteriograms. Report of a six-year experience. Am J Med 54: 735
59. Demaria AN, Lee G, Amsterdam EA, Low R, Mason DT (1980) The angina syndrome with normal coronary arteries: etiologic and prognostic considerations. JAMA 244: 826
60. Arbogast R, Bourassa MG (1973) Myocardial function during atrial pacing in patients with angina pectoris and normal coronary arteriograms. Am J Cardiol 32: 257
61. Boudoulas H, Cobb TC, Leighton RF, Wiet SM (1974) Myocardial lactate production in patients with angina-like chest pain and angiographically normal coronary arteries and left ventricle. Am J Cardiol 34: 501
62. Rosenblatt A, Selzer A (1977) The nature and clinical features of myocardial infarction with normal coronary arteriography. Circulation 55: 578
63. Thompson SI, Vieweg WVR, Alpert JS, Hagan AD (1977) Incidence and age distribution of patients with myocardial infarction and normal coronary arteriograms. Cathet Cardiovasc Diagn 3: 1
64. Cherrier F, Breton C, Bourdon JL, Neimann JL, Faivre G (1979) Profil épidémiologique des sujets porteurs d'un infarctus avec coronarographie normale. Arch Mal Coeur 72: 26
65. O'Reilly RJ, Spelberg RD (1974) Rapid resolution of coronary arterial emboli: myocardial infarction and subsequent normal coronary arteriograms. Ann Intern Med 81: 348
66. Oliva PB, Breckinridge JC (1977) Arteriographic evidence of coronary arterial spasm in acute myocardial infarction. Circulation 56: 366
67. Henderson RR, Hansing CE, Razavi M, Rowe GG (1973) Resolution of an obstructive coronary lesion as demonstrated by selective angiography in a patient with transmural myocardial infarction. Am J Cardiol 31: 785
68. Maseri A, L'Abbate A, Baroldi G, Chierchia S, Marzilli M, Ballestra AM, Severi S, Parodi O, Biagini A, Distante A, Pesola A (1978) Coronary vasospasm as a possible cause of myocardial infarction. A conclusion derived from the study of "preinfarction" angina. N Engl J Med 299: 1271
69. Jain AK (1976) Cigarette smoking, use of oral contraceptives and myocardial infarction. Am J Obstet Gynecol 126: 301
70. Reeves TJ, Oberman A, Jones WB, Sheffield LT (1974) Natural history of angina pectoris. Am J Cardiol 33: 423
71. Cohen MV, Gorlin R (1975) Main left coronary artery disease. Circulation 52: 275
72. Humphries JO (1977) Expected course of patients with coronary artery disease. In: Rahimtoola SH (ed) Coronary bypass surgery. Davis, Philadelphia
73. Kent KM, Rosing DR, Ewels CJ, Lipson L, Bonow R, Epstein SE (1982) Prognosis of asymptomatic or mildly symptomatic patients with coronary artery disease. Am J Cardiol 49: 1823
74. Burggraf CW, Parker JO (1975) Prognosis in coronary artery disease: angiographic, hemodynamic and clinical factors. Circulation 51: 146
75. Webster JS, Moberg C, Rincon G (1974) Natural history of severe proximal coronary artery disease as documented by coronary cineangiography. Am J Cardiol 33: 195
76. Gross H, Vaid AK, Cohen MV (1978) Prognosis in patients rejected for coronary revascularization surgery. Am J Med 64: 9

77. Proudfit WL, Bruschke AVG, Sones FM Jr (1978) Natural history of obstructive coronary artery disease: ten-year study of 601 non-surgical cases. Prog Cardiovasc Dis 21: 53
78. Proudfit WL, Bruschke AVG, Sones FM Jr (1980) Clinical course of patients with normal or slightly or moderately abnormal coronary arteriograms: 10-year follow-up of 521 patients. Circulation 62: 712
79. Friesinger GC, Perry TM (1978) Prognostic and therapeutic considerations in ischemic heart disease. Schweiz Med Wochenschr 108: 1667
80. Chaitman BR, Waters DD, Corbara F, Bourassa MG (1978) Prediction of multivessel disease after inferior myocardial infarction. Circulation 57: 1085
81. Campeau L (1976) Grading of angina pectoris. Circulation 54: 522
82. Mautner RK, Phillips JH (1981) Coronary angiography post first myocardial infarction in the asymptomatic or mildly symptomatic patient: clinical, angiographic and prospective observations. Cathet Cardiovasc Diagn 7: 1

VIII Angiographic Explorations: Surgical Problems

1 The Role of Coronary Arteriography in the Decision to Operate

Coronary arteriography is always useful and often even indispensable to the heart surgeon in many aspects of his work. It is obvious that myocardial revascularization surgery is entirely dependent on coronary arteriography and that surgery relative to mechanical complications of myocardial ischaemia almost always benefits from it. In the case of congenital cardiopathies, mainly in the presence of tetralogy of Fallot, it permits detection of a possible anomaly in the course of a large coronary branch in the conus arteriosus or of the abnormal origin of a coronary artery [the left anterior descending artery (LAD) taking off from the right coronary artery (RCA), for example] or of a coronary fistula. In patients with acquired valvular disease, it also helps in the search for an unusual anatomical configuration and, especially, associated atheromatous stenoses. The surgeon must be aware of the existence of these lesions or anatomical variations when considering the possibility of a bypass, and be certain that myocardial protection will be ensured during aortic or mitral valve replacement.

1.1 Coronary Arteriography and Bypass Surgery

The surgeon's essential requirement is to be given an objective appreciation of the degree of coronary stenosis and of its haemodynamic consequences. This presents no problem in the case of a complete occlusion or a subtotal stenosis (99%) with stasis or slowing down in the wash-out of the contrast medium and injection of the distal artery by the collateral circulation. It is essential for the surgeon to be able to analyse each important vessel in at least two orthogonal projections so as not to overlook a significant stenosis and not to undertake an incomplete myocardial revascularization. On the other hand, it would be a serious mistake to perform unnecessary bypass surgery. The nitroglycerin test makes it possible to distinguish an organic stenosis from a spasm.

The surgeon requires the radiologist to have a good knowledge of the classic pitfalls and problems. The most difficult stenoses to visualize or appraise exactly are those of the left main coronary trunk, of the origin of the LAD and of the ostia. The procedures and projections most favourable to their visualization have been described in Part II, Chap. II. In some cases, despite administration of nitroglycerin, a spasm in addition to a stenosis can present a difficult diagnostic problem. This situation relates mainly to the initial segment of the RCA. Sometimes an image of a possible stenosis may go undetected during video recording and only show up once the film is developed and viewed. The clinical context is important to the decision made by the surgeon and the radiologist. When anginal pain, the ECG during rest and exercise, and myocardial thallium scintigraphy suggest that the doubtful image may indeed reveal a stenosis, it is essential to repeat arteriography. In fact, it is impossible during the intervention to assess the severity of a stenosis without opening the suspect artery, which would practically be equivalent to opting for bypass surgery. A difficult problem is to appreciate the degree of severity of stenoses which appear to be borderline in haemodynamic terms. For example, when a stenosis of the vertical part of the RCA or of the proximal circumflex (Cx) reduces the calibre of the vessel by 50% in each of two orthogonal projections, it is apparent that this corresponds to a reduction in the cross-sectional area of around 75%. Does this stenosis have haemodynamic consequences? If not, that is if there is no pressure gradient or drop in coronary output during effort, it is clear that there would be no advantage in a surgical bypass, which would create a competing flow with turbulences favourable to thrombosis of the graft and even of the bypassed artery. On the other hand, if the stenosis disturbs coronary flow and has a potential for a greater degree of occlusion, it would be an error not to perform bypass surgery. In a few propitious cases it might be possible to consider transluminal angioplasty as a complementary procedure in the event of error or of delayed progression of the stenosis.

Locating the exact site of stenoses in the left coronary artery (LCA) and its branches is of particular advantage. When a proximal stenosis of the LAD affects the point of origin of a large first or second septal artery, some surgeons consider the feasibility of an additional bypass for the septal artery. When the point of origin of the main diagonal artery is either affected by a stenosis of the LAD or lies between two stenoses in this artery, the surgeon must revascularize the diagonal artery at the same time as the LAD by a double bypass or a sequential bypass [1]. Some surgeons systematically bypass all the diagonal branches, whereas others do not opt for the additional bypass if the diagonal artery appears spindly and morbid on the coronary arteriogram [2]. The same reasoning applies to the Cx and its marginal branches. Their distribution varies greatly from one subject to another, and it is important to know their number so as not to choose the wrong marginal artery during the intervention.

The number of bypasses depends on the assessment made by each surgeon, who takes into account the minimum calibre of a vessel suitable for bypass and the extent of the atheromatous lesions. The principle is generally admitted now that coronary revascularization must be as complete as possible [2]. Yet that does not mean that it is always efficient. The quality of the downstream network is of capital importance. The ideal artery is regular and has a good calibre downstream from the stenosis. However, this is not always the case, since rigid plaques and multiple stenoses to the periphery may pose problems as to the method to adopt. The surgeon must then choose among various procedures:

- a simple bypass, after exploration with a dilator, performed downstream from non-stenotic plaques; the existence of a morbid and spindly LAD is a good reason for considering anastomosis with the internal mammary artery rather than a saphenous vein graft

- a bypass located more distally than would be desirable, in order to avoid a morbid area; this procedure concerns the LAD in particular
- a double bypass upstream and downstream from a stenosis located in the mid-part of the LAD.
- complementary transluminal angioplasty of the artery performed either upstream or downstream from the bypass using balloon-tipped catheters
- complementary endarterectomy downstream from the bypass, a procedure proposed by some surgeons and used mainly for the RCA [3].

On the whole, it must be admitted that the attitude of surgeons towards the same coronary arteriographic images is not uniform. Some prefer to locate bypasses whenever possible in a healthy area, thus downstream from lesions. Others do not hesitate to perform complementary endarterectomy. Finally, when the RCA network is diffusely morbid, with inferior necrosis and akinetic plaque at that level, the present authors, among others, feel that a bypass has no functional value. In one particular, rather common condition, coronary arteriography does not visualize the coronary artery downstream from a total occlusion and there is no backflow of contrast medium as a result of collateral circulation (Fig. 1). In this case, what should the surgeon do? In our opinion, a bypass or an endarterectomy would not be useful as far as the RCA and the Cx are concerned, though it must be acknowledged that not all teams share this view. On the other hand, our approach is to explore the LAD during the intervention to determine whether a bypass is feasible.

1.2 Coronary Arteriography, Left Ventriculography and Other Surgical Problems

The surgeon appreciates the radiologist advising him, whenever possible, of the presence and sites of atheromatous or aneurysmal lesions of the ascending aorta which complicate implantation of saphenous vein grafts on the aortic wall. Likewise, it is of capital importance that left ventriculography or aortography ensure detection of associated valvular lesions, particularly minor aortic or mitral regurgitations, which disturb extracorporeal circulation and may compromise the results of the operation.

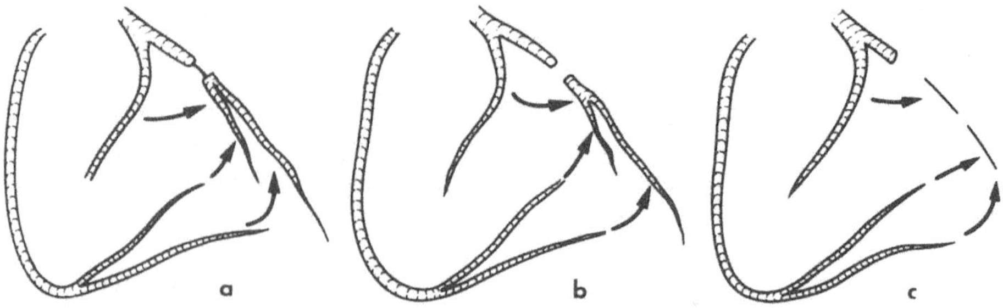

Fig. 1 a–c. The degree to which the downstream bed of an obstructed artery is visible may be **a** very good, **b** good or **c** very poor, depending on the efficiency of anastomoses as well as on the quality of the distal part of the artery. The first case **(a)** is the most frequent; the third **(c)** is the least common

Some anomalies of the course of coronary arteries are not easy to recognize, as in the relatively rare instance of an intra-atrial RCA or in the rather frequent cases of an intramyocardial LAD (5% of cases). This latter anomaly may easily be identified by coronary arteriography when the myocardial bridge squeezes against the LAD in systole. In the absence of this sign it is not unusual for the anomaly to go undetected until surgery.

The importance of angiographic assessment of left ventricular (LV) function is unanimously admitted. In particular, the postoperative prognosis is greatly influenced by LV condition. As far as possible, LV contraction anomalies should be filmed in two projections. The degree of alteration of wall contraction should be determined for each segment and correlated with the coronary artery stenoses. If necessary, the effect of β-blocking agents and other drugs should be taken into account. The ejection fraction (EF) is a valuable index for calculating operative risk. The mortality rate is less than 2% if the EF is greater than 50%, but is above 10% if the EF is below 30% [4]. Our practice is to advise against operation where there is a diffuse and considerable alteration in LV contraction, with clinical signs of LV insufficiency and no or minimal anginal symptoms.

Ventriculography gives useful guidance on the indications for LV resection, whether complementary to a bypass or not. In the case of a LV aneurysm, ventriculography indicates its site and size and, especially, the quality of the remaining ventricle and whether or not there is mitral regurgitation. The indication for operation is regarded as a function of the clinical signs: heart failure, angina and rhythm disturbances. The extent of the excision, the need for an associated mitral prosthesis, the operative risk and the long-term prognosis are appraised on the basis of ventriculographic data.

Non-aneurysmal akineses are often fortuitous discoveries made during assessment of an anginal condition with no clinical heart failure. Ventriculography reveals more or less significant anomalies: paradoxical expansion of the apex, or extensive akinetic plaque suggesting a need for complementary resection of the altered myocardium [5]. It is our personal practice to avoid such resections, in the belief that they have no influence on angina and that they cannot improve haemodynamic conditions in the absence of cardiac insufficiency [6]. Unlike other surgeons, we prefer not to resect akinetic plaques, for fear of worsening LV function or of performing a useless surgical act. On the whole, it is our opinion that removal of aneurysmal sacs must be limited to those which present a risk in the course of the disease.

2 Postoperative Evaluation of the Coronary Patient

Our knowledge of the postoperative course of the coronary patient relies mainly on the work of teams which have been able to carry out numerous follow-up coronary arteriographic examinations [7–23]. Non-invasive methods [pulsed Doppler and computed tomography (CT) scanner] can also provide valuable information.

It is easier to check on graft permeability if the surgeon has indicated the implant site with a metal marker, although such markers have the disadvantage of disrupting

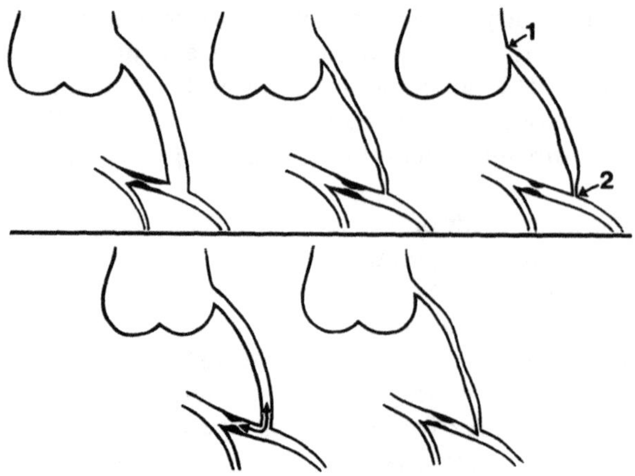

Fig. 2. Common anomalies observed in aortocoronary vein grafts. *Top,* from *left to right:* vein calibre too large in comparison to artery calibre; irregular and moniliform appearance of the graft; stenosis at the proximal end of the graft *(1)* or at its distal end *(2)*. *Bottom,* from left to right: opacification by backflow either into the graft from the artery or into the artery from the graft; iatrogenic stenosis of the proximal angle of the anastomosis resulting from surgical technique

ultrasound and CT studies. Before asserting that a graft has been obliterated, it is absolutely essential to demonstrate the existence of the graft stump or the small recessus of the ostial occlusion by selective opacification or general aortography.

2.1 Bypasses and Implants

2.1.1 Angiographic Evaluation

Venous Aortocoronary Bypass Grafts

General prospective studies of venous aortocoronary bypass grafts based on repeated examinations show that the permeability rate 1 month after surgery (around 85%) remains nearly stable until the 6th month and that deterioration is minimal beyond the 1st year. Examinations performed 4 or 5 years after grafting indicate that the permeability rate of the grafts drops by 4%–5% per year. Morphological anomalies of vein grafts (Figs. 2 and 3) are quite varied. Some may be ascribed to errors in surgical technique relative to implantation on the aorta or the bypassed artery: kinking, bending, local narrowings or tapering, angulations, and pulling on the coronary artery. In some patients there is a peculiar anomaly involving retraction of the vein graft and a diffuse narrowing of the lumen. In extreme cases the bypassed vessel may be drawn towards the aorta by the retracted vein graft. There is also what is referred to as "graft disease". Histologically, this is due to a process of intimal fibrous hyperplasia. In some cases an irregular graft may in time become reshaped and eventually take on the appearance of a true artery with a perfectly regular calibre.

The haemodynamic and angiographic modifications secondary to bypasses are well known (Fig. 4). The pre-existing anastomoses which supplied the bypassed ves-

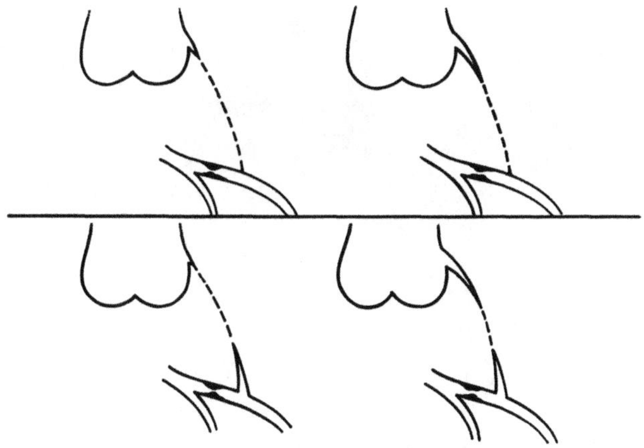

Fig. 3. Different types of vein graft obstruction depending on the site and extent of luminal obliteration

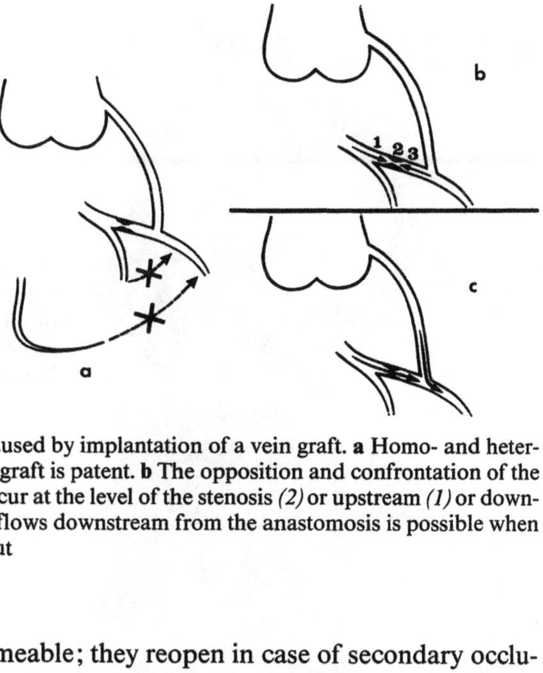

Fig. 4 a–c. Haemodynamic phenomena caused by implantation of a vein graft. **a** Homo- and heterolateral anastomoses disappear when the graft is patent. **b** The opposition and confrontation of the respective flows of the two vessels may occur at the level of the stenosis *(2)* or upstream *(1)* or downstream *(3)* from it. **c** An opposition of the flows downstream from the anastomosis is possible when both are of approximately the same output

sel disappear when the graft is permeable; they reopen in case of secondary occlusion of the graft, as has been demonstrated repeatedly by examinations. Four circulatory systems are possible at the level of the bypassed network:

1. The proximal stenosis is transformed into a complete occlusion and the graft supplies the coronary artery completely downstream from this occlusion (the case in approximately 50% of permeable bypasses).
2. The proximal stenosis remains permeable and there is a two-way flow, with a back-and-forth movement of the opacifying agent relative to the proximal stenosis when either the graft or the bypassed vessel is injected.

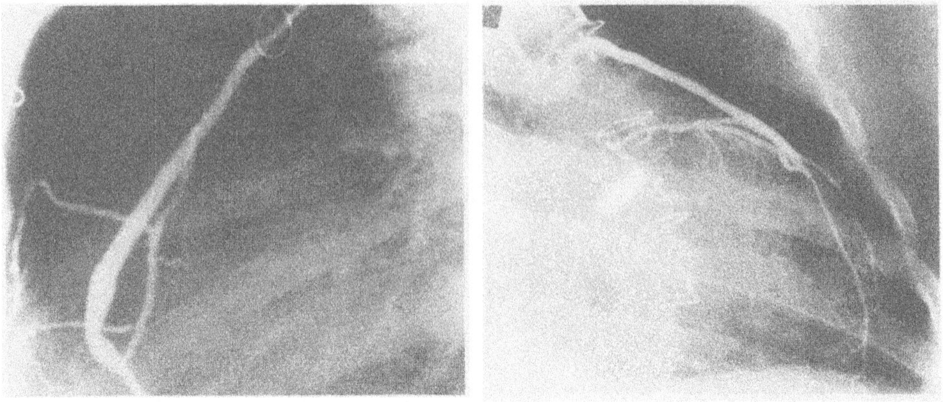

Fig. 5. Very good perfusion *(left):* of a right coronary artery and *(right):* of a left anterior descending artery, both of which are totally obstructed. Good graft appearance

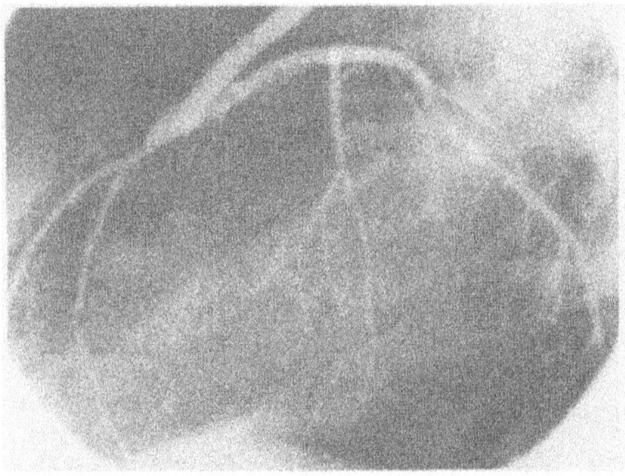

Fig. 6 *(upper).* Perfusion of an entire left coronary artery by a graft in a very severe case of ostial stenosis. At the point of the anastomosis the calibre of the vein graft is a little too large, which is quite often unavoidable

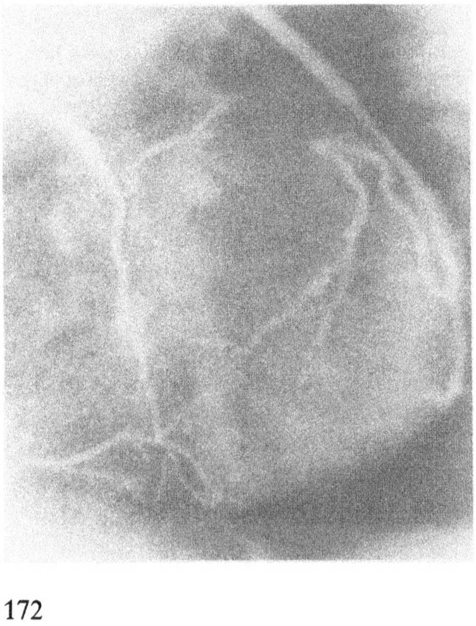

Fig. 7 *(lower).* Y-shaped aortocoronary venous bypass connecting to the left anterior descending artery and circumflex. Good revascularization with opacification of the distal part of an occluded right coronary artery thanks to anastomotic collateral circulation

3. The distal part of the bypassed network is opacified by the normal passage as well as by the graft: this condition ordinarily corresponds to a bypass downstream from a relatively slight stenosis (an unnecessary bypass?).
4. The graft is opacified upstream when the bypassed vessel is injected: this ordinarily indicates development of a stenosis downstream from the anastomosis.

Figures 5–12 illustrate various favourable or unfavourable aspects of venous aortocoronary bypass grafts as revealed in follow-up coronary arteriographic images.

Arterial Internal Mammary Grafts.
Mammary implantation is more surgically demanding and difficult than vein graft implantation. This operation is difficult to conceive of in an emergency involving a high-risk patient, and the cases in which two internal mammary arteries can be implanted on two different coronary vessels are rare. Moreover, certain very spindly internal mammary arteries are poorly suited to anastomosis, and the flow which they can provide is relatively low. Indeed, bypass longevity is in part related to the volume of blood flow allowed by the grafts, and it is known from intra-operative studies that vein grafts have a greater blood flow than mammary grafts. Yet, despite these reservations, repeated follow-up examinations of internal mammary grafts have shown us that this vessel is capable of dilatation when the downstream bed is good [24], and that its initially poor flow may improve with time [25]. The early permeability rate runs around 95%–98%, and the deterioration with time is slight [24–26]. The adaptation of the arterial graft to physical exertion seems greater than that of the vein graft. The exercise ECG shows greater improvement after revascularization surgery by mammary artery than after that by vein graft [26].

Our experience is based on 93 patients and a total of 100 mammary grafts: 60 early follow-up examinations (less than 2 years), 16 late (2–5 years) and 24 very late (beyond 5 years). Bypass permeability was assessed by opacification of the internal mammary artery from its ostium to the anastomosis and by opacification of the LAD downstream from the anastomosis. According to these criteria, 99 bypasses were permeable (99%), corresponding to 92 of the 93 patients examined (98.9%). The non-permeable bypass belonged to the early group: the obstruction of the internal mammary artery was detected in the 4th month following surgery. This artery was opacified over the greater part of its course and was uniformly thin, with no ostial stenosis and no parietal irregularity. It was totally obstructed immediately upstream from the anastomosis. In another case, the mammary artery, which was very spindly, presented successive wall irregularities along its entire course and a 50% stenosis of the right angle anastomosis. In 93 of the 99 remaining arterial grafts (93.9%), the appearance of the bypass walls was considered normal: regular, smooth and parallel. The angle between the mammary artery and the coronary artery at the point of the anastomosis was measured in 91 patients, and a significant correlation was found between the increasing degree of this angle and the frequency of stenoses at the graft-LAD junction. Finally, the ratio of the diameter of the arterial graft to that of the LAD was measured: it proved equal to 1 in 61 patients, less than 1 in 7 and greater than 1 in 31. The value of this ratio was independent of bypass longevity.

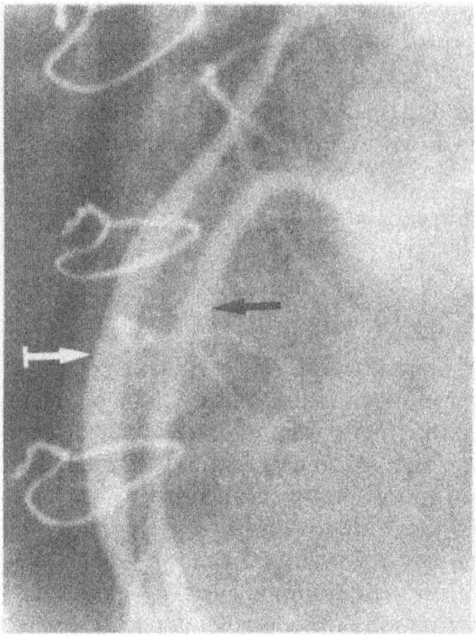

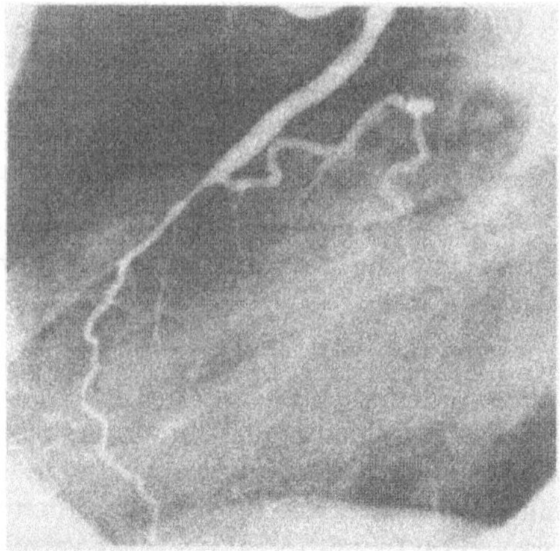

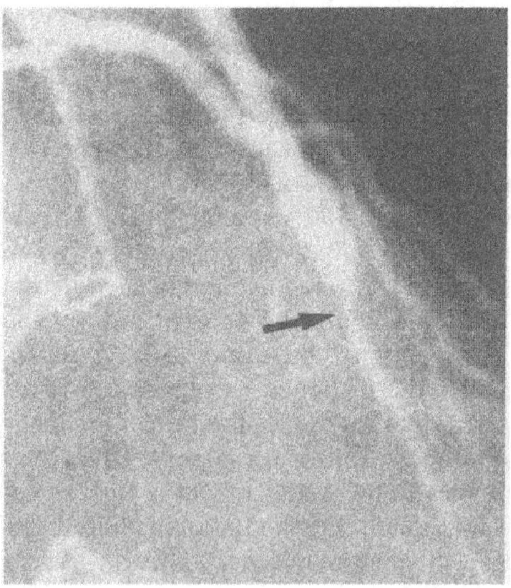

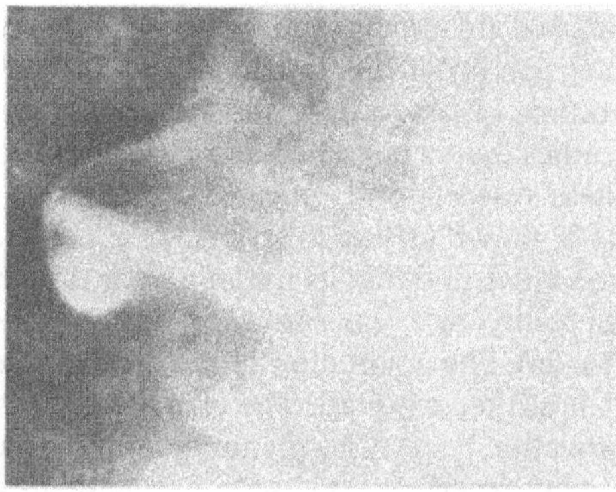

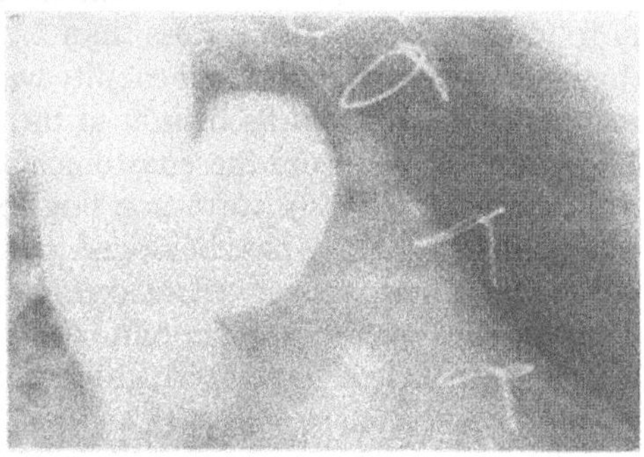

Fig. 8 *(upper left)*. Selective injection in a grafted right coronary artery *(black arrow)*. The contrast medium flows back into the vein graft *(white arrow)* as far as the aorta, indicating less severe coronary stenoses than were supposed

Fig. 9 *(upper right)*. Example of the pull of a vein graft exerted on a left anterior descending artery with an incipient stenosis downstream from the anastomosis

Fig. 10 *(lower left)*. Example of severe stenosis of the left anterior descending artery in the distal angle of the vein-to-artery anastomosis

Fig. 11 *(middle right)*. Example of proximal obstruction of a graft 5 mm from the aortic wall

Fig. 12 *(lower right)*. A rare complication: a false aneurysm has developed in the anastomosis between the aorta and the vein graft

Vineberg's Operation.
Vineberg's operation has been practically abandoned. The infrequent examinations performed show that the mammary artery implanted in the myocardium sometimes provides a vascularization of relatively great volume. The most favourable cases usually correspond to patients having a good intercoronary anastomotic network before surgery.

2.1.2 X-Ray Computed Tomography

Various studies have demonstrated the reliability of X-ray CT in the study of bypasses [27–32]. Our experience [27] is based on evaluation of 36 patients with a total of 59 aortocoronary bypasses: 20 single bypasses, 10 double, 5 triple and 1 quadruple. Angiographic and CT evaluation was performed on average 24 months after surgery. CT scans were performed the day before coronary arteriography in 36 patients, with 7-mm thick thoracic sections taken before and after intravenous injection of contrast medium. A permeable aortocoronary bypass was visualized as a para-aortic opacity with a density which increased after injection of contrast medium (Fig. 13). During coronary arteriography a bypass was considered to be permeable when it, as well as the bypassed vessel, was selectively opacified. The qualities of the anastomosis, the downstream bed, the distal coronary network and the collateral circulation were assessed. In addition, 23 patients with a total of 36 bypasses underwent myocardial scintigraphy on the same day as CT. A normal uptake of thallium-201 in the region of the bypass indicated that it was permeable.

Coronary arteriography revealed that 44 of 59 aortocoronary bypasses were permeable at 24 months. CT detected only 47 of 59 bypasses, either because of metal clips which caused striated artefacts or because of the impossibility of analysing CT sections (a total of 20% non-contributory CT scans). On analysable images CT assessed correctly 40 of 47 aortocoronary bypasses (85%), 30 of 32 being permeable (94%) and 10 of 15 occluded (67%). Myocardial scintigraphy was less reliable: 25 of 36 bypasses were correctly assessed (64%), 18 of 27 being permeable and five out of nine occluded. However, scintigraphy provided additional indications to those of CT scanning. In particular, it gave a better assessment of the condition of the coronary bed downstream from the bypass. The two techniques combined indicated correctly 15 out of 15 good results (permeable bypasses and good downstream beds) and six out of eight poor results (permeable bypasses but deficient downstream beds).

2.2 Left Ventricular Function

Left ventricular function is determined by measuring ventricular volumes and EF and by analysing segmental contraction. Improvement in LV function after revascularization surgery is not always apparent [33, 34]. There is no improvement in the subject whose pre-operative EF was normal, nor when there was pre-operative myocardial necrosis or fibrosis with extensive akinesis. On the other hand, in cases of hypokinesis or akinesis of non-necrosed sections of the LV wall, improvement in

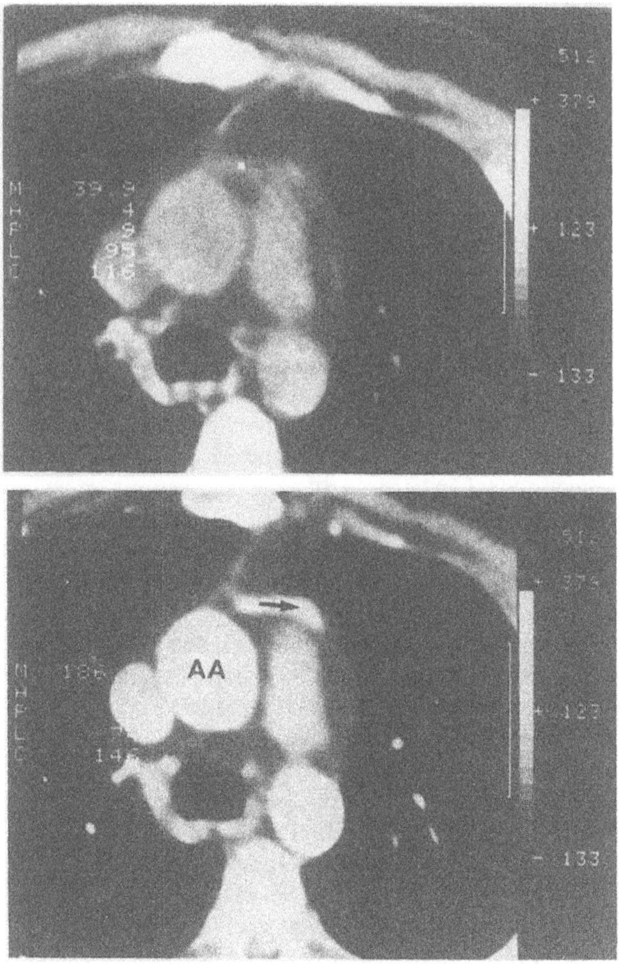

Fig. 13. X-ray computed tomography horizontal cross-section of the thorax *(upper):* before and *(lower):* after injection of contrast medium. The oblique course of the bypass *(black arrow)* directed from the ascending aorta *(AA)* to the left coronary artery is clearly visible

ventricular function is possible after surgery. About half the patients have improved postoperative LV function when all grafts are permeable. The increase is sometimes difficult to evaluate by ventriculography at rest and is better determined by postexercise ventriculography. Nitroglycerin and postextrasystolic potentiation of ventricular contraction are useful adjuvants in the identification of segments in which contractility has progressed after surgery (see Part II, Chap. V).

2.3 Coronary Arterial Network

Some studies have suggested that revascularization surgery may favour the progression of coronary atheromatous lesions undergoing stenosis. In effect, 30%–50% of stenoses located upstream from bypass anastomoses developed towards complete obstruction during the 1st postoperative year. This is not surprising in that a large number of these stenoses had been subocclusive. Moreover, there may be functional occlusion of the stenosis as a result of the good graft flow opposing the anterograde perfusion of the normal arterial route. The equalizing of pressures on both sides of the narrowing can also account for the occurrence of a thrombosis in situ. Analysis of the facts is relatively difficult [11, 13, 14, 19, 20]. In our experience [14], repeated examinations have shown that a stenosis upstream from a permeable graft, which arteriography indicates is totally occluded, may again prove permeable several months later when the graft is obstructed. In the case of an obstructed graft, precise analysis of the results leads to the conclusion that surgery is most often involved in the worsening of pre-existing lesions upstream or downstream from the anastomosis. With the exception of these iatrogenic aggravations, the progression of the coronary beds of bypassed vessels is no less favourable than that of vessels not operated upon.

References

1. Sewell WH (1974) Improved coronary vein graft patency rates with side to side anastomoses. Ann Thorac Surg 17: 538
2. McNeer JF, Lonley MJ, Starmer LF, Behar-Konte Y, Peter RH, Bartelag AG, Oldman NN, Young WH, Sabiston PC, Rosati RA (1974) Complete and incomplete revascularisation at aortocoronary by-pass surgery: experience with 392 consecutive patients. Am Heart J 88: 176
3. Cheanvechai C, Groves LK, Reyes EA (1975) Manual coronary endarterectomy – clinical experience in 315 patients. J Thorac Cardiovasc Surg 70: 524
4. Cosgrove DM, Loop FD, Irarrazaval MJ, Groves LK, Taylor PC, Golding LA (1978) Determinants of long survival after ventricular aneurysmectomy. Ann Thorac Surg 26: 357
5. Kitamura S, Echevarria M, Kay JM, Krohn BC, Redington JV, Mendez A, Zubiate P, Dunne EF (1972) Left ventricular performance before and after removal of the non-contractile area of the left ventricle and revascularisation of the myocardium. Circulation 45: 1005
6. Sesto M, Schwart F, Thiedeman KU, Flamente W, Schlepper M (1979) Failure of aneurysmectomy to improve left ventricular function. Br Heart J 41: 79
7. Amiel M, Mikaeloff P, Chassignolle C, Rubet A, Age C, Dupont JC, Janin A (1972) Les explorations angiographiques dans les pontages aorto coronariens: artériographie et ventriculographie. J Radiol 53: 611
8. Bourassa MG, Lesperance J, Campeau L, Simard P (1972) Factors influencing patency of aortocoronary vein grafts. Circulation 45 [Suppl I]: 79
9. Lesperance J, Bourassa MG, Saltiel J, Grondin CM (1972) Late changes in aortocoronary vein grafts: angiographic features. AJR 116: 74
10. Lesperance J, Bourassa MG, Saltiel J, Campeau L, Grondin CM (1973) Angiographic changes in aortocoronary vein grafts: lack of progression beyond the first year. Circulation 48: 633
11. Grondin CM, Lesperance J, Bourassa MG, Pasternac A, Campeau L, Grondin P (1974) Serial angiographic evaluation in 60 consecutive patients with aortocoronary artery vein grafts 2 weeks, 1 year and 3 years after operation. J Thorac Cardiovasc Surg 67: 1
12. Campeau L, Crochet D, Lesperance J, Bourassa MG, Grondin CM (1975) Postoperative changes in aortocoronary saphenous vein grafts revisited. Angiographic studies at two weeks and at one year in two series of consecutive patients. Circulation 52: 369
13. Itscoitz SB, Redwood DR, Stinson EB, Reis RL, Epstein SE (1975) Saphenous vein bypass grafts: longterm patency and effect on the native coronary circulation. Am J Cardiol 36: 739
14. Amiel M, Mikaeloff Ph, Chassignolle J, Delaye J, Allard D (1976) Angiographic studies after revascularization. In: Lichtlen PR (ed) Coronary angiography and angina pectoris. Thieme, Stuttgart
15. Lawrie GM, Lie JT, Morris GC, Beazley HL (1976) Vein graft patency and intimal proliferation after aortocoronary bypass: early and long-term angiopathologic correlations. Am J Cardiol 38: 856

16. Lawrie GM, Morris GC, Chapman DW, Winters WL, Lie JT (1977) Patterns of patency of 596 vein grafts up to seven years after aortocoronary bypass. J Thorac Cardiovasc Surg 73: 443
17. Lawrie GM, Morris GC, Howell JF, Ogura JW, Spencer WH, Cashion WR, Winters WL, Beazley HL, Chapman DW, Peterson PK, Lie JT (1977) Results of coronary bypass more than 5 years after operation in 434 patients. Clinical, treadmill and angiographic correlations. Am J Cardiol 40: 655
18. Campeau L, David PR, Lesperance J, Bourassa MG (1978) Perméabilité et modifications tardives des pontages aortocoronariens par greffe saphène: 5 à 7 ans après chirurgie. Arch Mal Coeur 71: 1195
19. Mikaeloff P, Perrin A, Delaye J, Milon H, Amiel M, Leoni F, Clerget JM, Willems P, Biron A (1978) Analyse des facteurs pronostiques après pontage aorto-coronaire et résultats des contrôles coronarographiques tardifs. Arch Mal Coeur 71: 33
20. Campeau L, Lesperance J, Hermann J, Corbara F, Grondin CM, Bourassa MG (1979) Loss of improvement of angina between 1 and 7 years after aortocoronary bypass surgery: correlation with changes in vein grafts and in coronary arteries. Circulation 60 [Suppl I]: 1
21. Bopp P, Fournet PC, Noble J, Moret P, Hahn C, Faidutti B (1979) Perméabilité à 5 ans des pontages veineux aorto-coronariens. Arch Mal Coeur 72: 139
22. Guthaner DF, Robert EW, Alderman EL, Wexler L (1979) Long term serial angiographic studies after coronary artery bypass surgery. Circulation 60: 250
23. Grondin CM, Campeau L, Lesperance J, Solymoss BC, Vouhe P, Castonguay YR, Meere C, Bourassa MG (1979) Atherosclerotic changes in coronary vein grafts six years after operation. Angiographic aspects in 100 patients. J Thorac Cardiovasc Surg 77: 24
24. Bardner HB, Mudd JG, Mark AL, Naseer A, Dickens JF (1976) Patency of internal mammary coronary grafts. Circulation 54: 70
25. Hamby RI, Aintablian A, Wisoff BG, Harstein ML (1977) Comparative study of the postoperative flow in the saphenous vein and internal mammary artery bypass grafts. Am Heart J 93: 306
26. Jones JW, Ochsner JL, Mills NL, Hughes L (1980) Clinical comparison between patients with saphenous vein and internal mammary artery as a coronary graft. J Thorac Cardiovasc Surg 80: 334
27. Vasile N, Usdin JP, Belloir C, Ferrane J, Galey JJ, Vernant P (1979) Perméabilité des pontages aorto-coronaires explorés par tomodensitométrie. Arch Mal Coeur 72: 1346
28. Brundage BH, Herfkens RJ, Berninger WH, Redington RW, Chatterjee K, Carlsson E (1980) Detection of coronary bypass grafts by computed tomography. Circulation 61: 826
29. Moncada R, Salinas M, Churchill R, Love L, Reynes C, Demos TC, Hale D, Schreiber R (1980) Patency of saphenous aortocoronary-bypass grafts demonstrated by computed tomography. N Engl J Med 303: 503
30. Kahl FR, Wolfman NT, Watts LE (1981) Evaluation of aortocoronary bypass graft status by computed tomography. Am J Cardiol 48: 304
31. Daniel WG, Dorhing W, Lichtlen PR, Stender HS (1980) Non-invasive assessment of aorto-coronary by-pass graft patency by computed tomography. Lancet 1: 1023
32. Perrenoud JJ, Hauser H, Bopp P, Hahn C, Rutishauer W (1981) Valeur de la tomoradiométrie transverse dans le contrôle de la perméabilité des ponts aorto-coronaires par rapport à la coronarographie. Arch Mal Coeur 74: 41
33. Swan HJC, Chatterjee K (1974) Objective evidence of improved left ventricular function following myocardial revascularisation. Adv Cardiol 11: 143
34. Levine JA, Bechtel DJ, Cohn PF, Herman MV, Gorlin R, Cohn LH, Collins JJ Jr (1975) Ventricular function before and after direct revascularization surgery. A proposal for an index of vascularization to correlate angiographic and ventriculographic findings. Circulation 51: 1071

IX Angiographic Explorations: Coronary Arterial Involvement in Various Diseases

1 Acquired Valvular Diseases

The actual frequency of association of a coronary artery disease with a valvular disease is not known with accuracy because published works concern either autopsy analyses after valve replacement [1] or non-randomized arteriographic studies [2], most often limited to aortic valvular diseases [3–6]. Coronary atheromatous lesions have been observed in 15%–40% of aortic [4–7] and 16% of mitral valvular diseases [2]. The association is found to be increasingly more frequent in relation to the subject's advancing age, a fact which in itself accounts for the difference in frequency between aortic (17.7%), mitro-aortic (21%) and mitral (8.6%) valvular diseases in the autopsy series of Coleman [1].

The clinical recognition of coronary artery disease associated with a valvular disease is difficult, if not impossible. Myocardial ischaemia together with angina pectoris, observed in more than 50% of aortic and in a lesser percentage of mitral valvular diseases, may be secondary to the simple increase in cardiac work resulting from valvular disease [3]. The severity of the valvular disease may limit the functional capacity of patients and thus prevent clinical detection of the underlying coronary artery disease during exercise, although this hypothesis is not acceptable to some authors [3, 5]. In any case, absence of anginal pain generally corresponds to less severe coronary afflictions.

In the absence of definite clinical criteria for detecting coronary involvement, the use of coronary arteriography in assessing a valvular disease before surgical treatment is generally acceptable. It is admitted in cases of exertional angina and, a fortiori, resting angina, in cases of ECG anomalies suggestive of previous myocardial infarction and, in most laboratories, in asymptomatic subjects from the fifth decade of life on, an age group in which coronary disease shows a significant increase in frequency in the general population. Finally, such indications concern more than 90% of patients with acquired aortic stenosis [7].

Exploration should be performed with special care to assess the respective severity of the two afflictions, study of left ventricular function being absolutely essential [7]. Technical difficulties are encountered in selective catheterization of coronary ostia and in the assessment of aortic valvular diseases. Following verticalization of the plane of the aortic orifice, the left ostium is frequently seen to originate from the roof of the left coronary sinus, the right ostium being displaced frontwards and downwards. The presence of an aortic jet or of a massive regurgitation makes the catheter unstable above the right coronary valve. In elderly subjects (over 70), it is not infrequently discovered that iliac arterial sinuosities limit catheter manoeuvering by the femoral approach; thus the brachial approach is preferable. The findings of coronary arteriography have fundamental therapeutic implications: a normal coronary network in the presence of angina constitutes a proof of the severity of the valvular disease; and the existence of significant coronary artery stenoses suggests the possibility of associating myocardial revascularization surgery with prosthetic valve replacement. The advantage of this treatment is still an important subject of controversy [8, 9]. In all cases, the angiographic exploration of coronary artery disease would seem to be the single reliable means of determining the surgical prognosis with reasonable accuracy [1–10].

2 Mitral Valve Prolapse

The prolapse of the posterolateral leaflet of the mitral valve can be found in asymptomatic subjects or as a consequence of rather specific clinical and ECG signs of Barlow's syndrome: palpitations, vertigo, thoracic pains, mid-systolic click and late systolic murmur, anomalies of the ST segment in leads II, III and aVF, arrhythmias, cerebral embolisms and, in rare cases, progression towards sudden death. Mitral valve prolapse is one of the most common cardiac anomalies (5%–10% of the population) and has been described in a variety of affections: Marfan's syndrome and other connective tissue disorders, cardiomyopathies, rheumatic diseases, ischaemic cardiopathy, etc. The pathology shows that this mitral anomaly is most often secondary to an idiopathic valvular myxomatous involvement. The diagnosis is based on clinical examination and ultrasonography. Left ventriculography [11, 12] in right anterior oblique (RAO) projection clearly shows the systolic protrusion of the little valve into the left atrium, behind the low part of the mitral ring and the fulcrum (Fig. 1). The tissue redundancy is sometimes evident in the distinctly scalloped edges of the prolapsed leaflet. The possible associated anomalies are protrusion of the posterior, and sometimes the anterior, papillary muscle into the ventricular cavi-

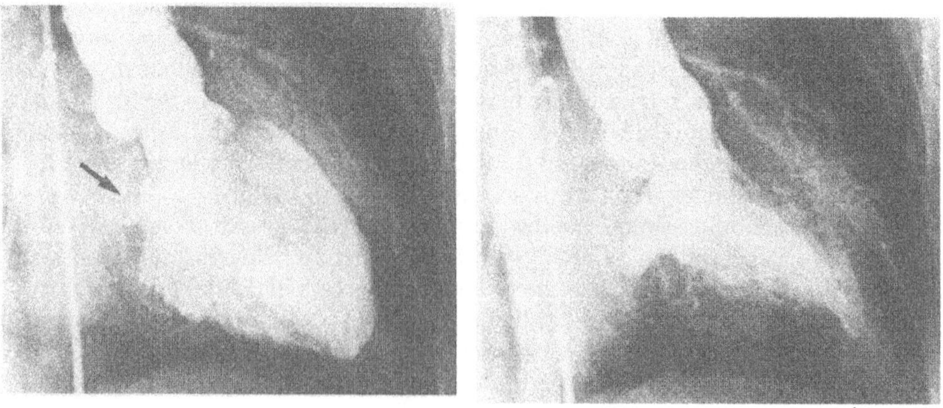

Fig. 1. Mitral valve prolapse. Right anterior oblique view of left ventricular angiogram. *(Left):* diastole: abnormal scalloped contour of the atrial limit of the mitral valve *(arrow)*; *(right):* systole; marked protrusion of the valve beyond the line joining the aortic valve to the posterior point of the inferior wall

ty, ventricular dilatation, and hypokinesis of the lateral and/or inferior basal part of the ventricle. Localized cardiomyopathy has been considered, but its nature, whether primary or secondary to the valvular anomaly itself, has not been made clear. Agenesia or hypodevelopment of the circumflex artery has been implicated as the cause [13]. The ischaemic pathogenesis is evident in patients who have suffered an infarction with dysfunction of a papillary muscle [14]. When the coronary arteries appear to be angiographically normal in patients afflicted with angina or infarction, coronary embolisms have been considered responsible [15], by analogy with the cerebral embolisms observed in this same syndrome. The overall frequency of mitral valve prolapse in coronary artery disease has been assessed as 31.6% [16] and 16% [17]. These high rates reinforce the hypothesis that valvular disease is secondary to a left ventricular segmental contraction anomaly, which sometimes shows a preference for papillary muscle involvement.

3 Myocardial Bridges

Although long familiar to anatomists, intramyocardial coronary artery routes were only described in angiographic terms by Amplatz in 1968 [18]. A normally epicardial artery is covered along part of its course (1–4 cm) by a bridge of myocardial fibres. This anatomical variation concerns mainly the proximal third of the left anterior descending artery (LAD) and, secondarily, its diagonal and left marginal branches or the right marginal branches (tetralogy of Fallot). The arteries of the atrioventricular grooves are not involved. The intramyocardial course entails an abnormal angulation of the artery, which momentarily loses its natural curvature before recovering it. In the most typical cases, and the easiest to identify, there is a systolic strangulation or "milking effect". For the anterior interventricular artery this systolic narrowing is clearly visible in left anterior oblique (LAO) projection free of superimposed features (Figs. 2 and 3). In lateral projection the intramyocardial LAD often leaves the anterior heart border, coursing behind its diagonal branch for 1–4 cm. A marked left ventricular hypertrophy, especially in obstructive hypertrophic cardiomyopathies, is certainly a factor revealing the anomaly. Its association with spasm is possible. Most myocardial bridges produce no symptoms, which is hardly surprising, since 75% of myocardial perfusion is ensured during diastole. In a certain number of cases, anginal manifestations indisputably occur, and sometimes rhythm disturbances, mainly during exercise, perhaps because of enhanced inotropism and shortening of the diastole. Aortocoronary bypass is likely to improve the condition of some patients and to make the biological signs of ischaemia disappear [19]. In any case, the logical solution is simply to eliminate the bridge whenever possible. Spontaneous or pacing-induced tachycardia and intensification of contraction by means of an extrasystole or a stimulating beta agent are factors contributing to marked increase in systolic strangulation, as is nitroglycerin, according to Ishimori [20], who has estimated the frequency of LAD bridges as 1.6% of the population subjected to coronary arteriography.

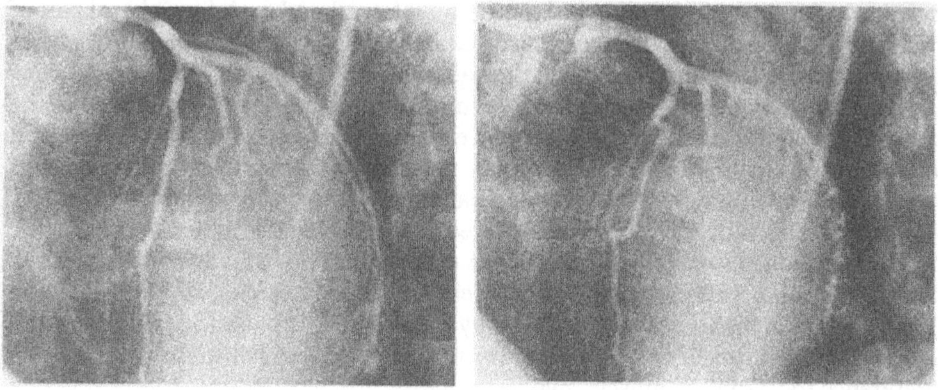

Fig. 2. Myocardial bridge. Left anterior oblique view of the left coronary artery. Desaxation of the left anterior descending artery *(left):* persisting in diastole and *(right):* strongly accentuated in systole, with rather moderate arterial narrowing

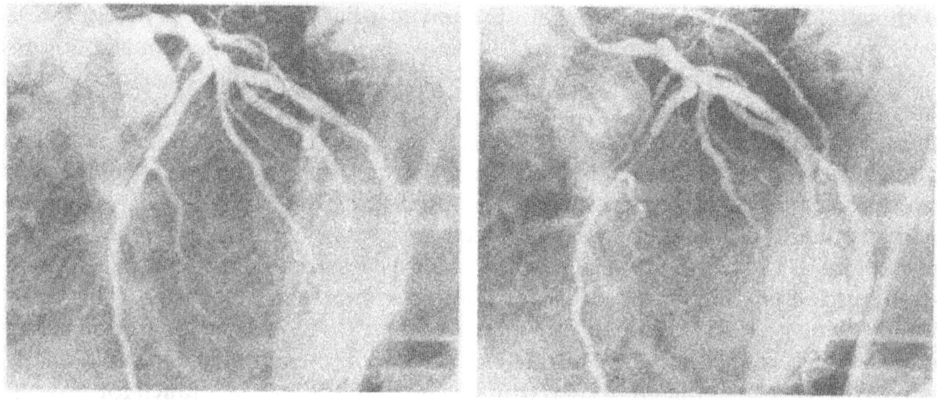

Fig. 3. Myocardial bridge. Left anterior oblique view of the left coronary artery. There is virtually no desaxation of the left anterior descending artery (LAD) when it passes under the bridge, either *(left):* in diastole or *(right):* in systole. Severe milking effect on the LAD in systole

4 Coronary Arterial Embolism

There are many causes of coronary arterial embolism [21–23]: acute and subacute infective endocarditis; left intracavitary thromboses in association with mitral valvular disease, atrial fibrillation, myocardial infarction, a valve prosthesis or a cardiomyopathy; fragmentation of the calcifications of a stenosed aortic valve or of a left intracavitary tumour; a paradoxical embolism which has passed through a defect in the interatrial septum or a distended foramen ovale; and iatrogenic embolisms [24]. The acute occlusion of a coronary artery has been a rare complication of coronary arteriography ever since systematic heparinization of the patient was recommended [25]. Fibrinocruoric or fibrinoplatelet embolisms are the most common types, but it is also possible for the catheter or metallic guide to carry fatty or muscle material from the point of skin puncture to the coronary artery. Initially, this complication occurred more frequently with Judkins' than Sones' technique. The perfecting of sheaths of the Desilets-Hoffman type, specially adapted to the arterial route, was a second decisive advance in eliminating these embolic complications almost completely. Angiographically, the coronary embolism is characterized by an image of abrupt and total arterial obstruction, with no variation in vessel calibre before the occlusion and no anastomotic collateral circulation. Most often the site of the occlusion is distal. These angiographic characteristics may be absent when the embolus is blocked by a pre-existing stenosis. According to histopathological reports, the left coronary artery is more affected than the right coronary artery and the LAD more than the circumflex [23] in cases of spontaneous embolism. This distribution may not be perfectly representative of reality because of the definitely higher mortality rate for LAD occlusions. With respect to accidents due to coronary arteriography, occlusion of the circumflex seems to be the most frequent. Emergency surgical treatment of these complications has been proposed only for patients whose rhythmic or haemodynamic condition is unstable [24], since an intervention cannot prevent formation of an infarct. Today, intracoronary thrombolytic treatment must, of course, be considered first. Despite customary technical precautions, any catheter manoeuver involves a certain degree of risk of coronary or other embolism in some affections: infective endocarditis, calcified aortic stenosis, infarction or cardiomyopathy with intracavitary thrombosis, friable tumour of the left cardiac chambers, and intra-aortic floating thrombus. A last cause very characteristic of coronary ostial embolism is papillary fibro-elastoma of the aortic valve, also called "fixed embolism".

5 Syphilitic Coronary Arterial Stenosis

It is well known that syphilis has a predilection for the ascending aorta during the secondary phase of the disease. By order of frequency, coronary ostial stenosis is the third-ranking cardiovascular complication after aortic aneurysm and aortic regurgitation. A significant coronary ostial stenosis is found in 26% of patients presenting a cardiovascular syphilitic affection upon autopsy [26]. In the living subject ostial stenosis is generally detected at the moment of pre-operative assessment of aortic regurgitation or of angina pectoris. In our experience its frequency is of the order of two out of 1000 coronary arteriography examinations; and it is curious to note that the diagnosis of syphilis is often suggested because of angiographic data. The presence of extensive calcifications of the thoracic aorta or, a fortiori, of a calcified aneurysm of the ascending aorta is very indicative of syphilitic aortitis. It is unusual to discover ostial stenosis complicated by angina in patients younger than 45. The risks for coronary arteriography are the same as for stenoses of the left main coronary trunk. Suprasigmoid aortography in LAO projection can visualize the ostial stenosis (Fig. 4), but the method is uncertain. In effect, either the oblique angle ideal for placing the X-ray beam parallel to the plane of the ostium may not be obtained, or the filling of the coronary arteries may be poor in the case of aortic insufficiency. Selective coronary arteriography is the only reliable method for making the diagnosis, detecting associated atheromatous lesions and confirming, if such is the case, the presence of pure functional angina caused by aortic insufficiency.

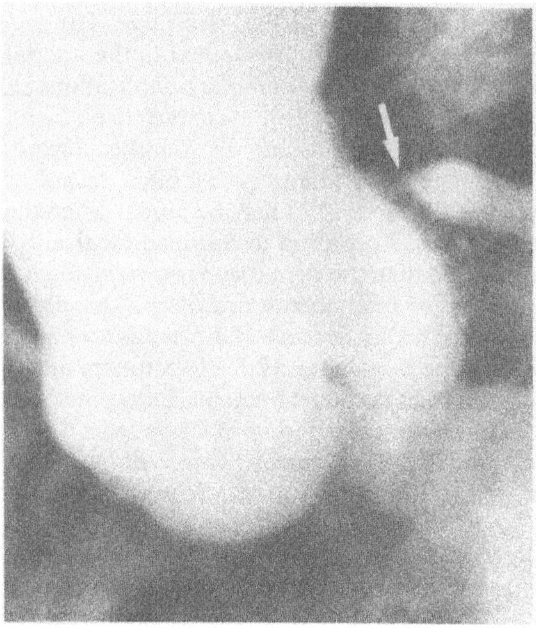

Fig. 4. Syphilitic left ostial coronary stenosis *(arrow)* evidenced by aortography in the left anterior oblique projection

6 Takayasu's Disease

The cause of this disease, described by an ophthalmologist in 1908 [27], is still a mystery. Asia and Africa are its principal domains. In effect, it is an inflammatory arteritis which has a preference for the thoracic and abdominal aortas, the brachiocephalic vessels and the renal arteries. It is especially a disease of young women (85% of cases). Coronary involvement is a possible complication of the disease. Clinically, it is revealed by anginal attacks or myocardial infarction [28, 29]. The stenoses, which are generally proximal, are more often located in the coronary ostia (60%–75%) than in the proximal arterial segments [28–30]. The true ostial stenosis is due to the compression and progressive obliteration of the orifice by proliferative fibrosis of the aortic intima. Para-ostial or proximal stenosis is caused by spread of the arteritic process to the coronary artery. The angiographic images are remarkably similar to those for syphilitic aortitis (Fig. 5).

7 Cardiac Tumours and Intracavitary Thrombi

Coronary arteriography plays a secondary role in the diagnosis of cardiac tumours. Alterations in the morphology of cardiac cavities detected by angiocardiography are generally sufficient indicators of tumour dimensions. It is only in the case of intramural tumours that angiographic study of the disorganization and compression of the coronary artery branches can be truly useful. There are no specific coronary arteriographic features to indicate whether a tumour is benign or malignant [31]. Myxomas, which are by far the most frequent tumours, are traversed by a very fine

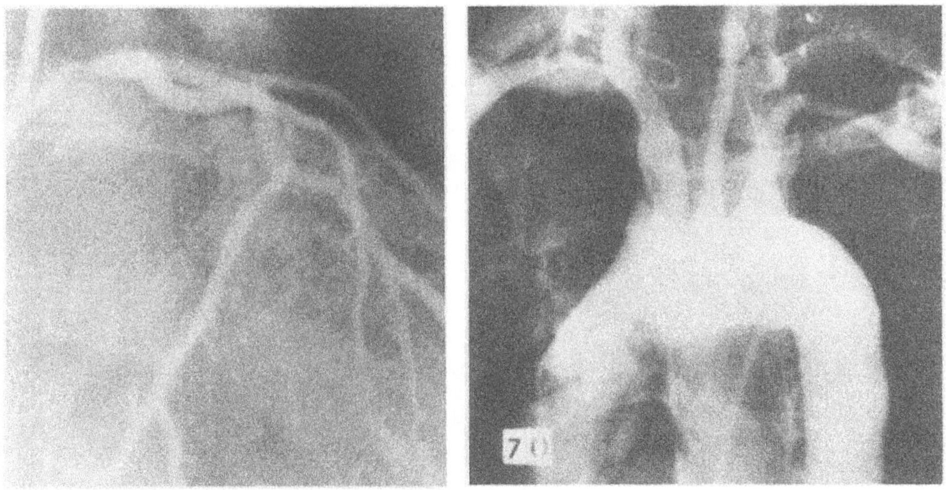

Fig. 5. Takayasu's disease in a 35-year-old woman. *(Left):* right anterior oblique view of a para-ostial stenosis of the left main stem; *(right):* left anterior oblique view of the aorta demonstrating the arteritic involvement of this vessel and its main branches, especially of the subclavian arteries

arteriolar network. Coronary arteriography can visualize this delicate vascular network, and sometimes also a more markedly hypervascularized area [32, 33]. Coronary arteriography can localize the pedicle of tumour implantation and show its relations with the coronary arteries. It can be useful in detecting a recurrence. By analogy with the myxomas, it is of interest to mention the neovascularizations of left intraventricular or intra-atrial mural thromboses observed by some authors [34, 35]. Coronary arteriography is an essential exploration in pre-operative assessment of a tumour capable of invading the myocardium. Pericardial cysts and tumours deform the cardiac silhouette and are the cause of more or less marked extrinsic compression of cardiac walls and coronary arteries, so that there is apparent alteration in the normal external heart contour (Fig. 6). The hydatid cysts have an intramural site such that they compress and deform the endocardial outline of the cardiac cavities and force up the epicardial arteries, pushing them away from the centre of the cardiac mass (Fig. 7).

8 Traumatic Coronary Injuries

During the early years of extracorporeal circulation the traumatic injury most often observed in coronary arteriography was stenosis following coronary cannulation (Fig. 8). The perfecting of cannulation material and the development of modern methods of intra-operative myocardial protection have eliminated this complication.

Injury to a coronary artery, whether a contusion or laceration, can be caused by blunt trauma or penetrating trauma of the thorax. The main causes are traffic accidents, crushing of the thorax due to falls or collisions and knife or bullet wounds.

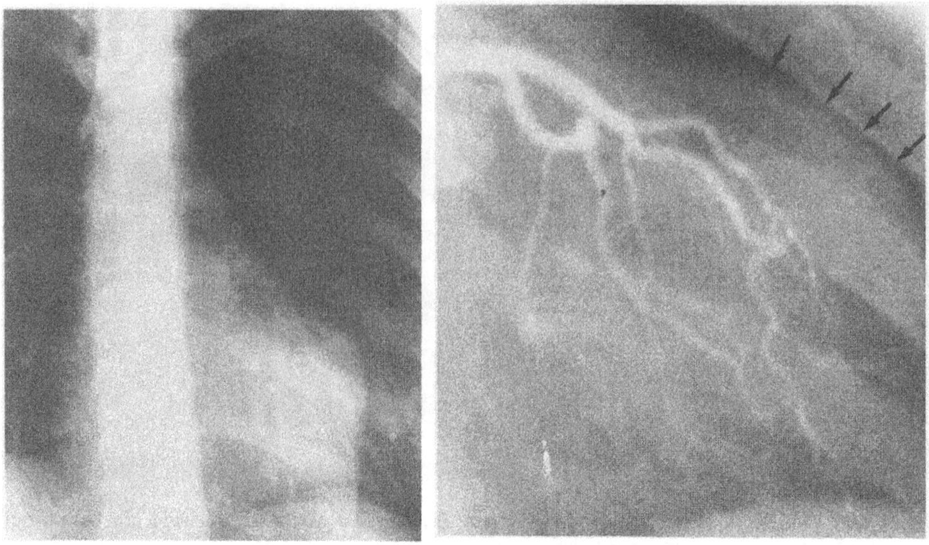

Fig. 6. Pericardial cyst. *(Left):* Presence of a bump on the left border of the heart. *(Right):* The nature of the bump is probably pericardial, as it appears outside the coronary arteries

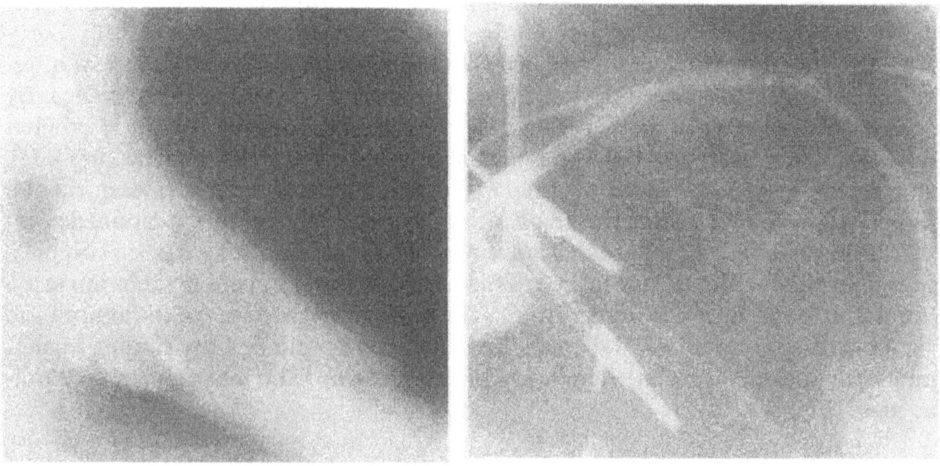

Fig. 7. Intramyocardial hydatid cyst. Right anterior oblique views of *(left):* the left ventricle and *(right):* the left coronary artery. Note the rectilinear aspect of the ventricular anterior wall and the raised, swollen course of the left anterior descending artery and its diagonal branch

Coronary contusion can be responsible for myocardial infarction, though the exact mechanism is often difficult to define (Fig. 9). In our experience, if the patient is young it is advisable to perform coronary arteriography as soon as possible. In fact, some time after the accident the coronary arteries often look normal, so that it is impossible to differentiate between infarction due to pure myocardial contusion and

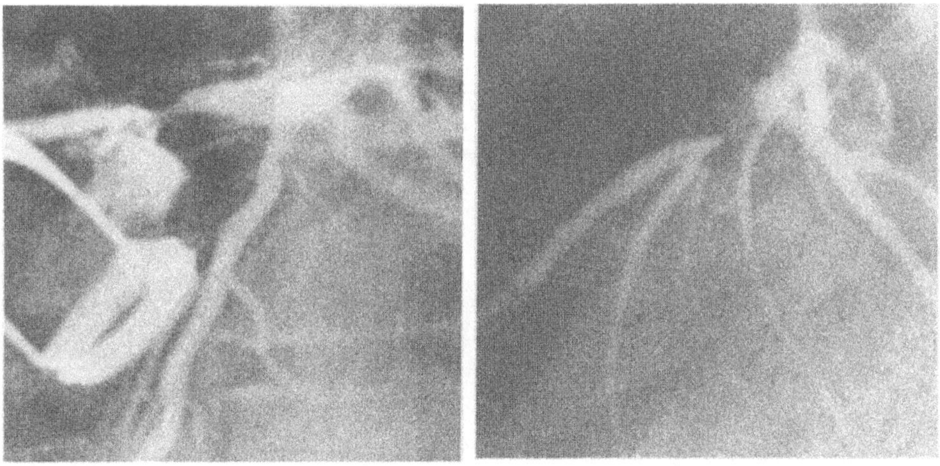

Fig. 8 *(upper)*. Left anterior oblique view of the left coronary artery. Typical postcannulation regular concentric stenosis of the left main trunk in a patient with aortic prosthetic valve replacement

Fig. 9 *(lower)*. Transverse view of the left coronary artery in a young man in the late phase of an anterior myocardial infarction following a chest trauma. Subtotal stenosis of the proximal left anterior descending artery interpreted as a sequela of a primary complete occlusion

that due to transient coronary occlusion. The occlusion would seem to be due to formation of a clot upon contact with an intimal fissure or a subintimal haemorrhage. We (Amiel) have observed three major angiographic features in a total of ten patients: total and abrupt obstruction of the artery, eccentric stenosis suggesting extrinsic compression by detachment of the intima, and irregular stenotic contours indicative of parietal dilaceration (a feature observed after intra-operative iatrogenic injury to the LAD). In all these cases there were associated signs of myocardial infarction. In the elderly subject significant atheromatous stenoses are often conducive to infarction. Other authors have provided proof of the total obstruction of normal arteries in young subjects during the early phase of traumatism [36]. In our angiographic experience there have been no cases of coronary arterial lacerations during the acute phase of the accident. In practice, such lacerations are treated by emergency operation [37]. At a late stage they may take the form of a coronarocardiac fistula (Fig. 10). In around two-thirds of cases these fistulae are located in the right coronary artery [38]. Among the traumatic coronary injuries which may occur are iatrogenic coronary artery dissections (see Sect. 9).

9 Coronary Artery Dissection

The vast majority of spontaneous coronary artery dissections are discovered upon autopsy in patients with a history of infarction, sometimes after sudden death or thoracic injury [39, 40]. Spontaneous dissections are rare, if the spread of an aortic dissection at the origin of the coronary arteries is excluded. Out of around 60 cases reported in the literature, most concern young women during the postpartum peri-

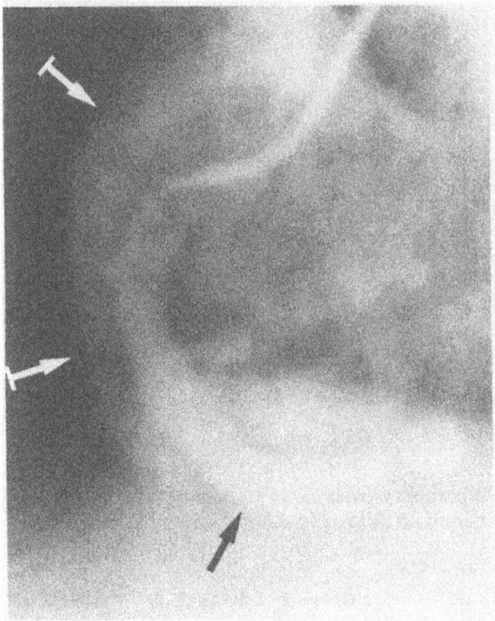

Fig. 10. Left anterior oblique view of the right coronary artery (RCA). Coronarocardiac fistula between the RCA *(black arrow)* and the right atrium *(white arrows)*, due to a penetrating gunshot wound

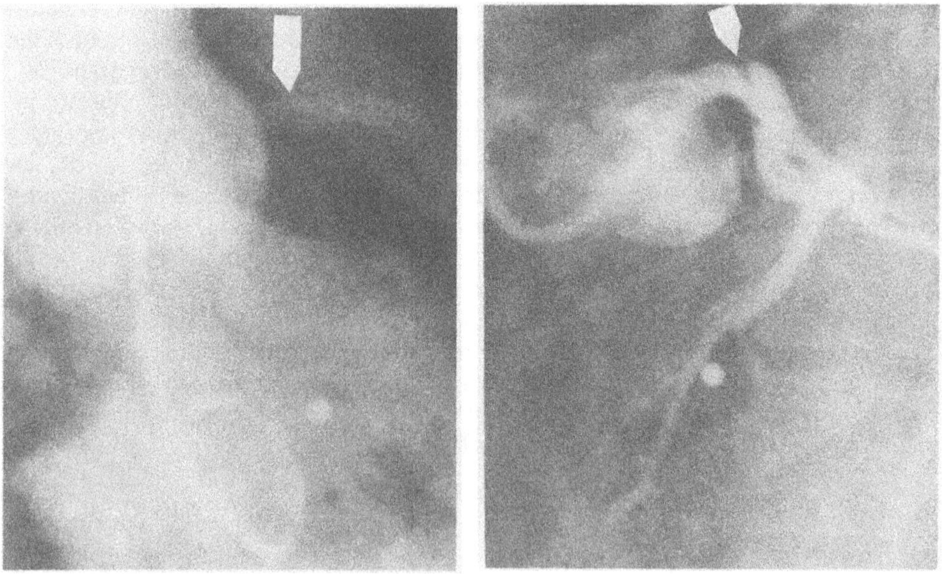

Fig. 11. Postpartum anterior myocardial infarction in a 25-year-old woman. The absence of risk factors led to systematic coronary arteriography. *(Left):* Right anterior oblique view of the left ventriculogram. The faint opacification of the left main trunk is sufficient to delineate the horizontal radiolucent dissected intima *(under the white arrow). (Right):* Left anterior oblique view of the left coronary artery. The radiolucency of the intima separates the arterial medial true channel from the external false one. The flow is severely delayed in the distal left anterior descending artery

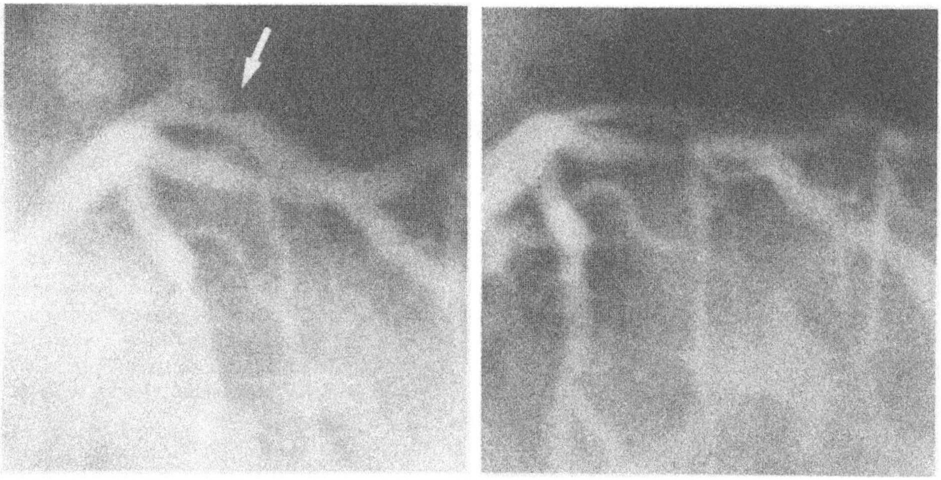

Fig. 12. Right anterior oblique views of the left coronary artery in a case of iatrogenic coronary dissection. *(Left):* The fine radiolucency of the dissected intima is clearly visible *(white arrow)* encircling the subintimal space, which retains dye. *(Right):* Later in the same examination the dissection is no longer detectable, but the left anterior descending artery is narrowed

od. Coronary artery dissection is a possible complication of Ehlers-Danlos syndrome. Some post-traumatic cases have been reported. In cases of spontaneous dissection only arteriography performed very shortly after the coronary accident allows diagnosis with certitude of the dissecting process; our observations include such a case in a young woman (Fig. 11).

Iatrogenic dissections, which were complications during the early years of coronary arteriography application, have become exceptional. They are facilitated by localized atheroma in the first centimetre of the artery and are due to detachment of an atheromatous plaque or of the adjacent intima. They are visualized in different ways: subintimal sequestration of the contrast medium over varying distances; eccentric pseudostenosis with stagnation of the contrast medium, which remains trapped in the subintimal space and disappears very slowly (Fig. 12); or, the most characteristic feature, a radiolucent image of the detached intima separating the true from the false channel, comparable to the image of aortic dissection (Fig. 13).

10 Cardiomyopathies

In cases of primary congestive cardiomyopathy, coronary arteriography is consistently normal. Artery calibre is generally greater than normal, in keeping with the increased myocardial mass. Coronary arteriography is rightly considered to be essential in confirming the idiopathic nature of the myocardial disease. Sometimes an ischaemic cardiomyopathy is discovered, with multiple significant coronary lesions which developed asymptomatically without pain until they led to extreme alteration of left ventricular contraction. Coronary arteriography is also useful in ruling out

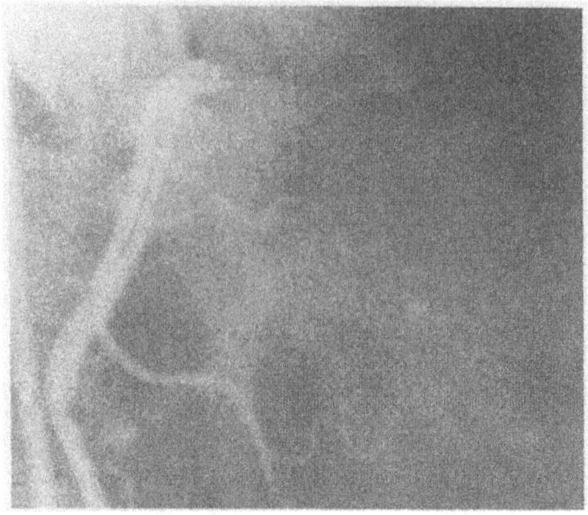

Fig. 13. Right anterior oblique view of the right coronary artery in a case of iatrogenic coronary dissection. The nearly vertical radiolucent line of the dissected intima is analogous to the image often seen in aortic dissection

the possibility of myocardial necrosis in cases with abnormal Q waves, either of dilated or hypertrophic cardiomyopathies.

Obstructive coronary atheroma is not infrequent in cases of hypertrophic cardiomyopathy, especially in its obstructive forms (idiopathic hypertrophic subaortic stenosis). According to some authors, coronary lesions conducive to stenosis are common in patients over 45 [41] and found in 40% of those over 40 [42]. The presence of angina does not allow the existence of such lesions to be diagnosed. A characteristic, though non-specific, angiographic feature of obstructive hypertrophic cardiomyopathies is the systolic narrowing of the septal arteries [43].

11 Other Diseases

Involvement of the coronary arteries is rare but possible in giant cell arteritis (Horton's disease or temporal arteritis) [44]. Occurrence of angina or infarction is a not infrequent possibility. As the patients are in general quite elderly, it is impossible to confirm that the coronary artery stenoses are due to arteritis as long as they have not been studied histologically. Atheroma is obviously the most common causal factor. Improvement in anginal symptoms following corticosteroid therapy provides evidence that the coronary lesions are caused by arteritis. Diagnosis of coronary artery involvement in rheumatoid arthritis is also based mainly on autopsy [45].

Among connective tissue diseases, coronary artery involvement is most frequent with periarteritis nodosa [46]. The clinical symptomatology is relatively scant; angina is infrequent and infarctions develop asymptomatically. This is due to the fact that the arterial lesions are distal and that they appear and multiply progressively. Angiographic detection of multiple small aneurysms is quite suggestive of periarteritis nodosa.

Kawasaki disease or mucocutaneous lymph node syndrome can be related to periarteritis nodosa. It is a disease of the newborn and the child observed mainly in Japan [47]. The coronary lesions consist in stenoses and aneurysms (Fig. 14). Death due to infarction or rupture of aneurysms is not unusual. Bypass surgery [48] must sometimes be performed. An at least partial regression of lesions has been noted in

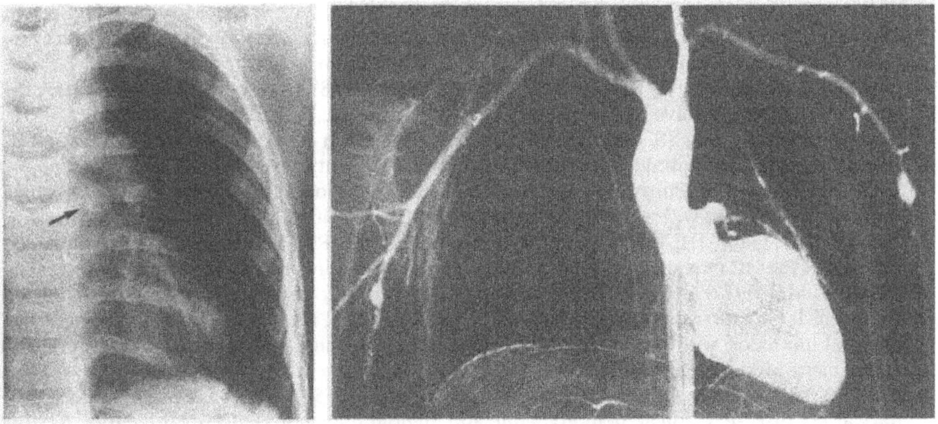

Fig. 14. Multiple aneurysms in a child suffering from Kawasaki disease. *(Left):* frontal chest roentgenogram: annular calcification *(arrow)* corresponding to a left main trunk aneurysm; *(right):* left ventricular angiogram: aneurysms of the left coronary stem and brachial arteries. (Courtesy of P. Chaumont)

survivors [49]. The nearly giant nature of certain coronary aneurysms is characteristic of the disease.

Angina, myocardial infarction and sudden death are possible complications of scleroderma or progressive systemic sclerosis. The autopsy shows that these myocardial ischaemic complications nearly always occur in normal coronary arteries [50]. The hypothesis of a spastic pathogenesis or coronary Raynaud's phenomenon is quite likely.

References

1. Coleman EH, Soloff LA (1970) Incidence of significant coronary artery disease in rheumatic valvular heart disease. Am J Cardiol 25: 401
2. Vacheron A, Metzger JP, Heulin A, Lafont H, Georges C, Di Matteo J (1978) La coronarographie dans l'exploration pré-opératoire des valvulopathies acquises non ischémiques. Arch Mal Coeur 71: 1233
3. Bonchek LI, Anderson RP, Rosch J (1973) Should coronary arteriography be performed routinely before valve replacement? Am J Cardiol 31: 462
4. Harris CN, Kaplan MA, Parker OP, Dunne EF, Cowell HS, Ellestad MH (1975) Aortic stenosis, angina, and coronary artery disease: interrelations. Br Heart J 37: 656
5. Paquay PA, Anderson G, Diefenthal H, Nordstrom L, Richman HG, Gobel FL (1976) Chest pain as a predictor of coronary artery disease in patients with obstructive aortic valve disease. Am J Cardiol 38: 863
6. Heulin A, Luxereau Ph, Ducimetiere P, Menuet JC, Bruntz JF, Valty J, Lablanche JM, Nicolas G, Bassand JC (1979) Les lésions coronaires des valvulopathies aortiques opérées. I. Fréquence et éléments cliniques de prévision. Arch Mal Coeur 72: 1108
7. Crochet D, Petitier H, De Laguerenne J, Wanlin P, Chiffoleau S, Grossetete R, Godin JF (1983) Le rétrécissement aortique de l'adulte: apport du cathétérisme pour l'étude des lésions associées. A propos de 137 cas. Arch Mal Coeur 76: 1057
8. Kirklin JW, Kouchoukos NT (1981) Aortic valve replacement without myocardial revascularization. Circulation 63: 252

9. Bonow RO, Kent KM, Rosing DR, Lipson LC, Borer JS, Mc Intosh CL, Morrow AG, Epstein SE (1981) Aortic valve replacement without myocardial revascularization in patients with combined aortic valvular and coronary artery disease. Circulation 63: 243
10. Linhart JW, De la Torre A, Ramsey HW, Wheat MW Jr (1968) The significance of coronary artery disease in aortic valve replacement. J Thorac Cardiovasc Surg 55: 811
11. Scampardonis G, Yang SS, Maranhao V, Goldberg H, Booch AS (1976) Left ventricular abnormalities in prolapsed mitral leaflet syndrome. Preview of eighty-seven cases. Circulation 54: 707
12. Smith ER, Fraser DB, Purdy JW, Anderson RN (1977) Angiographic diagnosis of mitral valve prolapse: correlation with echocardiography. Am J Cardiol 40: 165
13. Gentzler RD, Gault JH, Liedtke JA, Mc Cann WD, Mann RH, Hunter AS (1975) Congenital absence of the left circumflex artery in the systolic click syndrome. Circulation 52: 490
14. Crawford MH (1977) Mitral valve prolapse due to coronary artery disease. Am J Med 62: 447
15. Imaizumi T, Chandraratna PAN, Whayne TF Jr, Schechter E, Bhatia SK (1978) Transmural myocardial infarction with the prolapsing mitral-leaflet syndrome and normal coronary arteries. Arch Intern Med 138: 1354
16. Aranda LM, Befeler B, Lazzaro R, Embi A, Machado H (1975) Mitral valve prolapse and coronary artery disease. Clinical, hemodynamic and angiographic correlations. Circulation 52: 245
17. Verani M, Carroll R, Falsetti H (1976) Mitral valve prolapse in coronary artery disease. Am J Cardiol 37: 1
18. Amplatz K, Anderson R (1968) Angiographic appearance of myocardial bridging of the coronary artery. Invest Radiol 3: 213
19. Noble J, Bourassa MG, Petitclerc E, Dyrda I (1976) Myocardial bridging and "milking effect" of the left anterior descending artery: normal variant or obstruction? Am J Cardiol 37: 993
20. Ishimori T, Raizner AE, Chahine RA, Awdeh M, Luchi RJ (1977) Myocardial bridges in man. Clinical correlations and angiographic accentuation with nitroglycerin. Cathet Cardiovasc Diagn 3: 59
21. Cheitlin MD, Mc Allister HA, De Castro CM (1975) Myocardial infarction without atherosclerosis. JAMA 231: 951
22. Loire R, Dubreuil C, Perrin A (1977) Les embolies coronaires. Étude d'une série de trente cas anatomocliniques. Arch Mal Coeur 70: 1
23. Prizel KR, Hutchins GM, Bulkley BH (1978) Coronary artery embolism and myocardial infarction: clinicopathologic study of 55 patients. Ann Intern Med 88: 155
24. Guss SB, Zir LM, Garrison HB, Daggett WM, Block PC, Dinsmore RE (1975) Coronary occlusion during coronary angiography. Circulation 52: 1063
25. Adams DF, Fraser DB, Abrams HL (1973) The complications of coronary arteriography. Circulation 48: 609
26. Heggtveit HA (1964) Syphilitic aortitis. A clinicopathologic autopsy study of 100 cases, 1950 to 1960. Circulation 29: 346
27. Takayasu M (1908) Case with unusual changes of the central vessels in the retina. Acta Soc Ophthalmol Jpn 12: 554
28. Cipriano PR, Silverman JF, Perlroth MG, Griepp RB, Wexler L (1977) Coronary arterial narrowing in Takayasu's aortitis. Am J Cardiol 39: 744
29. Pasternac A, Lesperance J, Grondin P, Cantin M (1977) Primary arteritis in Takayasu's disease. A case studied by selective coronary arteriography. A JR 128: 488
30. Saito Y, Hirota K, Ito I, Yamaguchi H, Takeda T, Morooka S, Ueda H (1972) Clinical and pathological studies of five autopsied cases of aortitis syndrome. Part II: Pathological findings of the heart, coronary arteries and aortic valve with reference to prognosis of aortitis syndrome. Jpn Heart J 13: 107
31. Abrams HL, Adams DF, Grant HA (1971) The radiology of tumors of the heart. Radiol Clin North Am 9: 299
32. Marshall WH Jr, Steiner RM, Wexler L (1969) "Tumor vascularity" in left atrial myxoma demonstrated by selective coronary arteriography. Radiology 93: 815
33. Berman ND, Mac Laughlin PR, Bigelow WG, Morch JE (1976) Angiographic demonstration of blood supply of right atrial myxoma. Br Heart J 38: 764
34. Grollman JH Jr, Hoffman RB, Price JE Jr, O'Reilly RJ, Liley JM, Herman NP (1974) Abnormal vascularity in left ventricular mural thrombus demonstrated by selective coronary arteriography. Radiology 113: 591

35. Cipriano PR, Guthaner DF (1978) Organized left atrial mural thrombus demonstrated by coronary angiography. Am Heart J 96: 166
36. Oren A, Bar-Shlomo B, Stern S (1976) Acute coronary occlusion following blunt injury to the chest in the absence of coronary atherosclerosis. Am Heart J 92: 501
37. Espada R, Whisennard HH, Mattok KL, Beall AC Jr (1975) Surgical management of penetrating injuries to the coronary arteries. Surgery 78: 755
38. Anderson GP, Adicoff A, Motsay GJ, Sako Y, Gobel FL (1975) Traumatic right coronary arterial-right atrial fistula. Am J Cardiol 35: 439
39. Bulkley BH, Roberts WC (1973) Dissecting aneurysm (hematoma) limited to coronary artery: a clinicopathologic study of six patients. Am J Med 55: 747
40. Palank EA, Dawso NJT, Cowen GD, Tysinger JR (1977) Primary dissecting aneurysm of the right coronary artery. Chest 72: 774
41. Walston A II, Behar VS (1976) Spectrum of coronary artery disease in idiopathic hypertrophic subaortic stenosis. Am J Cardiol 38: 12
42. Lardani H, Serrano JA, Villamil RH (1978) Hemodynamics and coronary angiography in idiopathic hypertrophic subaortic stenosis. Am J Cardiol 41: 476
43. Pichard AD, Meller J, Teichholz LE, Lipnik S, Gorlin R, Herman MV (1977) Septal perforator compression (narrowing) in idiopathic hypertrophic subaortic stenosis. Am J Cardiol 40: 310
44. Klein RG, Hunder GG, Stanson AW, Sheps SG (1975) Large artery involvement in giant cell (temporal) arteritis. Ann Intern Med 83: 806
45. Lebowitz WB (1963) The heart in rheumatoid arthritis (rheumatoid disease). A clinical and pathological study of sixty-two cases. Ann Intern Med 58: 102
46. Holsinger DR, Osmundsen PJ, Edwards JE (1962) The heart in periarteritis nodosa. Circulation 25: 610
47. Kawasaki T, Kosaki S, Okawa S (1974) A new infantile, acute febrile mucocutaneous lymph node syndrome prevailing in Japan. Pediatrics 54: 71
48. Fukushige J, Nihill MR, Mc Namara DG (1980) Spectrum of cardiovascular lesions in mucocutaneous lymph node syndrome: analysis of eight cases. Am J Cardiol 45: 98
49. Glanz S, Bittner SJ, Berman MA, Dolan TF Jr, Talner NS (1976) Regression of coronary artery aneurysms in infantile polyarteritis nodosa. N Engl J Med 294: 939
50. Bulkley BH, Klacsmann PG, Hutchins GM (1978) Angina pectoris, myocardial infarction and sudden cardiac death with normal coronary arteries: clinicopathologic study of nine patients with progressive systemic sclerosis. Am Heart J 95: 563

X Contribution of Other Examination Techniques

Echocardiography

1 Introduction

At the present time the main role of echocardiography in the study of coronary artery disease is to assess the myocardial consequences of coronary lesions, that is, effects on left ventricular (LV) wall function and contraction. Analysis of regional wall kinetics also provides indirect information for localizing coronary obstructions. Improvements in ultrasonic imaging now make it possible to obtain direct viewing of proximal segments of the coronary arteries, and further progress is likely in this area.

Although time-motion (TM) echocardiography is still widely used, there is an increasing tendency to employ it as support for real time echocardiography, referred to as cross-sectional echocardiography, echotomography, or two-dimensional (2-D) echocardiography. The great advantage of these latter techniques is that they provide dynamic imaging of the cardiovascular structures which is more complete and closer to anatomical representation. Real time 2-D echocardiography makes use of various means of recording and producing the image: the electronic linear scanner, the mechanical sector scanner and the phased-array imaging system. The customary frequencies are 3 MHz for adults and 5 MHz for children. Good gray scale characteristics are necessary for optimal identification of all normal or abnormal echo-producing structures. Manufacturers of most machines provide continuous direct viewing of the image on a screen, slow-motion or stop frame features and video tape or cassette recording. The stroboscopic effect, which consists in continually freezing the same cardiac cycle image by means of a predetermined linkage with the ECG, is used mainly for study of the coronary trunks.

2 Left Ventricle

The two customary methods of LV ultrasonic study are the TM mode and the 2-D mode. The disadvantage of TM echocardiography is that it can explore only a part of the LV: the basal third of the septal and lateral walls using the subxiphoid route. 2-D echocardiography can explore the LV in cross-sectional slices either parallel or perpendicular to the long axis of the ventricle, thereby providing total imaging of the LV. This method is thus clearly preferable to the former for LV study of coronary patients. Because of their morphology, or of other reasons difficult to define, some patients are unsuitable for ultrasonic examination (up to 25% for the TM mode and around 10% for the 2-D mode), which constitutes a serious limitation of this method.

2.1 Contraction

During observation of modifications of the endocardial outline of LV walls, ultrasonography, like angiography, can identify the three main regional contraction anomalies: hypokinesis, akinesis and dyskinesis. It can also detect compensatory hyperkinesis of a normal area, such as that of the posterolateral wall in cases of anteroseptal infarction. TM echocardiography has good specificity because it analyses wall displacement and thickness variations remarkably well, but the sensitivity of the method is poor since it explores only one part of the LV. A fibrous sequela of transmural infarction is visualized as a thinned wall area of greater echo density with no variation in thickness during the cardiac cycle [1]. The neighbouring portion of the myocardium, partly healthy, partly fibrous, is moderately thinned, and its systolic thickening is reduced. Acute myocardial ischaemia, whether spontaneous or induced by an exercise test, is indicated by a very specific feature: the wall segment concerned becomes akinetic and thins during systole [2].

2.2 Function

Time-motion echocardiography makes it possible to measure the percentage of reduction in ventricular diameter and to evaluate an ejection fraction. Unfortunately, this technique measures the diameter between the septal and posterolateral walls in the basal part of the ventricle. The data obtained are thus not representative of the entire ventricle and should be regarded with caution in the case of coronary patients whose coronary and myocardial lesions vary greatly as to site. Nonetheless, an increase in ventricular end-diastolic diameter and of the distance between the septal wall and the anterior mitral valve, as well as a reduction in the opening of the mitral valve, are sure signs of severely altered LV function [3]. 2-D echocardiography provides more reliable information. The LV is analysed according to several cross-sectional planes, wall kinetics is assessed quantitatively and ventricular and ejection fraction volumes are calculated according to different mathematical models by analogy with angiography [4–6], correlations between the two methods being good. Determining the number of wall segments with abnormal contraction and the value of the ejection fraction provides a valid means of assessing the usefulness of complementary angiographic explorations, the advantages of surgical treatment and the general prognosis for the patient. Ultrasonography is an invaluable method, for it offers the possibility of repeating the examination as desired in order to follow the patient's progression, of performing exercise tests or volume or pressure overload tests, and of following up the effects of medical or surgical therapy.

3 Complications of Myocardial Infarction

3.1 Ventricular Aneurysms

Time-motion echocardiography shows little sensitivity in detecting ventricular aneurysms [7], failing to recognize many regardless of size. An increase in ventricular diameter when the ultrasonographic beam is moved from the base towards the apex is a fairly reliable sign of antero-apical aneurysm, provided that the aneurysm is large. 2-D echocardiography is, however, reliable and sensitive, being capable of detecting most aneurysms if the patient can be examined without difficulty [8]. Anterior and apical aneurysms are detected in all cases [9]. 2-D echocardiography is able to determine quantitatively the size of the aneurysm and the extent of the remaining ventricle; the correlation with angiography is good [9], and assessment of operability and prediction of the results of possible aneurysmectomy are often feasible [10].

3.2 False Ventricular Aneurysms

Left ventricular pseudoaneurysm is secondary to a rupture of the free wall retained by a partitioned pericardial sac. This quite infrequent complication most often concerns the posterodiaphragmatic wall. TM echocardiography reveals the presence of a vast, relatively echo-free space behind the ventricular wall, which must not be confused with a pericardial effusion. 2-D echocardiography is the ideal diagnostic method because it clearly visualizes the sac, which communicates by a narrow orifice with the LV [11].

3.3 Pericardial Effusions

The diagnosis of pericardial effusions is most often facilitated by TM echocardiography, which reveals an extramyocardial posterior echo-free space that does not change in systole and diastole. However, 2-D echocardiography is more reliable, providing better indication of the volume of the effusion and avoiding confusion with LV pseudoaneurysm. It demonstrates the respiratory variation in ventricular diameters and the impediment to ventricular wall movement during diastolic expansion.

3.4 Mitral Regurgitation

Most cases of postinfarction mitral regurgitation are due to dysfunction of a posterior papillary muscle, which then becomes highly echogenic and easily detectable with 2-D echocardiography because of its immobility at the level of a wall segment itself showing contraction. Other signs are more or less marked valve prolapse, abnormal echoes in the case of rupture of the chordae tendineae, LV volume overload and exaggerated left atrial wall kinetics when left heart function still remains rather good [12].

3.5 *Rupture of the Free Wall*

Rupture of the free wall can only be diagnosed by echocardiography when it develops subacutely, in which case signs of pericardial effusion and cardiac tamponade may be observed. According to some authors [13], it is possible during the acute stage of infarction to obtain localized images of intramyocardial sonolucency, which may correspond to parietal areas exposed to the rupture.

3.6 *Rupture of the Septal Wall*

Diagnosis of rupture of the septal wall is based on evidence of right ventricular dilatation associated with paradoxical septal motion and on direct 2-D echocardiographic imaging of the septal defect [12]. Septal motion is sometimes really non-existent or severely reduced; the septum may have an aneurysmal appearance.

3.7 *Intraventricular Thromboses*

Two-dimensional echocardiography is a good means of detecting and following up thrombi which form upon contact with an akinetic, dyskinetic or aneurysmal segment following infarction [14]. Such thrombi show a preference for the apical region. They are indicated by abnormal echogenic structures, which are rounded or elongated and protrude more or less into the ventricular cavity.

4 Coronary Arteries

Using ultrasonic techniques, it would be of particular advantage to examine the coronary arteries and localize surgically treatable lesions. However, this is not possible now because of the physical limitation of the method. It is quite apparent that the large wavelength of ultrasounds as compared to that of X-rays does not allow well-defined images of small arteries to be obtained. To improve image resolution it would be of interest to use high-frequency ultrasounds, except that unfortunately these are rapidly absorbed by the biological tissues. Ultrasonography offers the advantage of imaging vascular walls, unlike angiography, which reveals the vessel lumen. Theoretically, it would be possible to apply the pulsed Doppler technique to the measurement of coronary flow, but in practice this method encounters numerous difficulties, the greatest being the mobility of the coronary arteries. In effect, aortocoronary bypasses are more suitable to the technique. Although TM echocardiography makes it possible to localize the main coronary trunks, 2-D echocardiography has been used for this purpose ever since Weyman's initial publication on the subject [15].

4.1.1 Left Coronary Artery

The transducer is placed in a left parasternal position (Figs. 1 and 2) and rotated until parallel with the transverse axis of the aorta. The ultrasonic scan plane is adjusted so that it is parallel with the left main coronary trunk (LMCT) [16], which is in focus when its lumen appears in the form of two dominant linear echoes arising from the inferolateral border of the aorta. The ostium is in focus when there is continuity between the aortic and coronary lumina [15]. The angulation of the probe is then

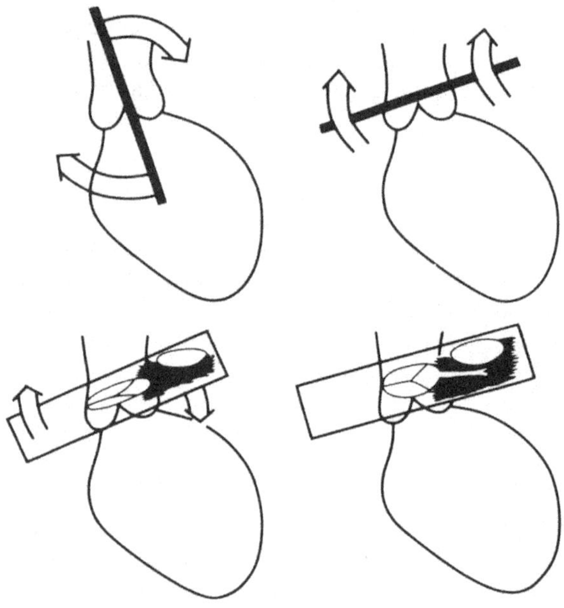

Fig. 1. Transducer positioning for left main coronary artery visualization in the parasternal position. The successive rotations of the ultrasonic transducer (see text) are shown above the frontal silhouette of the left ventricle and ascending aorta

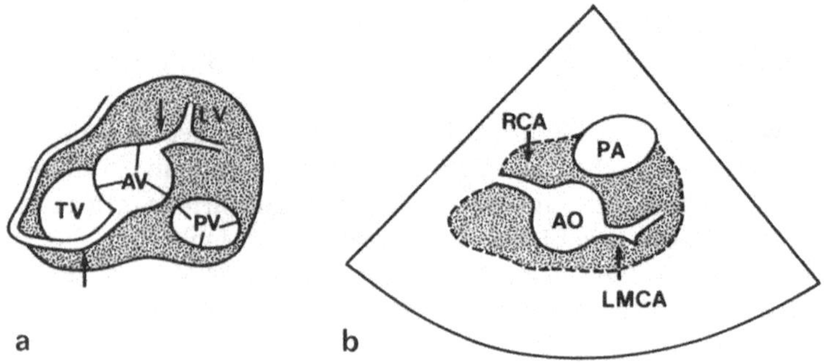

Fig. 2 a, b. Parasternal position. **a** schematic anatomical view of the heart (superior view). *LV:* left ventricle; *AV:* aortic valve; *PV:* pulmonary valve; *TV:* tricuspid valve; **b** schematic echocardiographic imaging of the coronary arteries. *LMCA* and *RCA:* left main and right coronary arteries; *AO:* aorta; *PA:* pulmonary artery

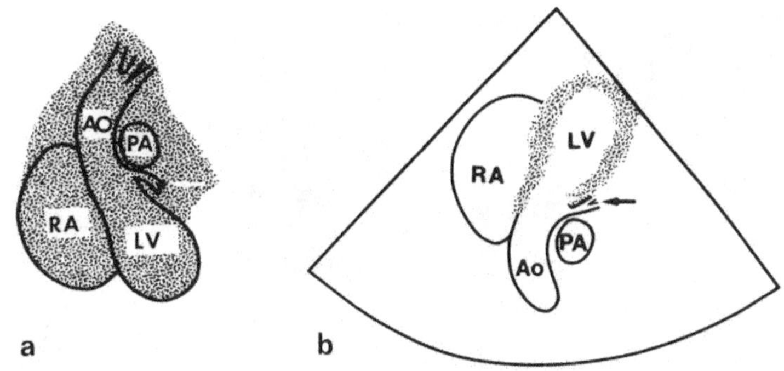

Fig. 3 a, b. Apical position. **a** Schematic anatomical view of the heart (long axis). *AO:* aorta; *PA:* pulmonary artery; *LV:* left ventricle; *RA:* right atrium. The *arrow* indicates the left main coronary artery. **b** Schematic echocardiographic imaging of the left main coronary artery *(arrow)*

slightly adjusted in an attempt to visualize the bifurcation of the trunk and the proximal part of the left anterior descending artery. For a patient in left lateral decubitus it is also possible to show the left coronary trunk when the probe is in the apical position (Fig. 3) [17–19]. Visualization of a Judkins catheter inserted into the left coronary ostium has provided in vivo demonstration of the validity of the ultrasonographic method [19]. A study on an anatomical specimen has shown that ultrasonography reveals only the common trunk, its bifurcation and sometimes the first millimeters of the left anterior descending artery and circumflex [20]. One source of difficulty in performing examinations is the existence of anatomical variants: a very short or virtually non-existent common trunk, the ectopic origin of the left coronary artery (LCA) and the initial division of the trunk into three or sometimes four branches instead of two. Aortic valve calcifications may also prevent visualization of the ostium and left trunk [19].

4.1.2 Right Coronary Artery

To visualize the right coronary orifice and trunk when the probe is in parasternal position, the ultrasonic scan plane should be adjusted so that it is parallel to a cross-sectional plane intersecting successively the aorta and the upper part of the tricuspid annulus. It is not possible to explore the right coronary artery (RCA) by the apical route.

4.1.3 Aortocoronary Bypasses [21]

Grafts branching from the LCA pass in front of or to the left of the infundibulum of the right ventricle. For a subject in left lateral decubitus they are searched for with the probe in left parasternal position in the second or third intercostal space. Grafts anastomosed with the RCA course in front and to the right of the aorta. For a subject in right lateral decubitus they are searched for with the probe in the right parasternal position.

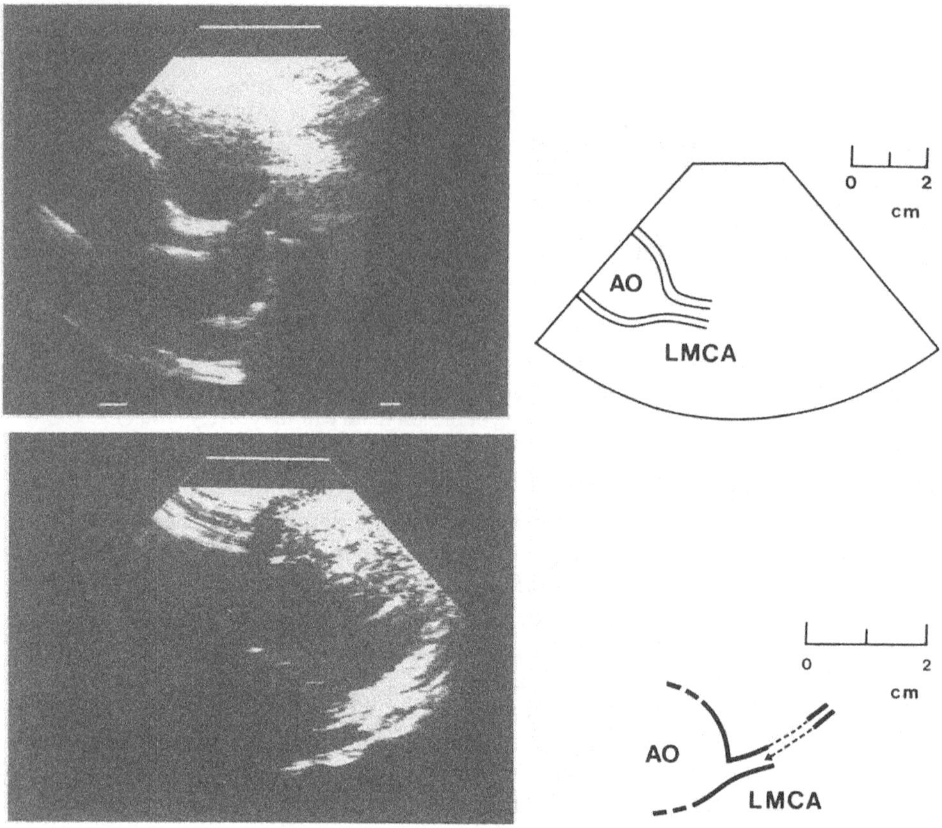

Fig. 4. Normal left main coronary artery and bifurcation. Parasternal position. *(Upper):* left coronary artery main stem; *(lower):* bifurcation. *AO:* aorta; *LMCA:* left main coronary artery

4.2 Normal Results

In a series of 108 subjects whose LMCT was angiographically normal, 2-D echocardiography, using the parasternal position, visualized this vessel correctly in only 57% of cases [16]. The main causes of failure were obesity, emphysema and a large thoracic anteroposterior diameter. Figure 4 shows a normal common trunk. The rate of successful examinations was higher for young adults. Feigenbaum identified the left trunk 71 times in a series of 72 patients explored consecutively [22]. The operator's greater experience and his use of more reliable equipment account for this better result as compared with those of other authors. In a group of 32 children, Yoshikawa identified the right and left ostia in all cases, the right trunk in only 12 subjects and the left trunk in 24 [23]. In general, the bifurcation of the LMCT is identifiable in almost all cases when the trunk itself is clearly visible. When the probe is in the apical position, the success rate is lower: the LMCT was viewed in only 69% of 52 subjects studied by Chen [19], and in another study the bifurcation was difficult to visualize [22].

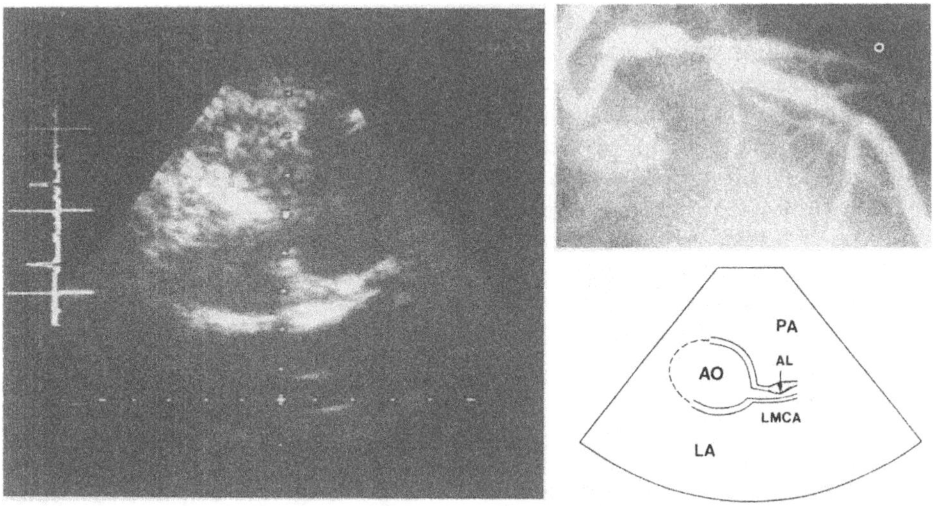

Fig. 5. Obstruction of the left main coronary artery. *(Left):* Cross-sectional echocardiography. High-intensity echoes are recorded in the region of the atherosclerotic lesion *(AL)*. *(Upper right):* Corresponding selective coronary arteriography. Courtesy of M. C. Malergue. *(Lower right):* Corresponding schematic drawing; *LA:* left atrium

4.3 Atheromatous Coronary Arterial Diseases

The first observations of stenosis of the LMCT were reported by Weyman [15], who clearly stressed the need to visualize the vessel lumen both upstream and downstream from the lesion. In a comparative study with coronary arteriography, ultrasonography using the parasternal approach detected greater than 50% stenoses of the common trunk in 60% [16] to 100% [21] of cases (Fig. 5). In some patients echoes suggestive of obstruction of the trunk corresponded in fact to stenoses of the LAD as determined by the coronary arteriographic examinations. The criteria for coronary stenosis are an image of partial or total obstruction of the lumen of the trunk and the presence of asymmetric high-intensity echoes (HIE) in the obstructive mass or the artery wall [19, 22]. These HIE apparently indicate the presence of calcium or dense substances and serve as good indicators of atheromatous alteration of the artery wall. After having studied HIE in 100 coronary patients, Rogers [24] concluded that they have good sensitivity and specificity for predicting the presence of coronary artery disease. According to Friedman [25], it is possible to improve detection of stenoses of the LMCT by suitable processing of the image, taking into account other factors as well as resolution.

4.4 Other Coronary Arterial Diseases

The abnormal origin of the LCA from the pulmonary artery can be diagnosed [26, 27] by direct or indirect signs: absence of a LCA arising from the aorta; RCA very dilated at its point of origin; a linear echo-free structure emerging from the pulmonary artery trunk.In 12 cases of coronary artery fistulae, 2-D echocardiography provided visualization of the enlarged lumen of the RCA eight times and of the LCA four times [28]. Weyman, in his preliminary study [15], reported the first case of coronary aneurysm identified by ultrasonography. This kind of lesion has most often been observed in the child afflicted with Kawasaki disease or mucocutaneous lymph node syndrome [23]. Coronary aneurysms, indicated by well-defined echo-free circular or fusiform spaces, are visible in the LCA or RCA. The diagnostic value of these images has been confirmed by coronary arteriography [23]; ultrasonography is used to observe the development of the aneurysms in the 2- to 4-week period after onset of the disease and to follow their progression. Disappearance of the aneurysms after a period of 10 months has occasionally been observed.

4.5 Aortocoronary Bypass Grafts

Aortocoronary grafts can be studied by the continuous wave or pulsed Doppler technique. Diebold [21] studied 163 grafts in 108 consecutive patients by the pulsed Doppler technique. When the bypass was permeable, a diastolic flow was recorded which was sometimes associated with a systolic component moving in the same or in the opposite direction. One hundred and thirty-eight out of 163 tests were positive, indicating a theoretically permeable graft. In 25 cases no diastolic flow was detected. However, the specificity of the method is poor: 22 tests yielded erroneous results, 11 being false negatives and 11 false positives. Factors contributing to error included natural sources of diastolic flow, such as the superior vena cava and the internal mammary veins.

5 Conclusion

It may be concluded from this review of the present contribution of ultrasonic techniques that they do not provide a sufficiently precise assessment of coronary pathology. Echocardiography is a planar imaging technique poorly adapted to three-dimensional spatial study of the coronary artery network. Only the main coronary arteries can be partially analysed. Too great a part of the coronary tree is not accessible to the method. It is probable that digital angiography will soon provide a better means of satisfying the demand for non-invasive exploration of the coronary arteries and aortocoronary bypasses.

Echocardiography, especially in the 2-D mode, is less disappointing with respect to the study of LV function and regional contraction and to detection of mechanical complications of infarction and intracardiac thromboses. Unfortunately, despite improved resolution and appreciable technical progress, there is still a high percentage of patients refractory to ultrasound for whom no reliable image can be obtained. There is no certainty that this limitation can be totally overcome in the future.

Computed Axial Tomography

1 Introduction

Since 1976, as a result of improvements in computer programming, it has been possible to apply computed tomography (CT) scanning to the thorax, allowing a reduction from 5 to 2 min in the time needed to analyse a section. Yet initially it was the stationary or nearly stationary structures of the thorax to which the technique was applied. From 1976 to 1982 technological efforts concentrated on increasing the number of detectors (to more than 600) and on bringing exposure time per section to around 1–2 s for the most efficient scanners. Thus morphological and densitometric analysis of the large vessels, the chambers and the walls of the heart has gradually become possible. Intravenous injection of contrast medium has improved visualization of the ventricular and atrial cavities. Currently, the spatial reconstruction of the heart is still inadequate for study of all its features, and the image obtained is generally a mean computed on the basis of the different phases of the cardiac cycle [29]. As a result, measurements of myocardial structures and ventricular cavities are possible but rather approximate. Comparative study with a technique improved by the gating process has shown that the mean cardiac configuration obtained without gating corresponds to a slightly smaller volume than that of the end-diastolic heart.

An ideal cardiac scanner should satisfy the following specifications: Production of very thin serial sections of the heart to reconstruct the configuration of the different cavities, if possible, in all spatial planes

- spatial resolution of a millimetre or less for clear visualization of the intercavitary septa and the walls of the aorta and of the pulmonary artery at their point of origin
- a very fine resolution to differentiate the respective densities of the blood and the myocardium
- excellent temporal resolution, of about 0.1 s, to eliminate the kinetic blur induced by the rapid and complex movements of the heart
- production of a minimum of 25 images per second to enable a kinetic study of the heart to be performed

2 Methods

Different research techniques are now available. *Dynamic cardiac computed tomography* involves the performance of several successive complete scans with data acquisition either during a sweep back and forth or in the continuous mode during several successive full revolutions. The limitations of this technique are the high radiation dose for the patient and the enormous amount of data to be acquired and stored [30].

The gating technique has several variations [31–34]. Retrospective gating consists in storing in memory all the sections as well as the ECG associated with each of them. The selection is made a posteriori. The operator can reconstitute the image of a given phase of the cardiac cycle. He can also effect a dynamic reconstitution using a chronological series of sections, that is, of temporally contiguous images. Prospective gating consists in selecting certain projections deemed useful at the data acquisition stage by means of an ECG-synchronized suppression of X-ray emissions. The advantage of this technique by comparison with retrospective gating is that it involves lower amounts of radiation; its disadvantage is the need for a regular heart rhythm.

Ultrarapid computed tomography, which is suitable to scanners with very fine temporal resolution, is capable of obtaining all the data necessary for image reconstruction in 0.01–0.05 s. Two great projects are currently under way in this field: the Dynamic Spatial Reconstructor being developed by the Mayo Clinic in Rochester, Minnesota, and the Cardiovascular Computed Tomographic Scanner being developed in the Department of Radiology of the University of California at San Francisco. The realization of such powerful systems is particularly advantageous because they will possess a temporal resolution practically equal to that of radio-cinematography today. The completion of these projects will provide equipment capable of simultaneous non-invasive analysis of cardiac morphology, density and dynamics, and will constitute a remarkable advance in this field.

3 Indications

At present, there are very few indications for CT in the assessment of coronary artery disease and myocardial ischaemia. However, in patients who have had myocardial infarction, CT following intracoronary injection of contrast medium provides good analysis of the peripheral coronary network. Myocardial filling defects can be shown more simply by intravenous injection of contrast medium according to the angioscanner technique. Acute myocardial infarction is indicated in the late phase by an accumulation of contrast medium in the area adjacent to the infarct [35, 36]. These densitometric measurements are in good agreement with histological observations as well as with images of radiolucent spaces provided by radio-nuclide studies. These early CT studies have mainly a theoretical value. Their practical application is limited by the impossibility of combining them with exercise tests and by the fact that CT detects only anomalies of the anterior, apical, lateral and septal walls. The anomalies of the diaphragmatic wall, which is confused with the mass of the liver, elude this technique. Moreover, it is still not sufficiently accurate to define the extent of the infarct very clearly.

For anomalies of LV contraction, the gating techniques provide satisfactory analysis by comparison of end-systolic and end-diastolic images. The prospect of three-dimensional reconstructions offers hope of a better approach to segmentary analysis of the LV walls. For interventricular communications due to septal rupture by infarction, there seems as yet to be no publication of a specific case, although morphological analysis of the septum is now possible. It is possible to detect left intraventricular thromboses by CT. In a few fortunate observations an intracavitary radiolucent space has been revealed.

The inspection of aortocoronary bypasses [37] is one of the best indications for the use of CT (see Part II, Chap. VIII and Fig. 13 in Chap. VIII). The predictability rate for graft permeability is 89.6% according to Lackner [33]. Finally, examinations performed after rapid intravenous injection of contrast medium sometimes reveal the proximal part of the coronary trunks, mainly the LMCT. However, the resolution is inadequate, so that the method is not competitive with coronary arteriography, which provides a far superior spatial resolution of 0.1 mm.

Videodensitometry

It is always difficult to estimate the degree of reduction in coronary flow, at rest or during exertion, resulting from arterial stenosis. Yet the exact measurement of this degree is important since, as Lipscomb's studies have shown [38], the flow of the vessel at rest is diminished only when the stenosis is extremely narrow, reducing the cross-sectional area of the artery by 95% or more. Between 85% and 95%, the decrease in flow only occurs during exertion, and there is a reduction in vasodilatation capacity in the downstream coronary bed during induced hyperaemia. In practice, exact measurement of a stenosis is difficult [39]. The methods of measuring coronary flow probably provide, directly or indirectly, the best means of assessing the effects of a stenosis on the myocardium downstream from it.

Among the various methods proposed for the measurement of coronary flow, videodensitometry has the advantage of being efficient and reproducible and of not requiring a very large investment. This technique, which applies the principle of densitometric measurements to angiographic video tape recording has been studied by Rutishauser [40], Lanz [41] and Erikson [42]. It can provide either absolute measurement of coronary flow based on calculation of the transit time of an opaque embolus through a determined artery segment, or relative measurement according to the method of Stewart Hamilton, that is, recording the densitometric curve for the passage of the contrast material through the vessel in question, using the same process as for other tracers.

Measurement of transit time [40] requires the use of two videodensitometer windows located at the level of two points along the vessel studied and separated by a distance L. Each window (photoelectric cell) records the transit of the opaque embolus, producing a distinctive upwards deflection of the videodensitometric curve (Figs. 6 and 7). The time t between the two deflections may easily be measured. The speed S of passage of the embolism is then calculated: $S = L/\Delta t$. Determination of the diameter of the vascular segment between the two windows makes it possible to calculate its cross-sectional area A, enabling the flow F through the vessel to be computed according to the formula $F = A \times S$.

There are several disadvantages to the use of this method. Coronary blood flow is not steady during the entire cardiac cycle, and it is also difficult to measure the exact cross-sectional area and length of a vessel embedded in the thorax, as its direction is more or less oblique in space and its magnification factor difficult to determine with accuracy. This method has been used by Rutishauser [40] and seems valid for measurement of the flow of aortocoronary vein bypasses. However, it is difficult to apply it to the coronary arteries themselves.

Lanz has proposed an original method applicable to other vessels [41] and offering two possible approaches: absolute measurement and relative measurement, the

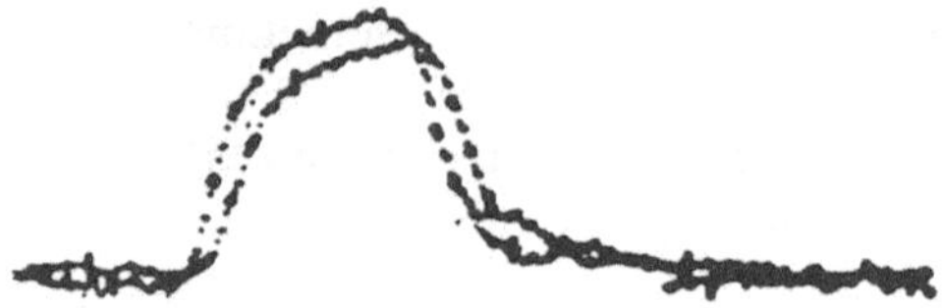

Fig. 6. Time-density curves recorded by the two electronic windows of a densitometer when the contrast medium passes through the examined vascular segment. Transit time is provided by the interval between either the two ascending limbs or the two density peaks of the curves. (Courtesy of U. Erikson)

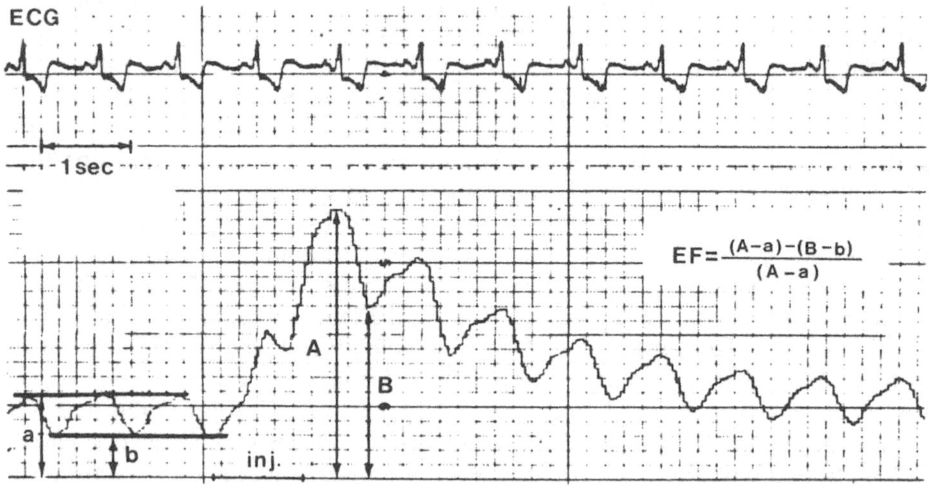

Fig. 7. Time-density curve recorded in a patient following left ventricular opacification. From this type of curve, the stroke volume, ejection fraction and aortic regurgitation fraction are obtainable. *A* and *B:* height of the density curve in diastole and systole after the injection *(inj.)* of contrast medium; *a* and *b:* same parameter before injection. (Courtesy of U. Erikson)

latter involving study of variations in flow subject to various influences. Absolute measurement consists in determination of cardiac flow by a conventional technique (Fick principle, dye dilution, isotopes) and then of videodensitometric evaluation of the fraction of this flow through the vessel under study. There are two phases to the videodensitometric procedure. The first consists in injecting a known quantity $Q1$ of contrast material into the LV and of recording the curve $C1$ of dilution in the vessel, e.g. the left anterior descending artery. The area $A1$ below the curve $C1$ is determined by planimetry. The second phase consists, under the same measurement and recording conditions, in selective injection of a known quantity $Q2$ of contrast material into the artery under study and recording of the curve $C2$. The area $A2$ below the curve $C2$ is then determined by planimetry. The value for coronary flow is expressed by the following equation:

$$\frac{F2}{F1} = \frac{Q2 \cdot A2}{Q1 \cdot A1}$$

where $F1 =$ cardiac flow and $F2 =$ the flow in the vessel under study;

hence $F2 = F1 \dfrac{Q2 \cdot A2}{Q1 \cdot A1}$

Thus $F2$ may be determined once cardiac flow is known.

The relative measurement method, which studies the flow variations in a coronary vessel before ($F1$) and after ($F2$) inducing hyperaemia downstream from a stenosis in this vessel, also has two phases. The first consists in selective injection of a quantity $Q1$ of contrast material into the vessel under study, which gives a curve $C1$ of the area $A1$. The second phase involves injection of a quantity $Q2$ of contrast material into the same vessel after having induced hyperaemia by an exercise test or by injection of a vasodilator. A curve $C2$ of the area $A2$ is recorded. The ratio of baseline flow to flow after hyperaemia is expressed by the formula

$$\frac{F1}{F2} = \frac{Q1 \cdot A1}{Q2 \cdot A2}$$

It is only necessary to use equal quantities, $Q1$ and $Q2$, of contrast material to simplify the calculation: $F1/F2 = A1/A2$.

This procedure provides a percentage of the variation of flow in a coronary artery, which may be used as an index of severity for the stenosis. Lanz's work [41] has demonstrated the validity of this method on both animal and human models and in normal and pathological cases.

References

1. Rasmussen S, Corya BC, Feigenbaum H, Knoebel SB (1978) Detection of myocardial scar tissue by M-mode echocardiography. Circulation 57: 230
2. Corya BC, Rasmussen S, Feigenbaum H, Knoebel SB, Black MJ (1977) Systolic thickening and thinning of the septum and posterior wall in patients with coronary artery disease, congestive cardiomyopathy, and atrial septal defect. Circulation 55: 109
3. Corya BC, Rasmussen S, Knoebel SB, Feigenbaum H (1977) M-mode echocardiography in evaluating left ventricular function and surgical risk in patients with coronary artery disease. Chest 72: 181
4. Carr KW, Engler RL, Forsythe JR, Johnson AD, Gosink B (1979) Measurement of left ventricular ejection fraction by mechanical cross-sectional echocardiography. Circulation 59: 1191
5. Folland ED, Parisi AF, Moynihan PF, Jones DR, Felkman CL, Tour DE (1979) Assessment of left ventricular ejection fraction and volumes by real-time, two dimensional echocardiography. A comparison of cineangiographic and radionuclide techniques. Circulation 60: 760
6. Gueret P, Corday E (1981) Etude quantitative de la fonction ventriculaire gauche par l'échocardiographie bidimensionnelle. Arch Mal Coeur 74: 329
7. Dillon JC, Feigenbaum H, Weyman AE, Corya BC, Peskoe S, Chang S (1976) M-mode echocardiography in the evaluation of patients for aneurysmectomy. Circulation 53: 657
8. Teichholz LE, Kreulen T, Herman MV, Gorlin R (1976) Problems in echocardiographic volume determinations: echocardiographic-angiographic correlations in the presence or absence of asynergy. Am J Cardiol 37: 7
9. Weyman AE, Peskoe SM, Williams ES, Dillon JC, Feigenbaum H (1976) Detection of left ventricular aneurysms by cross-sectional echocardiography. Circulation 54: 936

10. Barrett MJ, Charuzi Y, Corday E (1980) Ventricular aneurysm: cross-sectional echocardiographic approach. Am J Cardiol 46: 1133
11. Catherwood E, Mintz GS, Kotler MN, Parry WR, Segal BL (1980) Two-dimensional echocardiographic recognition of left ventricular pseudo-aneurysm. Circulation 62: 294
12. Chandraratna PAN, Balachandran PK, Shah PM, Hodges M (1975) Echocardiographic observations on ventricular septal rupture complicating acute myocardial infarction. Circulation 51: 506
13. Werner JA, Speck SM, Greene HL, Janko CL, Gross BW (1981) Discrete intramural sonolucency: a new echocardiography finding in acute myocardial infarction. Am J Cardiol 47: 404 (abstract)
14. Asinger RW, Mikell FL, Sharma B, Hodges M (1981) Observations of detecting left ventricular thrombus with two dimensional echocardiography: emphasis on avoidance of false positive diagnoses. Am J Cardiol 47: 145
15. Weyman AE, Feigenbaum H, Dillon JC, Johnston KW, Eggleton RC (1976) Non-invasive visualization of the left main coronary artery by cross-sectional echocardiography. Circulation 54: 169
16. Chandraratna PAN, Aronow WS (1980) Left main coronary arterial patency assessed with cross-sectional echocardiography. Am J Cardiol 46: 91
17. Ogawa S, Hubbard FE, Pauletto FJ, Chaudry KR, Chen CC, Moghadam AN, Dreifus LS (1978) A new approach to noninvasive left coronary artery visualization using phased array cross-sectional echocardiography. Circulation 58 [Suppl II]: 188 (abstract)
18. Ogawa S, Chen CC, Hubbard FE, Mardelli TJ, Morganroth J, Dreifus LS, Akaishi M, Nakamura Y (1980) A new approach to visualize the left main coronary artery using apical cross-sectional echocardiography. Am J Cardiol 45: 301
19. Chen CC, Morganroth J, Ogawa S, Mardelli TJ (1980) Detecting left main coronary artery disease by apical, cross-sectional echocardiography. Circulation 62: 288
20. Rogers EW, Feigenbaum H, Weyman AE, Godley RW, Vakili ST (1980) Evaluation of left coronary artery anatomy in vitro by cross-sectional echocardiography. Circulation 62: 782
21. Diebold B, Theroux P, Bourassa MG, Peronneau P, Guermonprez JL (1979) Noninvasive assessment of aortocoronary bypass graft patency using pulsed Doppler echocardiography. Am J Cardiol 43: 10
22. Feigenbaum H (1981) Visualization of the coronary arteries by two dimensional echocardiography. In: Rijsterborg H (ed) Echocardiology. Nijhoff, The Hague, p 61
23. Yoshikawa J, Yanagihara K, Owaki T, Kato H, Takagi Y, Okumachi F, Fukaya T, Tomita Y, Baba K (1979) Cross-sectional echocardiographic diagnosis of coronary artery aneurysms in patients with the mucocutaneous lymph node syndrome. Circulation 59: 133
24. Rogers EW, Feigenbaum H, Weyman AE, Godley RW, Johnston KW, Eggleton RC (1980) Possible detection of atherosclerotic coronary calcification by two-dimensional echocardiography. Circulation 62: 1046
25. Friedman MJ, Sahn DJ, Goldman S, Eisner DR, Gittinger NC, Lederman FL, Pockette CM, Tiemann JJ (1979) High frequency, high resolution cross-sectional echo for evaluation of left main coronary artery disease: is resolution alone enough? Circulation 60 [Suppl II]: 153
26. Cadwell RL, Weyman AE, Hurwitz RA, Girod DA, Feigenbaum H (1980) Cross-sectional echocardiographic evaluation of coronary artery abnormalities in children. Am J Cardiol 45 [Suppl II]: 467
27. Fischer EA, Sephri B, Lendrum B, Luken J, Levitsky S (1981) Two-dimensional echocardiographic visualization of the left coronary artery in anomalous origin of the left coronary artery from the pulmonary artery. Circulation 63: 698
28. Yoshikawa J, Kato H, Yanagihara K (1980) Ultrasonic visualization of the enlarged main coronary arteries in coronary artery fistulae. Circulation 62 [Suppl III]: 162
29. Ferrane J, Utzmann O, Le Cudonnec B, Vasile N (1979) Tomodensitométrie cardiaque. Anatomie normale. J Radiol 60: 169
30. Boyd DP, Gould RG, Quinn JR, Sparks R, Staley JH, Herrmannsfeld WB (1979) A proposed dynamic cardiac 3-D densitometer for early detection and evaluation of heart disease. IEEE Trans Nucl Sci 26: 2724
31. Harell GS, Guthaner DF, Breiman RS (1977) Stop-action cardiac computed tomography. Radiology 123: 515

32. Sagel SS, Weiss ES, Gillard RG, Housfield GN, Jost RGT, Stanley RJ, Ter-Pogossian MM (1977) Gated computed tomography of the human heart. Invest. Radiol 12: 563
33. Lackner K, Thurn P (1981) Computed tomography of the heart: E.C.G.-gated and continous scans. Radiology 140: 413
34. Morehouse CC, Bordy WR, Guthaner DF, Breiman RS, Harell GS (1980) Gated cardiac computed tomography with a motion phantom. Radiation Phys: 213
35. Higgins CB, Siemers PT, Schlidt W (1979) Evaluation of myocardial ischemic damage of various ages by computerized transmission tomography. Circulation 60: 284
36. Newell JD, Higgins CB, Abraham JL (1980) Computerized tomographic appearance of evolving myocardial infarctions. Invest Radiol 15: 207
37. Brundage BH, Lipton MJ, Herfkens RJ (1980) Detection of patent coronary bypass grafts by computed tomography. A preliminary report. Circulation 61: 826
38. Lipscomb K, Hooten S (1978) Effect of stenotic dimensions and blood flow on the hemodynamic significance of model coronary arterial stenoses. Am J Cardiol 42: 781
39. Derouen TA, Murray JA, Owen W (1977) Variability in the analysis of coronary arteriograms. Circulation 55: 324
40. Rutishauser W (1971) Application of roentgen densitometry to blood flow measurement in models, animals and in intact conscious man. In: Roentgen-, cine- and video densitometry. Thieme, Stuttgart, p 108
41. Lanz BMT, Foerster JM, Holcroft JW, Link DP, Mason DT (1981) Angiographic measurement of coronary blood flow by video dilution technique. Acta Radiol 22: 121
42. Erikson U (1982) Kymographie, cinédensigraphie, vidéodensitométrie. Traité de radiodiagnostic. Vol 3. coeur et aorte. Masson, Paris

XI Therapeutic or Interventional Coronary Radiology

1 Transluminal Coronary Angioplasty

In 1964, Dotter and Judkins [1] performed the first arterial angioplasties on iliofemoral arteriosclerotic lesions. In 1977, Grüntzig [2] performed the first successful dilatation of a human coronary artery. This method of treating coronary atheroma attempts to act directly on the lesion in order to restore adequate coronary blood flow. Its role falls between that of medical treatment to limit the consequences of myocardial ischaemia and that of revascularization surgery to bypass the coronary stenosis. Its advantages over surgery are its relative simplicity, its reliability and its immediate effectiveness. The aims of current research are to clarify the indications, improve the safety and efficiency of the method and assess the long-term course of dilated stenoses.

1.1 Indications

Only those patients are accepted for angioplasty who give their informed consent and agree to undergo immediate surgery (aortocoronary bypass) should the intervention be unsuccessful. The ideal conditions, approved by all authors, are as follows:

1. When the patient is suffering from recent angina pectoris (having begun less than 6 months previously, if possible) which has not responded to correct medical treatment combining nitrates, a β-blocking agent and/or a calcium antagonist, and for which confirmation of myocardial ischaemia has been provided by an exercise stress test and/or thallium-201 myocardial scintigraphy.
2. When the patient's left ventricular function is good and he has single-vessel involvement with only one severe, short, uncalcified, relatively concentric proximal stenosis located in a rather straight artery segment which has no important collateral branch taking off within the area of narrowing.

The chances of success are greater for very proximal stenoses and for those of the left anterior descending artery and right coronary artery than for those of the circumflex. Some authors, as a result of experience and greater skill and of improvements in equipment, have expanded the indications and apply the method to patients with a history of infarction and to those with double-vessel involvement when both stenoses present favourable anatomical conditions. Dilation of a stenosis in a vein graft bypass is possible. The major contra-indications are multiple stenoses in the same vessel, multivessel involvement, distal stenoses and stenoses of the left main coronary trunk (LMCT). In the last case, regardless of what the angiographic images show, stenoses of the trunk may well involve the origin of the left anterior descending artery or circumflex, which is why surgical treatment should be given priority. However, none of these supposedly absolute contra-indications has been entirely respected in recent years [8, 9]. The American Food and Drug Administration recognizes only two essential contra-indications: coronary arterial spasm and total coronary occlusion. It is estimated that 5%–10% of patients previously referred to surgeons for bypasses may now be treated by angioplasty.

1.2 Technique, Preparation and Procedure

Transluminal coronary angioplasty is derived from coronary arteriography, from which it borrows its means of approach (femoral route by percutaneous puncture or humeral route by arteriotomy) and its techniques of selective catheterization of the coronary arteries. It requires close collaboration between cardiologists, radiologists, surgeons and intensive care personnel.

Two types of catheter (USCI Grüntzig Dilaca) are employed:

1. a catheter guide (9–10.5 F) is used for selective catheterization of the coronary artery to be dilated;
2. a 5-F dilation catheter (Fig. 1) is introduced into the artery concerned by means of the first type.

This second catheter has a straight or J-shaped fixed guide at its distal end and contains two channels: one to inflate the balloon with a radiopaque solution and the other to measure post-stenotic pressure and opacify the distal artery to be sure of correct catheter positioning before the balloon is inflated. Two radiopaque markers, one on each side of the balloon, indicate its position (Figs. 1 and 2). The diameter of an inflated balloon is constant, measuring 2, 3 or 3.7 mm according to the size used. There is also another dilation catheter model available which has a preshapable movable central guide (Simpson-Robert, Advanced Catheter Systems). To avoid overinflation of the artery, it is very important to measure the diameter of the pre- and post-stenotic lumen and to choose an adequate balloon size.

The dilation catheter is inflated and deflated either manually or by means of a mechanical device. In both cases, a lateral passage connects the balloon to a manometer which controls inflation pressure.

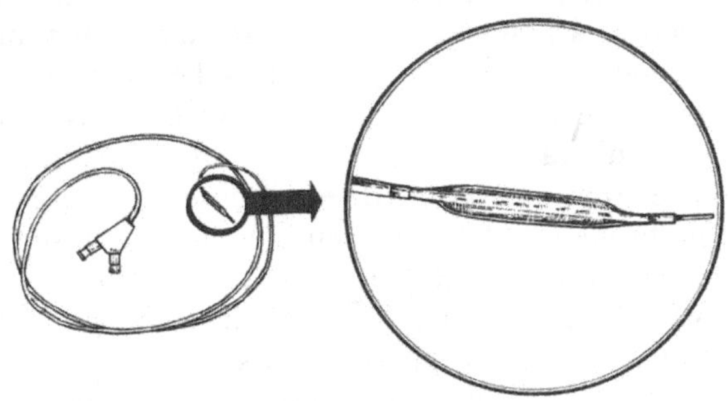

Fig. 1. Gruntzig-Dilaca dilation catheter with magnified presentation of distal part

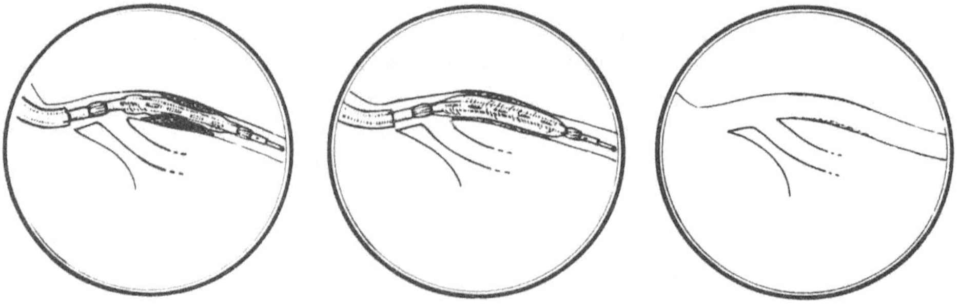

Fig. 2. The three main stages of transluminal angioplasty. *(Left):* The balloon is advanced through the stenosis. *(Middle):* Inflation of the balloon. *(Right):* Angiographic control

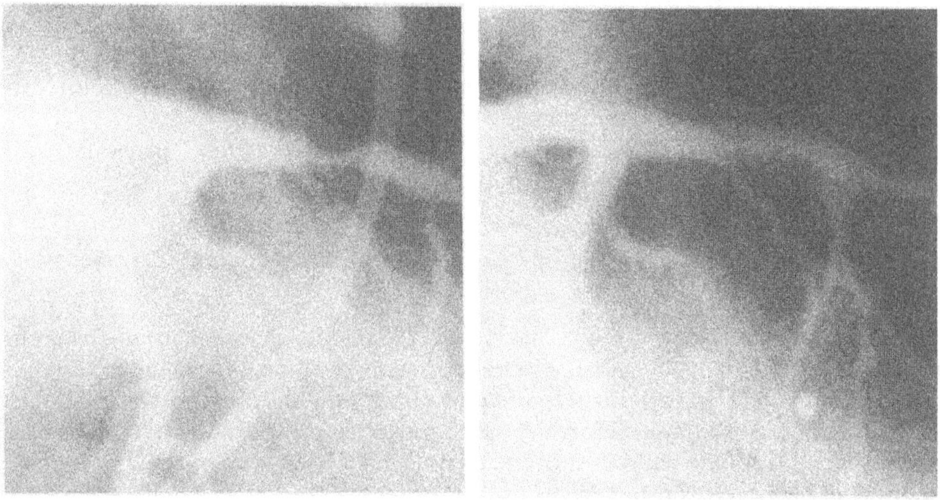

Fig. 3. Right anterior oblique views of the left coronary artery in a 51-year-old man suffering from severe exertional angina. *(Left):* Proximal 80% stenosis of the left anterior descending artery not influenced by intracoronary injection of 0.3 mg nitroglycerin. *(Right):* After angioplasty the stenosis has nearly disappeared

The therapy for a patient being prepared for angioplasty associates a β-blocking agent, a calcium antagonist and an anti-platelet-aggregation drug. The patient is regarded as a potential candidate for emergency myocardial revascularization surgery, and the usual precautions are taken in the event of this possibility. Angioplasty must not be attempted unless a surgical team is available to perform a bypass operation should failure or complication of the dilation occur.

The procedure outlined here is based on that recommended by Grüntzig [2, 3]. It is performed under mild neuroleptanalgesia and with continuous infusion of nitroglycerin. First, a catheter to monitor pressure is introduced into a peripheral artery, and then a stimulation catheter (Myler-Cordis type) is introduced into the pulmonary artery. The operator uses the latter catheter to locate the stenosis to be dilated (Fig. 3). He searches for the radiological projection allowing a segment of the catheter to be superimposed on the arterial stenosis. Control coronary arteriography is performed using the catheter guide after administration of nifedipine and intracoronary injection of nitroglycerin to eliminate risk of spasm and to ensure maximum dilation of the coronary arteries. The patient is heparinized (5000–10000 units). The dilation catheter is introduced, and its progression through the artery is controlled by injection of small amounts of contrast medium and monitoring of distal pressure. When the stenosis is crossed, the pressure gradient is recorded and successive dilations are performed by inflating the balloon under an increasing pressure of 3.5–6.5 atm (Fig. 2). At the end of the procedure, pressure is recorded during withdrawal of the catheter, and coronary arteriography is performed again in multiple projections. The dilated arterial segment often appears to lack homogeneity, showing an irregular, sometimes double-linear border immediately after the angioplasty procedure [4]. This image, which indicates the violent effects of the balloon on the intima, becomes normal in the weeks following the intervention. Technical reasons for failure of the procedure are inability to catheterize or penetrate the artery or vein graft, inability to advance as far as the stenosis or to cross it and inability to dilate the stenosis. The most common pitfall is turning aside into a collateral artery of the left anterior descending artery. Spasm, thrombosis and arterial dissection are the main risks of the procedure. They can result from a technical error on the operator's part, though they may simply be attributable to the fragility of the artery.

After the intervention, the patient is placed in an intensive care unit. Should myocardial infarction occur, signalled mainly by the failure of an elevation of the ECG ST segment to respond to nitroglycerin, the patient must be operated on immediately.

Later follow-up consists in assessing the effects of angioplasty. A recurrence of angina pectoris would suggest possible restenosis and require repeated coronary arteriography. In asymptomatic subjects, an exercise stress test and myocardial scintigraphy complement clinical examination. Systematic follow-up coronary arteriography is performed after 6 months. If results are still good, anticoagulant and/or anti-platelet-aggregation treatment is discontinued.

1.3 Results (Figs. 3–5)

Angioplasty is arbitrarily considered successful when it results in a decrease of at least 20% in the degree of the stenosis and in the pressure gradient [3]. The degree of the stenosis is determined by the diameter of the vessel lumen and not by the cross-sectional area. True success is attested by the disappearance of angina, by a negative maximal exercise stress test and by a normal myocardial scan in the absence of anti-anginal treatment. The effect of dilation is not always long term, and there is true risk of restenosis at short or middle term. Thus initial successes should be distinguished from long-term ones, depending on whether the enlargement of the artery is temporary or not.

The multicentre study undertaken in June 1979 by the National Heart, Lung and Blood Institute (NHLBI) groups the experience of 34 centres which treated a total of 631 patients by angioplasty. The population and the results of this study [9] appear in Tables 1 and 2. The rate of overall initial success was 59% for 663 attempts.

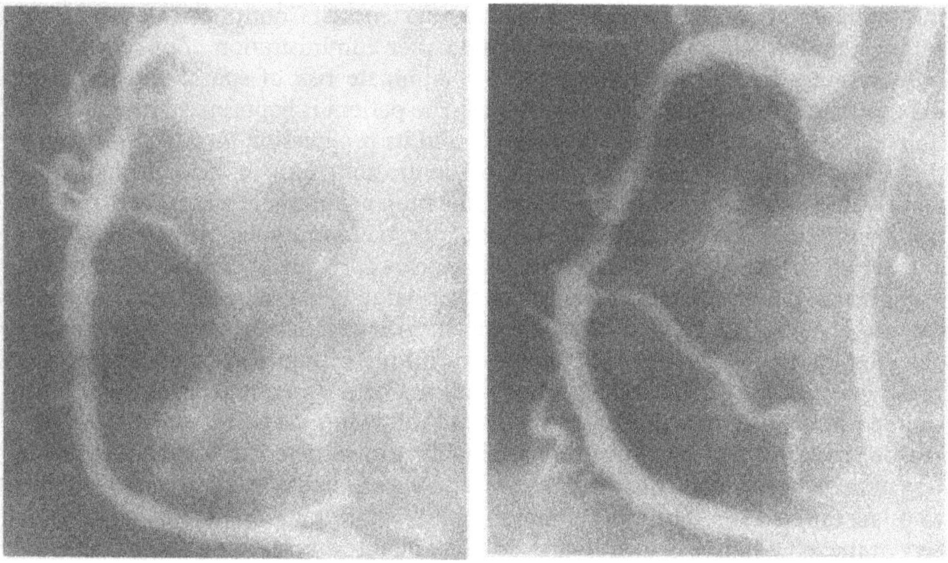

Fig. 4. Left anterior oblique views of the right coronary artery (RCA) in a 57-year-old patient suffering from unstable angina. *(Left):* Proximal 90% stenosis of the RCA. *(Right):* After angioplasty there is a clear arterial improvement in spite of persisting 50% stenosis

Table 1. Coronary angioplasty: population of the multicentre study conducted by the National Heart, Lung and Blood Institute [9][a]

	%
Men	78
Women	22
Chest pain [10]	
Canadian heart class II	38
Canadian heart class III or IV	60
Previous myocardial infarction	25
Vessel involvement	
Single	80
Double	15
Triple	2
Left main stem	3
Ejection fraction	
Over 0.70	30
Between 0.50 and 0.69	65
Site of dilation	
LAD	63
RCA	24
Cx	6
Left main stem	3

LAD: left anterior descending artery; *RCA:* right coronary artery; *Cx:* circumflex
[a] 631 patients: mean age 51 years

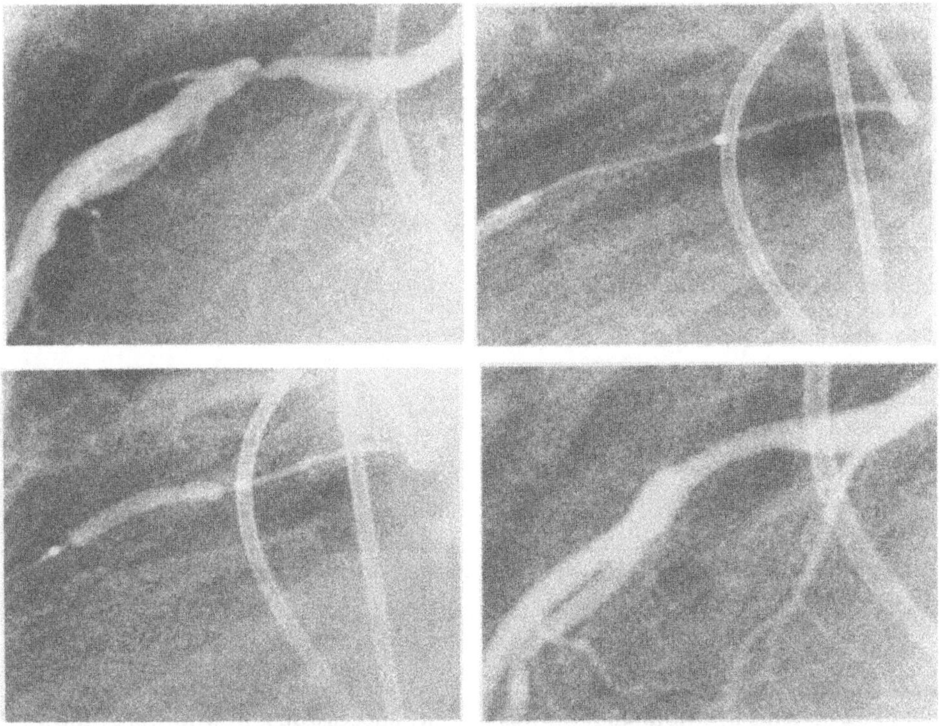

Fig. 5. Transverse views of the left coronary artery showing the main stages of transluminal angioplasty. *(Upper left):* Subtotal obstruction of the left anterior descending artery not influenced by intracoronary injection of 0.3 mg nitroglycerin. *(Upper right):* The balloon is advanced through the stenosis; the correct position of the catheter is controlled by means of the radiopaque markers and by a contrast medium injection. *(Lower left):* Inflation of the balloon. *(Lower right):* Angiographic control

The failures were due to the impossibility of reaching or crossing the stenosis (29%) or of dilating it (12%). The localization of the stenosis was one of the most inportant factors contributing to success: the success rate was 63% for the left anterior descending artery, 52% for the right coronary artery and 39% for the circumflex. Dilation of the LMCT was often successful (68%). Vein graft stenoses were impossible to dilate in about 50% of cases. The mean degree of severity of the stenoses was reduced overall from 83% to 31%. Complications with the method were encountered in 18.5% of patients. Six patients died (0.95%), all during or after an attempt at myocardial revascularization surgery, which was performed three times in emergency conditions because of an occlusion or coronary dissection.

These results are close to those published in the preliminary NHLBI report [5]. They are also close to those of Grüntzig [3], who recorded 66% initial success, a reduction in mean degree of stenosis from 84% to 34%, an emergency bypass operation in 12% of cases and no deaths. In 1981, Grüntzig and Myler reported 62% initial success for 163 patients [6]. The first French series published by Marco [7] is also in agreement with the preceding studies.

Table 2. Coronary Angioplasty: Results of the multicentre study conducted by the National Heart, Lung and Blood Institute [9][a]

	%
Main complications	
Prolonged angina	5.7
Coronary occlusion	4.4
Myocardial infarction	4.4
Coronary dissection	2.1
Hospital death	0.95
Emergency coronary bypass operation	
Because of coronary occlusion	2.85
For other indications	3.5
Overall initial success rate	59
Success rate according to site	
LAD	63 (n=426)
RCA	52 (n=157)
Cx	39 (n= 36)
Left main stem	68 (n= 19)
Venous graft	56 (n= 25)

LAD: left anterior descending artery; *RCA:* right coronary artery; *Cx:* circumflex
[a] 631 patients: 663 attempts

The long-term course of angioplasty has not yet been clearly assessed. In 1979, out of 32 patients in whom dilation was initially successful, and who were followed up for a mean period of 9 months, Grüntzig [3] found 25 functional improvements, 6 deteriorations and 2 late deaths, 1 from non-cardiac causes. He noted three arterial and three vein graft restenoses, all having occurred within the first 3 months. In 1982, out of 186 patients in the NHLBI study followed up for a mean period of 12 months, Kent [9] reported that functional symptoms improved in 79% of cases, remained unchanged in 9%, worsened in 3% and could not be specified in 9%. A second angioplasty was performed in 4% of patients. In 2% of patients, an aortocoronary bypass was necessary secondarily more than 30 days after angioplasty. Over a 3-year period, three late deaths occurred in the total group of 631 patients, two being related to dilations of the LMCT. In a series reported by David [8], the restenosis rate reached 29%. These restenoses were always early, and their frequency was significantly greater for calcified arteries and for initially eccentric stenoses.

The following approximate figures give a general idea of the risks and results of the coronary angioplasty technique: 60%–80% initial success, 10% total coronary occlusion, 5%–10% myocardial infarction, 5%–10% emergency bypass due to complications, 0 to 2% hospital mortality, 80% long-term functional improvement in subjects treated successfully and 15%–25% early restenosis.

1.4 The Present and Future Role of Angioplasty

Coronary transluminal angioplasty is an interesting therapeutic alternative to surgery, and its effectiveness has now been clearly demonstrated [3–9]. The advantages of this treatment in psychological, social, professional and economic terms are evident. A patient treated successfully by dilation can resume his normal active life within a week's time, and his medical treatment can be reduced and sometimes discontinued. The total cost of angiography is one-fifth to one-sixth that of surgery. The major advantage of the method for the patient is that it avoids surgery. The major drawback is that the patient may end up with more complications and less functional improvement than if he had undergone surgery. In view of the results previously cited, the superiority of dilation over surgery seems far from certain. The indications and rules of application specified initially by Grüntzig were perhaps transgressed to disadvantage from 1979 to 1982, at the risk of compromising the reliability of the method. Nonetheless, it should be noted that the results for this period necessarily include as an unfavourable statistical factor the initial experience of many centres with the technique [9]. It would seem preferable to rely on surgical treatment for stenoses of the LMCT, for eccentric and/or calcified stenoses and for triple-vessel involvement. Vein graft stenoses are usually poor indications. Quite severe subtotal stenoses (greater than 90%) very often entail failure with the method [8], so that this condition may soon be recognized as a preferential indication for surgery. Angioplasty is best indicated by 70%–90% stenoses meeting the angiographic criteria of Grüntzig and located in one or two vessels. Each centre should designate one, or possibly two, operators for application of this technique. The limited number of candidates for dilation and the great importance of the skill, experience and good sense of the operator justify this restrictive attitude. It is of capital importance that the patient undergoing angioplasty should not be exposed to complications greater than those of surgery, and especially that he should not be subject to a less satisfactory functional result if an operation is required because of a complication of the dilation. From this point of view, it is absolutely essential to respect the rule of having a surgical team ready to intervene without delay. Failure to respect this rule has been a cause of increase in the number of infarctions [3, 8]. In our opinion, it is still too early (in 1983) to pass a definitive judgement on this new form of therapy. The great number of patients who have benefited from lasting improvement, the possiblity of success with a second angioplasty and the reduction, albeit modest, in the number of surgical interventions are substantial reasons for continuing the methodical study of the possibilities and limitations of the method. A judicious selection of cases is essential to ensure that this study will lead to valid conclusions. Two pitfalls must be avoided:

1. choosing those patients who are "too easy", that is for whom angioplasty is not really justified, and
2. choosing those who are "too difficult", that is who clearly require multiple revascularization surgery, who present a very high risk factor (LMCT) or in whom probable causes of technical failure are evident (sinuous and angulated artery, eccentric or calcified lesion).

The method can sometimes replace surgery, but it is not a competitor; there are probably fewer real indications than initial estimations suggested [3, 7, 11] and these concern less than 5% of patients who undergo coronary arteriography.

The mechanism by which angioplasty acts has been demonstrated rather well in experimental studies and on human anatomical specimens [2, 3, 12, 13]. When anatomical conditions are favourable, the various tunicae of the artery are distended by the "controlled microtraumatism" induced by the balloon, causing fissure of the intima, modification of the atheromatous plaque, disorganization of the elastic and muscle fibres of the media and enlargement of the external diameter of the vessel. The degree of such alterations depends on the size of the balloon and the pressure and duration of inflation [12]. The atheromatous plaque itself is subject to little or no compression. Poor anatomical conditions (fibrosis, calcifications, arterial diameter of less than 1.5 mm) are conducive to more severe intimal lesions and coronary dissection [13]. Angiographic observations indicate that the artery is capable of forming its own scar tissue, with probable development of a new endothelium. In fact, it is not unusual during follow-up coronary arteriographic examinations to note that artery walls are smoother and that there is sometimes even additional enlargement of the lumen. During and after dilation, patients are treated by anticoagulants and/or anti-platelet-aggregation drugs in order to avoid complications of intimal lesions. Studies are now under way to assess the preventive value of this treatment with respect to restenosis.

2 Selective Intracoronary Thrombolysis

That coronary artery thrombosis plays a predominant role in the onset of acute myocardial infarction is now quite certain. Buja's anatomical study [14] of 55 subjects who died shortly after suffering infarction and DeWood's work [15] concerning 322 patients explored by coronary arteriography within 24 h after the onset of infarction have demonstrated that myocardial necrosis is most often due to occlusion of an artery caused by a thrombus. It is clear that the earlier coronary arteriography is carried out, the higher the percentage of thromboses is, and that the later the examination is performed, the more often arteries are found to be permeable. These observations testify to the value of recanalization induced by spontaneous fibrinolysis of the thrombus.

These ideas are apparent to those who since 1979 have been applying the intracoronary thrombolytic treatment advocated by Rentrop [16], and who have thus acquired experience in the performance of coronary arteriography within the first 6 h of myocardial infarction. In a series of 70 patients, Cribier [17] has noted that *transmural* necrosis is indeed associated with coronary artery thrombosis in 90% of cases, a finding in agreement with those of many other authors. If a controversy still exists, it concerns the respective roles of factors contributing to thrombosis. The very great reduction in coronary blood flow due to a very high-grade arterial stenosis is not always the sole cause. Other factors may also contribute: arterial spasm, a drop in the trans-stenotic perfusion gradient secondary to haemodynamic alterations, hypovolaemia, highly thrombogenic wall lesions and hypercoagulability. These factors cannot be overlooked because thrombosis may recur if they go untreated.

Table 3. Contra-indications to thrombolysis

Heart failure prior to infarction
Infective endocarditis and septicaemia
Serious liver or kidney disease
Life-threatening cancerous disease
Contra-indication to anticoagulant treatment
Surgical operation within the last 2 months
Cerebral vascular disorder within the last 2 months
Biopsy or arterial puncture within the last 2 weeks
Recent gastroduodenal ulcer
Pregnancy
Mental illness
Allergic disease
Previous streptokinase treatment

2.1 Indications for and Aims of the Treatment

Animal experiments have shown that the size of an infarct induced by arterial occlusion can be reduced if the jeopardized myocardium is revascularized early enough. In man, emergency myocardial revascularization surgery is a complicated and often disappointing therapeutic method. The first attempts at coronary fibrinolysis were made by intravenous administration of thrombolytic drugs. Though encouraging results with this method have recently been reported [18, 19], its true effectiveness remains unknown. On the other hand, the selective intracoronary thrombolytic technique initiated by Rentrop [16] has the advantage of a necessary association with coronary arteriography study immediately before and after treatment. It can be performed in patients under 75 years of age with clinically and electro-cardiographically convincing myocardial infarction, provided that they are admitted to the catheterization room no later than 4–6 h after onset of the infarction. The contra-indications are summed up in Table 3. The essential aims of the treatment are to maintain good left ventricular function and to reduce the rate of complications and mortality.

2.2 Technique and Protocol

The method itself is relatively simple, since it is derived directly from selective coronary arteriography. The catheter to be used in injecting the fibrinolytic drug should be chosen with care, as its distal end must remain perfectly stable in the coronary ostium. The methodology of intracoronary thrombolysis varies slightly from one centre to another because the technique is still in its testing stage. Table 4 gives the protocol used by our team (Petitier) for our first 60 patients. The main differences in the technical modalities practised in other centres are:

- total dose of streptokinase of over 250000 IU
- complementary use of plasminogen [20]

Table 4. Protocol for intracoronary thrombolysis

Prethrombolytic management

1. Record the 12-lead ECG.
2. Introduce a venous catheter.
3. Treat pain, hypotension and shock in customary fashion.
4. Ask the patient for informed consent.
5. Draw blood for conventional laboratory tests and those specific to thrombolysis.
6. Transfer the patient to the cardiac catheterization room.

Thrombolytic treatment

1. Perform right heart catheterization (femoral vein).
2. Introduce a pacing catheter in the IVC or the PA.
3. Perform left heart catheterization (femoral artery).
4. Inject 10000 IU heparin.
5. Perform biplanar left ventriculography.
6. Perform arteriography of the vessel perfusing the infarcted area. Inject 0.3 mg nitroglycerin into the occluded artery.
   Perform an arteriographic control.
7. Give 4–8 mg betamethasone or dexamethasone intravenously.
8. Inject a 1-ml bolus containing 12500 IU streptokinase in the thrombosed artery every 3 min.
9. Repeat coronary arteriography of the treated vessel every 9 min.
10. Continue the treatment
    For 30 min in the case of early recanalization
    Or until the total dose of 250000 IU is reached.
11. Perform arteriography of the non-thrombosed vessel.
12. Transfer the patient to the coronary intensive care unit.

IVC: inferior vena cava; *PA:* pulmonary artery

- use of urokinase in place of streptokinase
- more frequent boluses: every 1 or 2 min
- continuous streptokinase infusion at a rate of 4000 IU/min
- perforation of the thrombus using a flexible guide-wire with a movable core [16, 21]
- a second coaxial 3-F catheter advanced along the artery as close as possible to the clot [20].

In some randomized studies [22] the artery presumed not to be occluded is opacified first. Theoretically, the technique chosen should be the one best suited to providing therapy in view of the characteristics of the arterial occlusion: whether the trombus is proximal or distal, whether the contrast medium is stagnant or not when it comes into contact with the clot, and whether or not there are collaterals diverting a considerable part of the coronary blood flow.

Streptokinase is the product most often used today. Selective intracoronary injection offers the advantages of enabling a dosage much lower than that for the venous route and of limiting the effects of systemic proteolysis. After treatment, the catheters with their sheaths are left in place. When serum fibrinogen concentration reaches between 1 and 1.5 g/l, heparin treatment is begun in order to avoid coronary rethrombosis. After a few hours the catheters are withdrawn and the vein and artery are compressed.

2.3 Results

A coronary occlusion caused by a thrombus is found in 80%–90% of patients explored by coronary arteriography within the first 6 h of infarction [17, 20, 21, 23]. Recanalization of an artery by means of streptokinase is effected in 67%–80% of cases [17, 20, 21, 23–25]. In Ganz's series [20], the rate of arterial recanalization reached 90%, possibly because a microcatheter and/or plasminogen was used. When recanalization occurs, there is often a sudden disappearance of pain and a drop in the elevation of the ECG ST segment [16, 17, 20, 21], both of which are good signs of improvement of myocardial ischaemia. After recanalization, Q waves practically never disappear and may even appear. Thus thrombolysis is in effect a technique which limits the size of the infarct but does not prevent its occurrence. Study of enzyme release (CPK and CPK-MB) and late follow-up left ventriculography both confirm this notion of inescapable myocardial necrosis. Cases of reinfarction due to reocclusion of recanalized arteries confirm that thrombolysis allows myocardium to be saved if intervention comes early enough. Cases of reduction or disappearance of signs of cardiogenic shock [17, 26] also demonstrate that the treatment has an effect on left ventricular function. To assess this effect, studies of left ventricular function have been carried out 10–30 days after thrombolysis, with comparison made of patients treated with and without success [16, 17, 20, 21, 23–26]. When the overall results for a treated group are taken into consideration, these studies leave no doubt that an effective thrombolytic treatment leads to reduced deterioration of left ventricular function. However, for a given patient it is impossible to predict the outcome of treatment with certainty because it depends on too many variables: how long the occlusion has existed, the site of the thrombus, uncertainty about the initial phase of subtotal occlusion, the existence of collateral arteries perfusing to some extent the jeopardized artery, and the severity of the residual stenosis and of the reduction in coronary blood flow after recanalization.

In the long term it is not certain that thrombolysis reduces the morbidity and mortality of coronary artery disease. In the short term it improves the chances of survival of some patients suffering from cardiogenic shock. The complications of the technique are essentially haemorrhages [27].

There are often benign rhythm disturbances when myocardial reperfusion occurs: sporadic or multiple ventricular extrasystolic beats, ventricular tachycardia of very short duration and sinus bradycardia. These disappear spontaneously or under the effect of lidocaine or atropine. Serious arrhythmias (prolonged ventricular tachycardia, ventricular fibrillation, third-degree atrioventricular block) are rare and require electric cardioversion or ventricular pacing. When not associated with cardiogenic shock, these arrhythmias are normally curable. They may be complications of the infarction itself as well as of fibrinolytic reperfusion.

Angiographic features vary from one patient to another (Figs. 6–9). In our series of 60 patients no total arterial reopening was observed as the result of injection of intracoronary contrast medium or nitroglycerin alone, though such effects have been reported. After injection of nitroglycerin the thrombus causing the occlusion is sometimes more visible and partially surrounded by the opacifying product. Clot images are clearly visualized, especially during the initial phase of recanalization, just at the moment when the flow begins to be restored. The largest clots are found

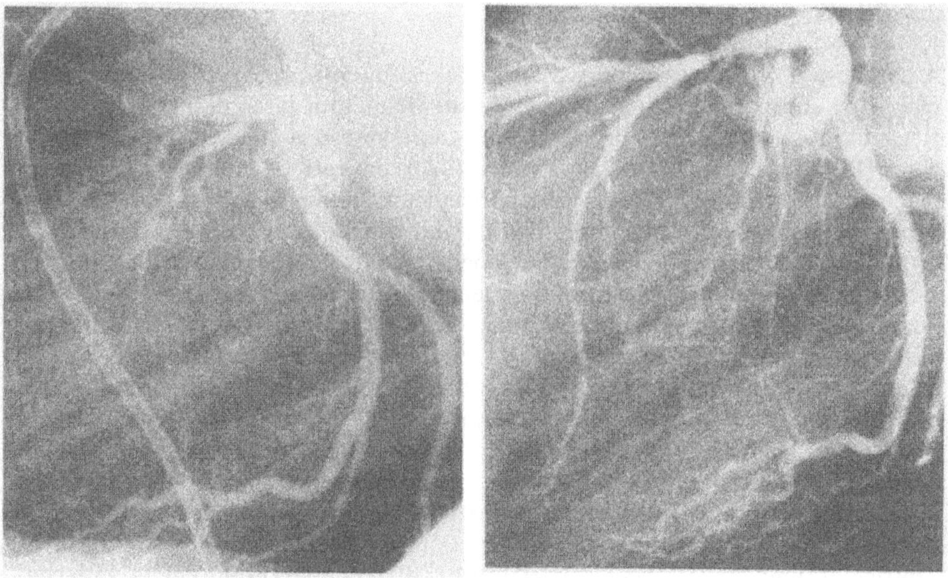

Fig. 6. Acute anterior myocardial infarction. *(Left):* Transverse view of the left coronary artery showing the totally occluded left anterior descending artery (LAD). *(Right):* Successful recanalization of the LAD by means of direct repeated intracoronary injections of streptokinase. Complementary transluminal angioplasty is suitable for treatment of the residual stenosis

mainly in the second segment of the right coronary artery (Fig. 7). The smallest clots are not always identified: the artery is first seen totally obstructed, then suddenly recanalized, showing an image of residual stenosis which does not vary during successive coronary angiographic controls. Very spectacular images of thrombus fragmentation and migration are occasionally filmed. These migrations are the cause of coronary embolisms which lead to amputations of the distal branches of the occluded artery (Fig. 8). As far as possible, lysis should be continued until these amputations and any visible sign of thrombus have disappeared. Sometimes, at the end of the thrombolytic procedure, a clot simulates a severe residual stenosis, so that the operator is surprised to discover during the follow-up examination in the 2nd or 3rd week that the artery is nearly normal (Fig. 9). This is still another reason for not discontinuing thrombolytic treatment too early.

2.4 The Present and Future Role of Thrombolysis

It is incontestable that selective intracoronary thrombolysis is a safe therapeutic method capable of saving myocardium if it is applied early enough in the phase of acute infarction. Randomized studies have been undertaken to quantify exactly the degree of improvement in left ventricular function in subjects undergoing fibrinolysis and compare it with that in subjects receiving conventional treatment. The results, soon to be published, will certainly be favourable from this point of view. But determining whether there is middle- or long-term benefit from thrombolytic treat-

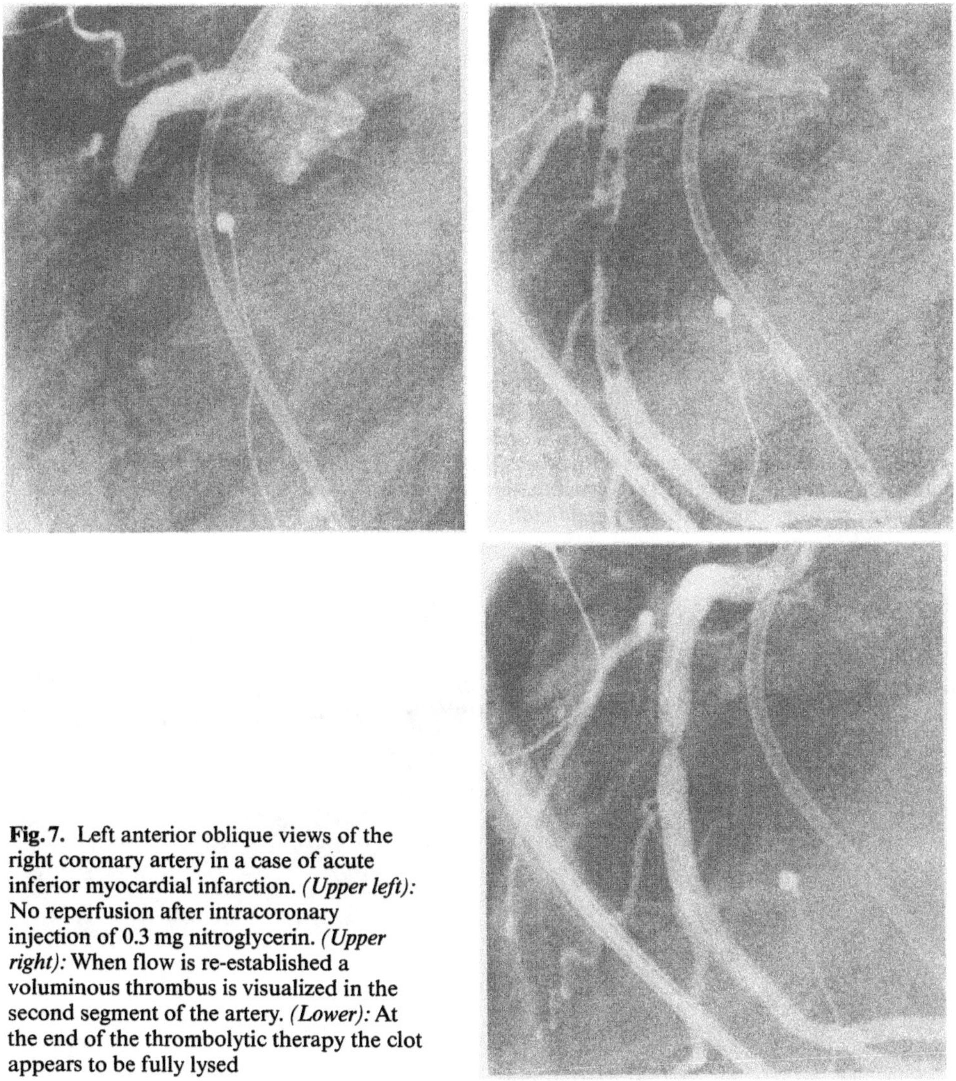

Fig. 7. Left anterior oblique views of the right coronary artery in a case of acute inferior myocardial infarction. *(Upper left):* No reperfusion after intracoronary injection of 0.3 mg nitroglycerin. *(Upper right):* When flow is re-established a voluminous thrombus is visualized in the second segment of the artery. *(Lower):* At the end of the thrombolytic therapy the clot appears to be fully lysed

ment is a more delicate affair. What are the risks of reinfarction, heart failure and death? Most patients in whom thrombolysis is performed have one or more surgically significant stenoses [27]. In Ganz's series [20], about one-third of the patients underwent complementary surgical treatment. Mathey [28] suggests that early revascularization surgery may be associated with thrombolysis. In the same vein, Meyer [29] recommends transluminal angioplasty together with the thrombolytic procedure whenever the former is anatomically feasible. The combination of the two procedures would presumably increase coronary flow to the reperfused myocardium and to the adjacent ischaemic myocardium and reduce the risk of rethrombosis, reinfarction and death. Another advantage of the treatment would be a saving in

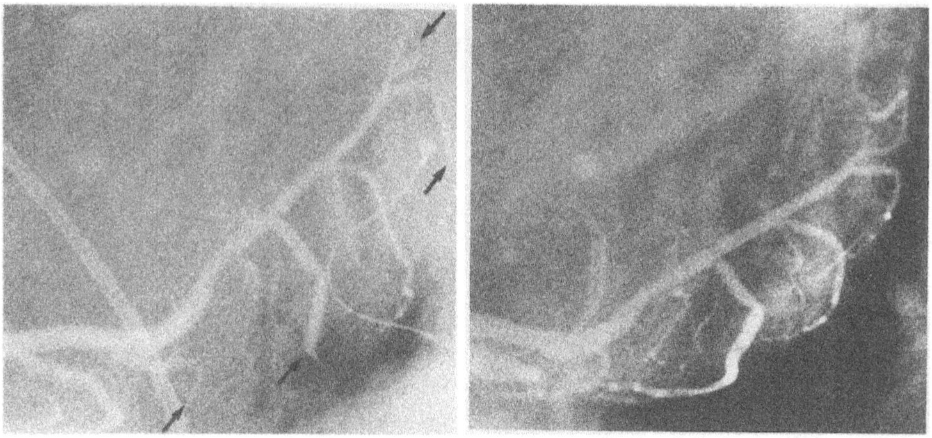

Fig. 8. Left anterior oblique views of the distal part of the right coronary artery in a case of acute inferior myocardial infarction. *(Left):* amputations *(black arrows)* of the terminal branches immediately after proximal recanalization; *(right):* full lysis at the end of the streptokinase therapy

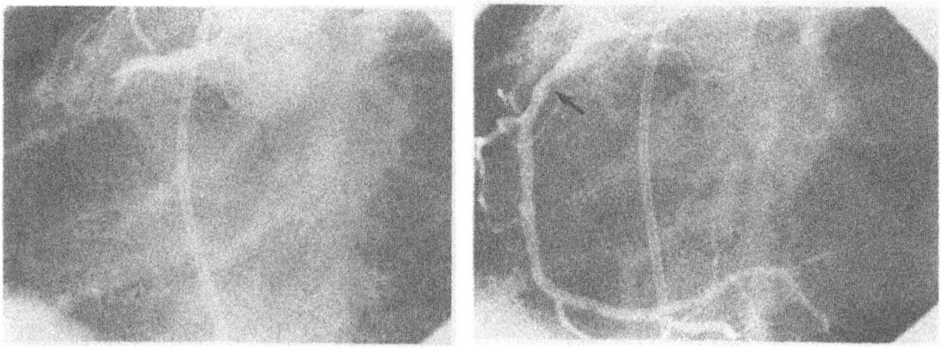

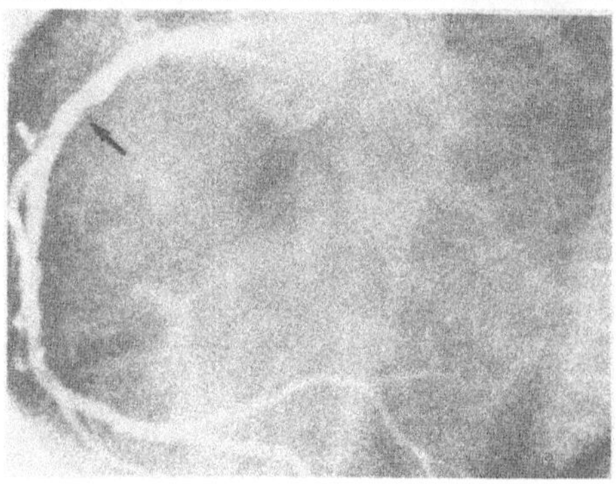

Fig. 9. Left anterior oblique views of the right coronary artery. *(Upper left):* thrombotic occlusion of the artery; *(upper right):* moderate residual stenosis at the end of the fibrinolytic procedure; *(lower):* nearly normal artery at the 10th day control

time and money, as both procedures could be performed during the same session. Swan [30] believes that these proposals should be taken seriously and studied thoroughly. He thinks it would be wise to place the severest cases of stenosis (greater than 90%) and the patients with multivessel disease in the hands of the surgeon as early as possible. In his opinion it is also advisable, when the patient's condition warrants it, to have angioplasty for stenoses of less than 90% performed by skilled and experienced operators immediately after recanalization.

References

1. Dotter CT, Judkins MP (1964) Transluminal treatment of arteriosclerotic obstruction. Description of a new technic and a preliminary report of its application. Circulation 30: 654
2. Grüntzig A (1978) Transluminal dilatation of coronary-artery stenosis. Lancet 1: 263
3. Grüntzig AR, Senning A, Siegenthaler WE (1979) Nonoperative dilatation of coronary-artery stenosis. Percutaneous transluminal coronary angioplasty. N Engl J Med 301: 61
4. Block PC (1980) Percutaneous transluminal coronary angioplasty. AJR 135: 955
5. Levy RI, Mock MB, Willman VL, Passamani ER, Frommer PL (1981) Percutaneous transluminal coronary angioplasty – a status report. N Engl J Med 305: 399
6. Grüntzig AR, Myler R, Stertzer S (1979) Percutaneous transluminal coronary angioplasty. Present state of the art. Circulation 60 [Suppl II]: 264 (abstract)
7. Marco J, Gouel Y, Fournial G, Alibelli MJ, Bernies M, Berthoumieu F, Bernadet P (1981) Angioplastie transluminale des coronaires. Résultats préliminaires. Arch Mal Coeur 74: 1131
8. David PR, Bourassa MG, Lesperance J, Scholl JM, Grepeau J, Dyrda I, Hudon G, Chaitman BR, Dupras G, Pelletier C, Maille JG, Paquet E (1981) Percutaneous transluminal coronary angioplasty: initial results in our first 110 patients. Can Med Assoc J 111: 23
9. Kent MK, Bentivoglio LG, Block PC, Cowley MJ, Dorros G, Gosselin AJ, Gruntzig A, Myler RK, Simpson J, Stertzer SH, Williams DO, Fisher L, Gillespie MJ, Detre K, Kelsey S, Mullin SM, Mock MB (1982) Percutaneous transluminal coronary angioplasty: report from the registry of the National Heart, Lung and Blood institute. Am J Cardiol 49: 2011
10. Campeau L (1976) Grading of angina pectoris. Circulation 54: 522
11. Hamby R, Katz A (1980) Percutaneous transluminal coronary angioplasty: its potential impact on surgery for coronary artery disease. Am J Cardiol 45: 1161
12. Castaneda-Zuniga WR, Formanek A, Tadavarthy M, Vlodaver Z, Edwards JE, Zollikoffer C, Amplatz K (1980) The mechanism of balloon angioplasty. Radiology 135: 565
13. Lee G, Ikeda RM, Joye JA, Bogren HG, De Maria AN, Mason DT (1980) Evaluation of transluminal angioplasty of chronic coronary artery stenosis. Value and limitations assessed in fresh human cadaver hearts. Circulation 61: 77
14. Buja LM, Willerson JT (1981) Clinicopathologic correlates of acute ischemic heart disease syndromes. Am J Cardiol 47: 343
15. De Wood MA, Spores J, Notske R, Mouser LT, Burroughs R, Golden MS, Lang HT (1980) Prevalence of total coronary occlusion during the early hours of transmural myocardial infarction. N Engl J Med 303: 897
16. Rentrop P, Blanke H, Karsch KR, Kreuzer H (1979) Initial experience with transluminal recanalization of the recently occluded infarct-related coronary artery in acute myocardial infarction. Comparison with conventionally treated patients. Clin Cardiol 2: 92
17. Cribier A, Berland J, Richard C, Redonnet M, Champoud O, Behar P, Saoudi N, Letac B (1983) Revascularisation myocardique en urgence par fibrinolyse intracoronarienne. Aspects méthodologiques et résultats immédiats. Arch Mal Coeur 76: 241
18. Schröder R, Biamino G, v. Leitner ER, Linderer T, Brüggemann T, Heitz J, Vöhringer HF, Wegscheider K (1983) Intravenous short-term infusion of streptokinase in acute myocardial infarction. Circulation 67: 536
19. Stampfer MJ, Goldhaber SZ, Salim Y, Peto R, Hennekens CH (1982) Effect of intravenous streptokinase on acute myocardial infarction. Pooled results from randomized trials. N Engl J Med 307: 1180

20. Ganz W, Buchbinder N, Marcus H, Mondkar A, Maddahi J, Charuzi Y, O'Connor L, Shell W, Fishbein MC, Kass R, Miyamoto A, Swan HJC (1981) Intracoronary thrombolysis in evolving myocardial infarction. Am Heart J 101: 4
21. Rentrop P, Blanke H, Karsch KR, Kaiser H, Köstering H, Leitz K (1981) Selective intracoronary thrombolysis in acute myocardial infarction and unstable angina pectoris. Circulation 63: 307
22. Kennedy JW, Fritz JK, Ritchie JL (1982) Streptokinase in acute myocardial infarction: western Washington randomized trial-protocol and progress report. Am Heart J 104: 899
23. Mason DT (1981) International experience with percutaneous transluminal coronary recanalization by streptokinase-thrombolysis reperfusion in acute myocardial infarction: new, safe, landmark therapeutic approach salvaging ischemic muscle and improving ventricular function. Am Heart J 102: 1126
24. Reduto LA, Freund GC, Gaeta JM, Smalling RW, Lewis B, Gould KL (1981) Coronary artery reperfusion in acute myocardial infarction: beneficial effects of intracoronary streptokinase on left ventricular salvage and performance. Am Heart J 102: 1169
25. Rutsch W, Schartl M, Mathey D, Kuck K, Merx W, Dorr R, Rentrop P, Blanke H (1981) Percutaneous transluminal coronary recanalization: procedure, results, and acute complications. Am Heart J 102: 1178
26. Mathey DG, Kuck KH, Tilsner V, Krebber HJ, Bleifeld W (1981) Nonsurgical coronary artery recanalization in acute transmural myocardial infarction. Circulation 63: 489
27. Merx W, Dorr R, Rentrop P, Blanke H, Karsch KR, Mathey DG, Kremer P, Rutsch W, Schmutzler H (1981) Evaluation of the effectiveness of intracoronary streptokinase infusion in acute myocardial infarction: post-procedure management and hospital course in 204 patients. Am Heart J 102: 1181
28. Mathey DG, Rodewald G, Rentrop P, Leitz K, Merx W, Messmer BJ, Rutsch W, Bucherl ES (1981) Intracoronary streptokinase, thrombolytic recanalization and subsequent surgical bypass of remaining atherosclerotic stenosis in acute myocardial infarction: complementary combined approach affecting reduced infarct size, preventing reinfarction and improving left ventricular function. Am Heart J 102: 1194
29. Meyer J, Merx W, Schmitz H, Erbel R, Kiesslich T, Dörr R, Lambertz H, Bethge C, Krebs W, Bardos P, Minale C, Messmer BJ, Effert S (1982) Percutaneous transluminal coronary angioplasty immediately after intracoronary streptolysis of transmural myocardial infarction. Circulation 66: 905
30. Swan HJC (1982) Thrombolysis in acute myocardial infarction: treatment of the underlying coronary artery disease. Circulation 66: 914

Recommended General Reference Books

Baltaxe HA, Amplatz K, Levin DC (1973) Coronary angiography. Charles C. Thomas, Springfield Illinois

Bourassa MG, Cachera JP (1980) La maladie coronarienne. Flammarion, Paris; Presses Université, Montreal

Gensini GG (1975) Coronary arteriography. Futura publishing Co, New York 1975

McAlpine WA (1975) Heart and coronary arteries. An anatomical atlas for clinical diagnosis, radiological investigation and surgical treatment. Springer, Berlin Heidelberg New York

Pujadas G (1977) The coronary angiography in the medical and surgical treatment of ischemic heart disease. Hospital Italiano de Buenos Aires, Buenos Aires

Vlodaver Z, Amplatz K, Burchell HB, Edwards JE (1976) Coronary heart disease. Clinical, angiographic and pathologic profiles. Springer, Berlin Heidelberg New York

Yang SS, Bentivoglio LG, Maranhao V, Goldberg H (1978) From cardiac catheterization data to hemodynamic parameters. Second edition. F. A. Davis Co, Philadelphia Pensylvania

Rigo P (1981) Applications de la scintigraphie à l'étude des fonctions cardiaques et de la maladie coronarienne. Thesis. University of Liege, Belgium

Subject Index

Contrast Media in Radiology

Appraisal and Prospects

First European Workshop – Proceedings – Lyon 1981

Editor: **M. Amiel**
With the collaboration of J.F. Moreau

1982. 141 figures. XXI, 353 pages.
ISBN 3-540-11534-X

Contents: General Toxicity. – Effect on the Heart. – Effects on the Nervous System. – Effects on the Kidney. – Various Topics. – Contrast Media and CT. – New Molecules and New Images. – Subject Index.

The scientific papers presented at the international workshop on contrast media in radiology held in Lyon are contained in this work. Evaluating new developments made in the field since the 1977 Colorado Springs workshop, the papers concentrate on

- new molecules of uroangiographic media with low osmolarity, either already in use or about to be marketed
- new molecules currently under investigation
- the toxicity of contrast media.

The book brings together information scattered throughout the literature up to now. It also offers the reader an account of the work of the world's leading specialists in the area, providing an up-to-date and comprehensive summary of the status of contrast media.

Springer-Verlag
Berlin
Heidelberg
New York
Tokyo

Iatrogenic Thoracic Complications

Editor: **P.G.Herman**
1983. 256 figures. XIX, 243 pages
(Radiology of Iatrogenic Disorders)
ISBN 3-540-90729-7

Percutaneous Transluminal Angioplasty

Technique, Early and Late Results

Editors: **C.T.Dotter, A.R.Grüntzig, W.Schoop, E.Zeitler**
1983. 179 figures. XV, 369 pages
ISBN 3-540-12654-6

Prognosis of Coronary Heart Disease. Progression of Coronary Arteriosclerosis

International Symposium Held in Bad Krozingen
October 22–23, 1982
Editor: **H.Roskamm**
1983. 94 figures, 80 tables. XI, 248 pages
ISBN 3-540-12367-9

Radiological Functional Analysis of the Vascular System

Contrast Media – Methods – Results

Editor: **F.H.W.Heuck**
1983. 195 figures. XIV, 296 pages
ISBN 3-540-12185-4

Transluminal Coronary Angioplasty and Intracoronary Thrombolysis

Coronary Heart Disease IV

Editors: **M.Kaltenbach, A.Grüntzig, K.Rentrop, W.-D.Bussmann**
With contributions by numerous experts
1982. 210 figures. XVIII, 442 pages
ISBN 3-540-11219-7

L.Jeanmart, A.L.Baert, A.Wackenheim

Computer Tomography of Neck, Chest, Spine, and Limbs

With the collaboration of M.Osteaux
With contributions by numerous experts
1983. 545 figures. XI, 194 pages
(Atlas of Pathological Computer Tomography, Volume 3)
ISBN 3-540-11439-4

Radiology Today

Volume 2
Editors: **F.H.W.Heuck, M.W.Donner**
1983. 306 figures, 44 tables. XII, 362 pages
ISBN 3-540-11754-7

Contents: Gastrointestinal Radiology. – Urogenital Radiology. – Cardiovascular Radiology. – Radiology of Lymphatic System. – Chest Radiology. – Skeletal and Soft Tissue Radiology. – Neuroradiology. – Selected Chapters on New Imaging Techniques. – Missed Diagnosis Conference. – Subject Index.

Springer-Verlag
Berlin
Heidelberg
New York
Tokyo

GPSR Compliance
The European Union's (EU) General Product Safety Regulation (GPSR) is a set of rules that requires consumer products to be safe and our obligations to ensure this.

If you have any concerns about our products, you can contact us on

ProductSafety@springernature.com

In case Publisher is established outside the EU, the EU authorized representative is:

Springer Nature Customer Service Center GmbH
Europaplatz 3
69115 Heidelberg, Germany

www.ingramcontent.com/pod-product-compliance
Lightning Source LLC
Chambersburg PA
CBHW061206240926
51846CB00006B/1128
* 9 7 8 3 6 4 2 6 9 6 0 6 0 *